THE NEURON

Cell and Molecular Biology

THIRD EDITION

IRWIN B. LEVITAN

University of Pennsylvania

LEONARD K. KACZMAREK

Yale University

OXFORD
UNIVERSITY PRESS
2002

OXFORD
UNIVERSITY PRESS

Oxford   New York
Athens   Auckland   Bangkok   Bogotá   Buenos Aires   Cape Town
Chennai   Dar es Salaam   Delhi   Florence   Hong Kong   Istanbul   Karachi
Kolkata   Kuala Lumpur   Madrid   Melbourne   Mexico City   Mumbai   Nairobi
Paris   São Paulo   Shanghai   Singapore   Taipei   Tokyo   Toronto   Warsaw

and associated companies in
Berlin   Ibadan

Copyright © 2002 by Oxford University Press.

Published by Oxford University Press, Inc.,
198 Madison Avenue, New York, New York, 10016
http://www.oup-usa.org

Oxford is a registered trademark of Oxford University Press.

Library of Congress Cataloging-in-Publication Data
Levitan, Irwin B.
The neuron : cell and molecular biology /
Irwin B. Levitan, Leonard K. Kaczmarek.—3rd ed.
p.   cm.
Includes bibliographical references and index.
ISBN 0-19-514522-4 (cloth)—ISBN 0-19-514523-2 (pbk.)
1. Molecular neurobiology.   2. Neurons.
I. Kaczmarek, Leonard K.
II. Title.
QP356.2 .L48 2001   573.8'536–dc21   2001021591

1 2 3 4 5 6 7 8 9
Printed in the United States of America
on acid-free paper

To the Sheilas

Preface

The passage of a mere five years since the second edition of *The Neuron* has rendered several statements that were made in the last two editions completely inaccurate. It is not that we are acknowledging any major errors of scientific fact in the past editions (although time will certainly show that some of what we now believe about the functioning of the brain is wrong). Rather, the arrival of a new millennium has made nonsense of most of the statements that began "Earlier in this century. . ." This by itself, however, was insufficient to induce us, yet again, to rent a room at the Marine Biological Laboratory in Woods Hole, to prepare a manuscript that represents a substantial revision of both the organization and content of the prior editions. It was, instead, the continuing rapid march of progress in neuroscience that provided the major incentive.

The third edition of *The Neuron* continues to provide a comprehensive first course in the cell and molecular biology of nerve cells, and the overall approach matches that of previous editions. The recent mapping of the human genome and those of other species has, however, led to the discovery of numerous new proteins that regulate the development, excitability, and other functions of neurons. These have been incorporated into the new edition in nearly all of the chapters. The first section of the book, which deals with neuronal excitability, has been reorganized substantially, so as to make it more readable for those students with less background in the physical sciences. This section has also been endowed with an additional chapter, prompted by the spectacular growth in our knowledge of the molecular nature of proteins that regulate excitability. A new chapter, on the "Birth and Death of Neurons," has also been added in the section on Behavior and Plasticity. In addition to covering new discoveries about the early development of neurons, this chapter describes the recent discovery that new neurons are continually being formed in certain parts of the adult mammalian brain. It also describes research on stem cells, which holds the therapeutic potential for the repair of damaged or diseased brain tissue. Finally, the use of imaging technologies in the study of the brain has expanded enormously in the past few years. The new edition describes some of these new approaches. Moreover, the introduction of full color plates in the new edition now allows many new images to be presented in their original form.

In addition to acknowledging again all of our colleagues and coworkers who read earlier editions and who were instrumental in providing materials for those editions, we now would also like to recognize the invaluable contributions of Thomas Kuner, Vincent Pieribone, Paul Forscher, Jim Trimmer, Matt Rasband, Phil Haydon, and Rod MacKinnon. Finally, we must say that it has been delightful, as always, to work with Fiona Stevens and Jeff House at Oxford University Press. In the last millennium, Fiona and Jeff worked for different publishers, and in fact were competitors for the first edition of *The Neuron*. It is our fantasy that it was this early competition that brought them together and that led to their eventual marriage. Even neuroscientists must be permitted the occasional romantic fantasy.

Woods Hole, Summer 2001   I.B.L.
                                                             L.K.K.

Preface to the Second Edition

There have been enormous advances in neuroscience in the five years since the first edition of *The Neuron* was published. Neuroscience remains one of the most dynamic research areas in modern biology, with cellular and molecular approaches to understanding brain function leading the way. This progress in cellular and molecular neurobiology has paralleled equally exciting advances in other areas of basic cell and molecular biology, which have been instrumental in helping us to understand how nerve cells work. Indeed, in the first edition of this book we emphasized the features that cells of the brain have in common with other cells, and these are becoming more and more apparent as time passes.

This rapid progress has led us to revise *The Neuron* thoroughly for this second edition. What was formerly the first chapter has been expanded substantially and divided into two separate chapters, to emphasize features of the cell biology of neurons and glia and their commonalities with other kinds of cells. The section on intracellular communication has also been expanded and reorganized. We now introduce the concept of ion channels as specialized membrane proteins at an early stage, making it easier to understand the idea of selective membrane permeability in terms of the properties of particular ion channel proteins. In addition, we emphasize the astonishing diversity of the voltage-dependent ion channels that has become evident in recent years, and discuss the implications of this diversity for neuronal physiology. In the section on intercellular communication, the chapter on secretion of neurotransmitters has also been rewritten to reflect the new level of understanding of secretion that has resulted from identification of many of the molecular players in vesicle fusion and exocytosis. Here again, information from many kinds of cells, including lower eukaryotes, has been instrumental in advancing our understanding of secretion. The remaining chapters in the section on intercellular communication have also been revised thoroughly, to include new information resulting from the cloning and characterization of the multitude of glutamate receptors, as well as to describe novel elements of intracellular signalling pathways in neurons and other cells. Finally, the substantial revision of the last section reflects the fact that cellular and molecular studies of development and plasticity have also been exceptionally fruitful during the last five years. As more and more of the molecular entities that are essential for neuronal development and adult plasticity are identified and characterized, phenomena that previously could be studied only at the descriptive level are now becoming understood in molecular detail.

It is an exciting time to be a neuroscientist. As was the case when we wrote the first edition of *The Neuron*, we enjoyed learning many new things from our friends and colleagues and from the burgeoning literature in cellular and molecular neurobiology. Many thanks to all who helped and encouraged us, particular our assistants Joyce Chase and Paula Shelly for dealing with a myriad of details, and our editor Jeffrey House of Oxford University Press for his constant encouragement and advice. It was fun the first time, and it was fun again this second time. We might even consider doing it again!

Summer 1996   I.B.L.
                                                                          L.K.K.

Preface to the First Edition

A fundamental goal of neuroscience is to understand the way neurons generate animal behaviors. This requires, among other things, a knowledge of how many neurons are involved in the control of a specific behavior, where these neurons are located, and how they are connected. All this information, however, is of no avail if we do not understand the intrinsic properties of the individual neurons themselves. Just as each individual human provides his or her unique contribution to society, the properties, abilities, and "personalities" of different cells in a neuronal circuit all play roles in the output of that circuit. They also determine how that output alters with time to change the behavior of an animal.

Neuroscience has come of age. Its practitioners are no longer simply a hodge-podge of physiologists, biochemists, and anatomists who stumbled across the brain and decided to study it. Rather it is a mature discipline in its own right. This is evidenced in part by the appearance of several textbooks of neurobiology, some aimed at medical students, others designed to give undergraduates a broad overview of the field. By necessity such treatments must emphasize breadth at the expense of depth, and we have found ourselves frustrated in looking for a textbook that can be used to communicate in detail to students the principles of cellular and molecular neurobiology. Hence this book.

The text reflects our own training, research interests, and biases. It is unabashedly reductionistic, in line with our conviction that understanding the elements of the nervous system—individual neurons and the molecules that regulate neuronal activity—is essential for even the most rudimentary understanding of how the brain works. We recognize that,

although understanding the elements is essential, it is not in itself sufficient for a complete description of brain function, and where appropriate
we place cellular and molecular principles in the context of the nervous
system in which they function. However, for the reasons given above we
have preferred to emphasize depth, and this is not intended to be a comprehensive text covering all of neuroscience. Rather it is designed for a
first course in cellular and molecular neurobiology, for undergraduate or
beginning graduate students who already have a basic grounding in biochemistry and cell biology. Students who have mastered the material in
this book can move on readily to more specialized courses in neural systems, development, behavior, and computational neurobiology.

We had fun writing this book. It gave us the opportunity to interact
with and tap the expertise of knowledgeable and stimulating colleagues
from whom we learned a great deal. Many of them read portions of the
manuscript and pointed out (occasionally with great glee) our miscon-
ceptions and murky writing style. Eve Marder, Chris Miller, and Jimmy
Schwartz undertook the heroic task of reading the entire book, and their
suggestions were invaluable. Others who read several (sometimes many)
chapters were Spyros Artavanis-Tsakonas, Bill Catterall, Arlene Chiu,
Martha Constantine-Paton, Pietro DeCamilli, Dorothy Gallager, Scott
Kasper, John Lisman, Joanne Mattessich, John Perkins, Jan Rosenbaum,
Larry Squire, and Kate Turtle. We are grateful to all of them. Much of the
treatment of resting and action potentials in Chapter 3 was inspired by a
wonderful little book titled *Neurophysiology: A Primer*, written by Chuck
Stevens many years ago (J. Wiley and Sons, New York, 1966). We are also
grateful to John Dowling, Paul Forscher, Steven Hunt, Andrew Matus,
Tom Reese, Bruce Schnapp, Toni Steinacker, Masatoshi Takeichi, Asa
Thureson-Klein, Monte Westerfield, and especially Dennis Landis for providing us with original photographs for some of the figures. Mike Lerner
gave us the idea for, and the chemical structures of, the different odorants
in Figure 13–16a. Maureen Ferrari and Joyce Chase did yeoman duty at
the keyboard and in dealing with endless administrative details, and Paula
Shelly helped with the preparation of the index. As always it was a pleasure to interact with our editor Jeffrey House and his colleagues Edith Barry,
Donna Grosso, and Susan Hannan at Oxford University Press. Finally we
thank our friends and colleagues for their encouragement, for telling us
over and over again that a text of cellular and molecular neurobiology is
sorely needed.

October 1990   I.B.L.
                                                                        L.K.K.

Contents

The Neuron

I

INTRODUCTION

The purpose of this book is to describe the cellular and molecular properties of neurons that allow them to carry out their assigned task in an animal. We begin in Chapter 1 with an overview of *neuronal signaling* to emphasize that the primary function of neurons is information transfer. This includes both *intra*cellular signaling, from one part of a neuron to another, and *inter*cellular signaling, from one neuron to another or to a muscle cell. Chapter 2 goes on to describe features of *neuronal* and *glial cell* biology. We emphasize here that neurons share many properties with other cell types in the organism, but at the same time are exquisitely specialized to carry out their signaling functions. For example, the *cytoskeleton*, a cellular scaffolding present in all cells, plays a particularly critical role in the organization and maintenance of neuronal form. Each of the themes introduced here will be elaborated in more detail in later chapters.

Signaling in the Brain

Tell me where is Fancy bred,
Or in the heart, or in the head?

*A*lthough Shakespeare asked this question near the end of the sixteenth century, the answer had been known, at least to some, for more than two millennia. Many ancient Greek scholars, Hippocrates and Plato among them, appreciated that there is something special about the brain, and argued that the brain is responsible for behavior in humans and other animals. We now take it for granted that the brain is the organ that obtains information about the environment, processes and stores this information, and generates behavior. In addition, it is the brain that is responsible for such vaguely defined aspects of behavior as feelings, aspirations, and abstract thoughts, those qualities we consider—with more than a touch of hubris—quintessentially human. Diseases of the brain, which often are associated with aging and hence are on the increase as the human life span lengthens, cause untold suffering for individuals, families, and society as a whole. In essence then, it is the brain that makes us what we are, and indeed it can be argued that all other organs are there simply to support the brain. For this reason understanding the biology of brain function is a major goal of modern science. The brain is one of the last great frontiers in the biological sciences, and the unraveling of its mysteries is comparable in complexity and intellectual challenge to the search for the elementary particles of matter or the effort to explore space.

Levels of Organization

One can study the functioning of the nervous system at a number of levels of organization (Fig. 1–1). Biochemists and molecular biologists, and

5

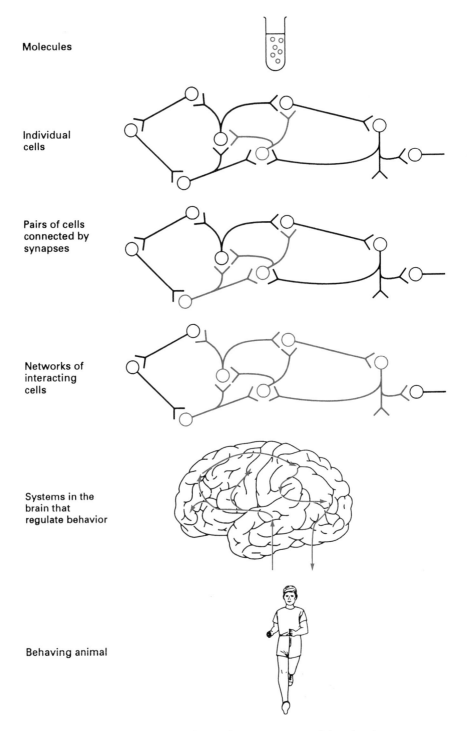

Molecules

Individual
cells

Pairs of cells
connected by
synapses

Networks of
interacting
cells

Systems in the
brain that
regulate behavior

Behaving animal

Figure 1-1. Levels of organization for studying structure and function in nervous systems. Depending on their background and training, different scientists may take different approaches to the study of the nervous system.

more recently structural biologists, investigate the properties of molecules that perform tasks important for brain function. Physiologists may study the characteristics of individual nerve cells or collections of cells that are functionally related. Behavioral psychologists explore patterns of behavior and its modification—learning—in experimental animals ranging from lower invertebrates to humans. Computational neuroscientists attempt to put it all together, to model higher brain functions in terms of the known properties of molecules, cells, or collections of cells.

In this book we will focus on the top part of Figure 1–1, on the cells of the brain and the molecules that control their function. Although where appropriate we will discuss these cells and molecules in the context of the nervous system to which they belong, our major emphasis will be on *signaling*, or *information transfer*, within and between nerve cells. We shall see that such signaling is essential for an organism to (*1*) sense information about its environment, (*2*) import this information into its brain where it can be processed, and (*3*) generate a behavioral response. Chapters 3 through 7 will explore the ways in which nerve cells are specialized for *intracellular signaling*, the movement of information from one part of the cell to another. Chapters 8 through 14 will consider *intercellular signaling*, the mechanisms by which nerve cells communicate with each other and the outside world. Finally, in Chapters 15 through 20 we will address *neuronal plasticity*, changes in the properties of a neuron. This section will include cellular and molecular aspects of *development*, the processes by which nerve cell number, position, shape, and patterns of connectivity (and hence signaling) are set down during embryonic and early postnatal life. In addition, we will discuss *behavior* and its modification at the level of signaling in individual nerve cells, collections of nerve cells, and behaving animals.

Although our focus will be on cellular and molecular mechanisms of brain function, we emphasize that cellular and molecular neurobiology does not exist in a vacuum. First, many of the mechanisms we will discuss in the context of brain cells have their counterparts in other cell types—that is, there is an emerging awareness of a satisfying unity in cell biology. Second, it is becoming evident that understanding the brain requires study at *all* the levels of organization depicted in Figure 1–1, from behaving human beings to single brain cells and the molecules that regulate cellular activity. No single level is inherently more important than any other, and information from all of them will be necessary for even the most rudimentary understanding of normal and abnormal brain functions. Thus, by its very nature, the problem demands a multidisciplinary attack, one that bridges traditional scientific disciplines and facilitates collaboration among scientists with very different training and experimental approaches. History has amply shown that it is at the boundaries between disciplines where the most significant advances are likely to be made.

The Cellular Hypothesis

We have grown so accustomed to thinking of the brain as a cellular organ that it is easy to forget how recently this view was the subject of intense debate. By 1840 it was evident, from the work of the anatomists Jacob Schleiden and Theodor Schwann, that discrete entities called cells are the basic architectural units of living tissues. It was, however, to be another 50 years and more before it was accepted that this principle also applies to the brain. Around the end of the nineteenth century the great neuroanatomists Santiago Ramón y Cajal and Camillo Golgi argued passionately about whether the brain consists of enormous numbers of discrete cells or is a continuous syncytium of tissue. The answer to this question is, of course, of enormous significance for understanding how signals spread from one part of the nervous system to another. Ramón y Cajal made elegant use of a technique, which had been discovered fortuitously by Golgi, for staining tissue. For reasons that are not understood to the present day, this technique, known as *silver impregnation*, results in the staining of only a small subset of the neurons present in a brain section. As a result, individual neurons show up clearly in tissue sections that actually contain a large number of neurons (Fig. 1–2). Using other staining methods that stain all the neurons, these same sections would have appeared only as "tangled thickets." Ramón y Cajal correctly identified these discrete entities as individual nerve cells, although Golgi never accepted this interpretation and continued to put forward his "reticular theory" of a continuous meshwork. The debate was finally won by the advocates of the cellular hypothesis, and it is now universally accepted that the brain, like other organs, is cellular. In retrospect it is clear that one reason for the long confusion over this issue is the complexity of brain tissue. As we shall see in this book, there are a large number of different cell types in the brain, and many of these cells have a complex asymmetric, three-dimensional structure that makes it extremely difficult to ascertain where one cell ends and the next begins.

Unique Structures of Neurons

Although in the next chapter we will also discuss those structures and organelles that neurons have in common with other cells, the remainder of this chapter will emphasize the features that make the neuron unique. It must be remembered that the essence of nervous system function is *signaling*, or *information transfer*, both *intra*cellularly from one part of a cell to another, and *inter*cellularly between cells. It is a fundamental premise of cellular neurobiology that a great deal will be learned about how the nervous system works by investigating

1. those aspects of neuronal structure that specialize them for information transfer;

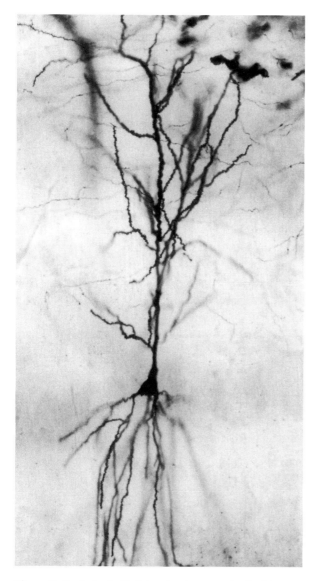

Figure 1–2. A single Golgi-stained neuron in the hippocampus. The Golgi stain allows the shape of the cell body and the complex dendritic arborization of this hippocampal pyramidal neuron to be resolved from the "tangled thickets" seen when all surrounding neurons are also stained. (Micrograph courtesy of Kristin Harris.)

2. the mechanisms of intracellular neuronal signaling;
3. the patterns of neuronal connectivity and mechanisms of intercellular signaling;
4. the relationship of various patterns of neuronal connectivity to different behaviors; and
5. the ways in which neurons and their connections can be modified by experience.

All of these will be discussed in this book. We begin now with a description of three structural elements unique to neurons: the *axon*, which is specialized for intracellular information transfer; the *dendrite*, which is often the site at which information is received from other neurons (but which also has other functions); and that most highly specialized structure of all, the *synapse*, which is the point of information transfer between neurons (Fig. 1–3).

The axon. The axon is a thin, tube-like process that arises from the neuronal cell body and travels for distances ranging from micrometers to meters before terminating (at a synapse—see below). As we shall see in Chapters 3 through 7, specialized proteins in the axonal plasma membrane allow the axon to transmit electrical signals rapidly along its length, from soma to terminal. The axon originates at a cone-shaped thickening on the cell body called the *axon hillock* (Fig. 1–3). It is often (but not always) unbranched until just before it terminates, but it may branch many times in its terminal region. The diameter of the axon remains more or less unchanged throughout its length. Its structure, like that of the dendrite, is formed and maintained by the *cytoskeleton*, a cellular scaffolding that is present in all cells but that exhibits certain unique properties in unusually shaped cells such as neurons. The role of the cytoskeleton in the formation and maintenance of neuronal form will be discussed briefly in Chapter 2.

The dendrite. Dendrites are neuronal processes that tend to be thicker and much shorter than axons and often are highly branched, giving rise to a dense network of processes known as the *dendritic tree* (Fig. 1–3). In addition, the dendritic cytoskeleton differs from that of axons (see Chapter 2). Dendrites often originate from the cell body, but in some neurons in invertebrates they arise from the proximal regions of the axon. A three-dimensional computer reconstruction, from images taken with a *confocal microscope*, reveals the presence of numerous finger-like projections or thickenings on the dendrites of some neurons. These projections, called *dendritic spines*, arise from the main shaft of the dendrite (Fig. 1–4). These spines are the synaptic input sites at which the neuron receives information from another cell. Like the axonal membrane, the plasma membrane of the dendrite contains a particular set of proteins that allows the dendrite to carry out its assigned functions (see Chapters 11 and 12). In this case, the proteins specialize the membrane in a way that allows the dendrite to receive and integrate information from other nerve cells or from elsewhere in the body. However, the role of the dendrite is not exclusively the receipt of information. Some dendrites share with axons the ability to transmit electrical signals, and in many nerve cells both information input and output occur on the same set of dendrite-like fine processes.

Interestingly, dendritic structure is not always fixed and immutable. Under some physiological conditions, the size and shape of dendritic spines

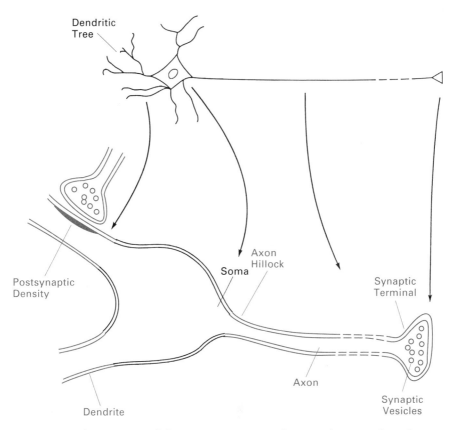

Figure 1–3. Ultrastructure of the neuron. Drawing of a typical nerve cell to show its overall shape. Structures and organelles that are found exclusively in nerve cells are shown in blue.

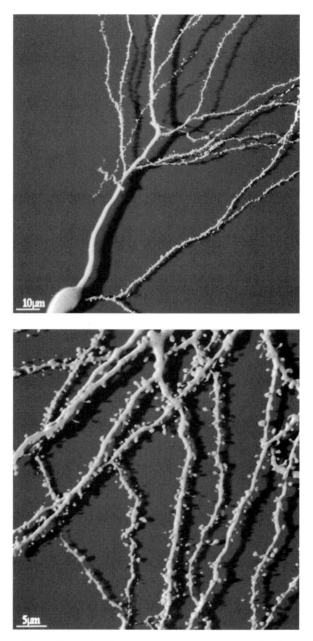

Figure 1–4. Dendritic spines. Three-dimensional computer reconstruction of a hippocampal pyramidal neuron, injected with the fluorescent dye *Lucifer yellow* and photographed with a confocal laser scanning microscope. Note the spiny projections arising from the apical dendrites (*top panel*); the dendritic region and its spines are shown at higher magnification in the *bottom panel*. (Micrographs courtesy of Anne McKinney, Scott Thompson, and Beat Gähwiler.)

can exhibit dynamic changes on a rapid time scale (Fig. 1–5 and Plate 1). It is thought that such alterations of spine morphology may contribute to long-lasting plastic changes in neuronal properties, of the kind that we shall discuss extensively later in this book.

Intercellular Communication

The synapse. We have emphasized that intercellular communication, which results in the passage of information from one part of the nervous system to another, is the essence of nervous system function. It is this information transfer that most clearly distinguishes the brain from other organs, and thus it is not surprising that the neuron has evolved a unique and highly specialized structure, the synapse, to carry out this task (Fig. 1–3). The term *synapse*, derived from a Greek word meaning "connect," was introduced by the British physiologist Charles Sherrington near the end of the nineteenth century. Sherrington was studying *spinal cord reflexes* (Fig. 1–6). Such reflexes are invariant behavioral responses to a particular kind of stimulus to the animal; they do not require the brain itself but are mediated via the spinal cord. One often-cited example is the rapid withdrawal of the arm when the fingers encounter a hot stove.

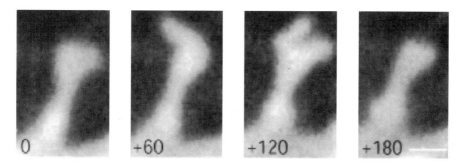

Figure 1–5. Dendritic spines are dynamic. Images of a single dendritic spine in a living hippocampal neuron, taken 60 sec apart (time in seconds is marked on each image). The neuron is from an animal that had been genetically engineered to express in its cells another fluorescent dye called *green fluorescent protein*, such that the fluorescent image represents the neuronal plasma membrane. Note that the shape and position of the spine head (top of images) is highly dynamic, whereas the base of the spine (where it meets the dendritic shaft) changes little during the 3-min observation period. A pseudo-color representation of spine movements such as these is shown in Plate 1. White bar = 2 μm. (Images courtesy of Martijn Roelandse and Andrew Matus [see also Fischer et al., 1998].)

Sherrington's studies on reflexes coincided with the time when the neuron doctrine was becoming well established as a result of the work of Ramón y Cajal and his followers. He defined a set of neuronal connections, a *pathway*, responsible for the reflex, and noted that information always travels through the reflex pathway in one direction only. More specifically, input is via the *sensory* component of the pathway (black in Fig. 1–6), which provides information about the outside world. Output is through the *motor* component (blue in Fig. 1–6), which drives muscles to provide an appropriate behavioral response to the sensory input. Sherrington also became convinced from his detailed anatomical and physiological studies that the pathway is not unicellular, but that there is a discontinuity between the sensory and motor components. In many reflex arcs there may also be an additional neuron called an *interneuron* in the spinal cord, which provides the link between the sensory and motor neurons.

With remarkable insight Sherrington proposed that at the point of contact between the sensory and motor neurons there might be a structure— the synapse—that allows unidirectional information transfer between the neurons. It is important to emphasize that Sherrington's definition of the

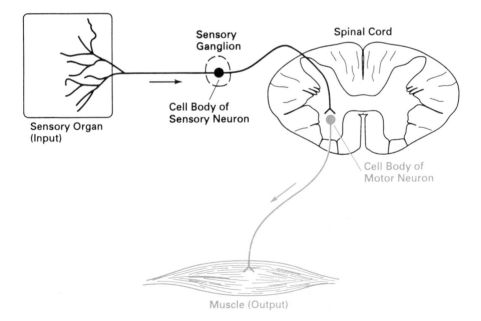

Figure 1–6. A reflex arc. The classic reflex arc, with its sensory neuron input and motor neuron output. The arrows indicate the direction of information flow in the reflex pathway.

synapse was a functional one, and it was to be many years before the anatomical correlate of this functional connection was identified.

Sherrington's pioneering work established the idea that understanding synaptic structure and function is essential for understanding how the brain works. This emphasis on the synapse in cellular neurobiology has been maintained throughout the twentieth and now into the twenty-first century. We know now that the strength of synaptic transmission—information transfer at synapses—is not fixed. This is in contrast to information transfer along the axon, which has been thought of (not entirely correctly, as we shall see) as *all-or-none*. Accordingly, one widely held belief in modern neurobiology is that changes in the properties of synapses underlie the plasticity of nervous system function, including learning and memory (see Part IV). In addition, it is becoming evident that malfunctioning synapses are associated with a whole range of debilitating diseases, among which are Parkinson's disease, manic-depressive illness, and schizophrenia. As our understanding of synaptic structure and function has increased, it has become possible to think about designing rational treatments for these diseases, but the relatively limited success to date emphasizes how far we still have to go. It is these considerations, together with the sheer intellectual excitement of trying to understand how intercellular communication works in the nervous system, that continue to motivate research on synaptic transmission.

Two kinds of synapses. Through the first half of the twentieth century there was a bitter controversy about the nature of information transfer at synapses. The school of neuropharmacologists, led by Sir Henry Dale, insisted that synaptic transmission is mediated by a chemical substance liberated from the terminal of one neuron (the *presynaptic* cell), which interacts with and influences the properties of the follower neuron or muscle cell (the *postsynaptic* cell). The first convincing piece of evidence for this idea came from the study of a classical neuron-to-muscle synapse in the frog. It had been known that electrical stimulation of the vagus nerve leads to slowing of the heart rate. In a classic experiment carried out in 1921, the Austrian pharmacologist Otto Loewi placed a frog heart, innervated by the vagus nerve, in a chamber containing physiological saline, and connected the chamber with another that contained a second, noninnervated heart (Fig. 1–7). The experimental arrangement allowed the saline solutions in which the two hearts were sitting to exchange freely. He then stimulated the vagus nerve, which of course resulted in slowing of the first heart. Loewi noted that, after some delay, the second heart slowed as well (Fig. 1–7). He concluded correctly that some chemical released by the firing of the vagus nerve results in slowing of the heart rate, and that this chemical diffused through the saline solution to the second chamber where it acted on the second heart. The chemical responsible for this phenomenon was subsequently isolated and identified as acetylcholine, the first chemical to be characterized as a *neurotransmitter*. Although this is a neuron-to-muscle synapse, it is now clear that neuron-to-neuron chemical synapses operate in the same general way, and that acetylcholine is an important neurotransmitter in the brain as well as in the peripheral nervous system.

The conflicting point of view, put forward most forcefully by the electrophysiologist Sir John Eccles, held that synaptic transmission is electrical and results from the movement of ions from one neuron to another

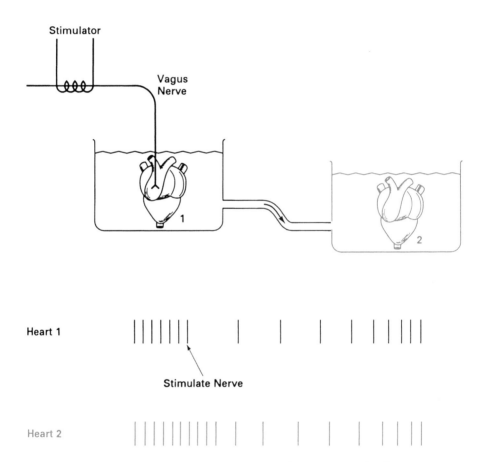

Figure 1–7. Chemical transmission at a nerve–muscle synapse. In this famous experiment performed in 1921, Otto Loewi placed an innervated (*1*) and a noninnervated (*2*) heart in two separate chambers connected by a bridge of physiological saline. At the bottom is shown the rate of beating of both hearts before and after stimulation of the vagus nerve connected to the first heart.

via direct physical connections between the neurons. Again, a variety of evidence supported this contention. The arguments between the two factions were often acrimonious because each believed that there is a single global mechanism of synaptic transmission. We know now that they were wrong in this belief, and that both points of view were correct. Chemical and electrical modes of synaptic transmission exist side by side in most and probably in all nervous systems.

Properties of chemical and electrical synapses. Although both chemical and electrical synapses mediate intercellular information transfer, they do so by very different mechanisms. It is instructive to consider those features that distinguish the two types of synapses in the context of the different functional roles that they may play. We know a good deal more about chemical than electrical synapses, but this may reflect historical accident rather than the relative importance of the two kinds of synapses. Convenient experimental preparations for the investigation of chemical synaptic transmission have been available for many years, but only more recently have conceptual and technical advances allowed a more thorough examination of the properties of electrical synapses. It is worth mentioning in this context that, until quite recently, much of what we know about chemical synaptic transmission had been gleaned from studies of the vertebrate *neuromuscular junction*, which is a neuron-to-muscle rather than a neuron-to-neuron synapse (see Fig. 9–1). This has arisen in part because the frog sciatic nerve–gastrocnemius muscle synapse is such an accessible and convenient experimental preparation, far more accessible than neuron-to-neuron synapses in the complex cellular networks of the central nervous system (Fig. 1–8). In addition, a number of gifted investigators, most notably Sir Bernard Katz and his collaborators in London, exploited this preparation brilliantly to elucidate the details of synaptic transmission between nerve and muscle cells.

Accordingly, the picture many neurobiologists hold of the "typical" chemical synapse is the neuromuscular junction. However, as recent technological advances have enabled more detailed mechanistic investigation of central nervous system synapses, it has become evident that this picture is inappropriate in many ways. For example, many central nervous system chemical synapses operate on a time scale orders of magnitude slower than that of the neuromuscular junction, and the molecular mechanisms involved in the transduction of the chemical signal into an electrical response in the postsynaptic cell can be very different (see Chapters 11 and 12). Although we will be referring often to studies on the neuromuscular junction in discussing various aspects of chemical synaptic transmission in subsequent chapters—and indeed, this is reasonable because (with apolo-

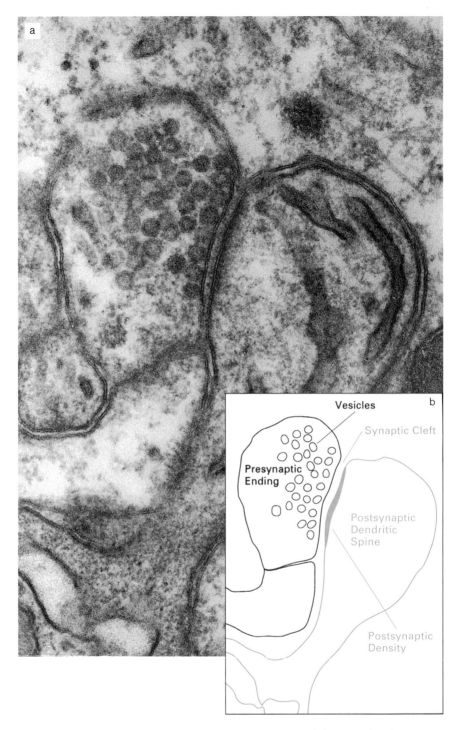

Figure 1–8. A chemical synapse. Electron micrograph (*a*) and drawing (*b*) of a synapse onto the spine of a Purkinje cell dendrite (micrograph from Landis, 1987).

18

gies to Gertrude Stein) a synapse is a synapse is a synapse—these caveats must be kept in mind.

Chemical synapses. The most obvious difference between chemical and electrical synapses is in their structure as seen in the electron microscope. Chemical synapses have an *asymmetric* morphology, with distinct features found in the presynaptic and postsynaptic parts or "elements" of a synapse (Figs. 1–3 and 1–8). The presynaptic ending is a swelling of the axon terminal, containing mitochondria and, most important, a variety of vesicular structures. As will be discussed in Chapter 8, the vesicles contain the neurotransmitter, for example, acetylcholine, that is released from the presynaptic terminal and produces some change in the postsynaptic cell. The vesicles are often clustered adjacent to the membrane of the presynaptic terminal at its point of closest contact with the postsynaptic cell (see Fig. 1–8). This clustering may be related to the association of vesicles with specialized cytoskeletal filaments.

The electron microscope also reveals that the pre and postsynaptic elements of a chemical synapse are separated by a 200 to 300 Å gap, the *synaptic cleft* (Fig. 1–8). This gap is somewhat larger than the normal extracellular space between cells, and its presence emphasizes that there are not direct membrane connections between the pre and postsynaptic cells at chemical synapses. Stains that bind to sugars reveal that the synaptic cleft is loaded with carbohydrate, presumably associated with glycoproteins in the pre and/or postsynaptic membranes. The function of this extracellular carbohydrate is not well understood, although one idea favored by many investigators is that it provides a matrix for some molecules that are important for synapse formation (see Chapter 18).

Just as most presynaptic endings are axon terminals, most postsynaptic elements of central nervous system synapses are dendrites, giving rise to the term *axodendritic synapse.* However, like most rules, this one has exceptions. *Axosomatic synapses* (where the postsynaptic target is a neuronal cell body or soma) and (more rarely) *axoaxonic synapses* exist. Moreover, as we have already mentioned, it is becoming evident that dendrites can also act as presynaptic elements (dendrodendritic synapses). In fact, in some nerve cells there are fine dendrite-like processes at which both input and output of information take place.

Virtually the entire somatic and dendritic surface of most central nervous system neurons is covered with presynaptic terminals (Fig. 1–9; see photomicrograph in Plate 2). In other words, there can be enormous *convergence*, onto a single neuron, of input information from hundreds or even thousands of presynaptic cells (Fig. 1–10). As we will see in subsequent chapters, neurons are constantly integrating these multiple synaptic inputs, and the location of any given postsynaptic site can be very important in determining its contribution to the neuron's overall activity. When we consider, in addition, that a single presynaptic axon may branch many times and provide input to dozens or hundreds of postsynaptic targets (*divergence*; see Fig. 1–10), we can begin to appreciate the complexity of the computations that even the simplest of nervous systems carry out.

In contrast to the presynaptic terminal, the postsynaptic element is usually characterized by the absence of vesicles adjacent to the plasma membrane. There is often a highly electron-dense structure, the *postsynaptic density*, associated with the postsynaptic membrane immediately opposite the accumulation of vesicles on the presynaptic side (Figs. 1–3 and 1–8). The functional significance of this distinctive morphological specialization is the subject of much investigation and is beginning to be understood. Among its functions is to help anchor receptors for neurotransmitters in the postsynaptic membrane. It also contains molecules that are involved in *transduction*, the conversion of the chemical signal into an electrical response in the postsynaptic cell (see Chapters 11 and 12).

Associated with the morphological asymmetry of chemical synapses is a fundamental functional asymmetry: chemical synapses are *unidirectional*.

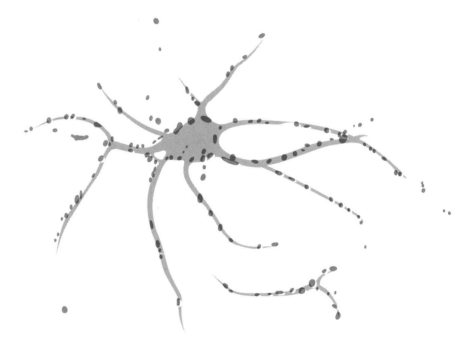

Figure 1–9. Convergent synaptic inputs (*blue*) on a cultured hippocampal neuron (*gray*). (drawn from a micrograph by Pietro de Camilli). See Plate 2.

That is, rapid transfer of information only occurs from the pre to the post-synaptic cell (see Fig. 1–6). Like most rules, this one too has an exception; we shall see that a different kind of information does appear to flow from the post- to the presynaptic cell via *retrograde messengers*. However, this is very different from the more or less symmetrical *bidirectional* information transfer characteristic of most electrical synapses. In addition, at chemical synapses, there is a delay that may be a millisecond or longer between the arrival of information at the presynaptic terminal and its transfer to the postsynaptic cell. This delay reflects the several steps required for the release and action of the chemical neurotransmitter (Chapter 9). Furthermore, the response of the postsynaptic neuron may outlast the presynaptic signal that evokes it, sometimes by a very long time. The transduction mechanisms that may be responsible for such long-lasting changes in the target cell will be considered in detail in Chapters 11 and 12.

Electrical synapses. The striking asymmetry in structure and function of chemical synapses may be contrasted with the symmetrical morphology and bidirectional information transfer characteristic of electrical synapses. First, there are no morphological specializations that allow pre- and postsynaptic elements to be distinguished. Indeed, since signals can move in both directions through electrical synapses, each cell may be pre- *or* postsynaptic at different times. Instead of the synaptic cleft that separates the two elements of the chemical synapse, electrical synapses are characterized by an area of very close apposition between the membranes of the pre- and postsynaptic cells. Within these areas of the membrane are found

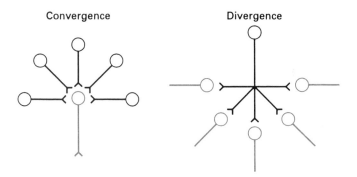

Figure 1–10. Convergence and divergence in nervous system function. *Left*: Any given nerve cell can receive convergent synaptic inputs on its dendrites from a large number—perhaps as many as thousands—of other neurons. *Right*: The axon of a neuron may branch many times, and thus divergent information may be provided to a large number of postsynaptic targets of this single neuron.

gap junctions, cell-to-cell pores that allow ions and small molecules to pass freely from the cytoplasm of one cell to the next. Gap junctions exist in many types of cells. One test that is often used to establish whether a pair of cells is connected by gap junctions is *dye coupling*—that is, a low-molecular-weight dye such as *Lucifer Yellow* injected into one of the cells can spread rapidly into the cytoplasm of its synaptic partner (Fig. 1–11). As is the case for gap junctions in other cell types, molecules with a molecular weight up to about 1000–1500 can be transferred through most neuronal gap junctions. The structure and function of gap junctions will be discussed in more detail in Chapter 8 (see Figs. 8–1 to 8–3).

It is the movement of small ions from one cell to another through cell-to-cell gap junction channels that mediates intercellular signaling at electrical synapses. These channels provide a low-resistance pathway for ion flow between the cells without leakage to the extracellular space, and thus signals can be transmitted with little attenuation. Two important functional properties follow immediately from this mode of transmission. First, as referred to above, information transfer can be bidirectional—that is, a *functional* symmetry accompanies the *structural* symmetry. There are examples where the efficacy of electrical synaptic transmission is higher in one direction than in the other (so-called rectifying synapses); in fact, the first electrical synapse whose properties were investigated in detail, between two large axons in the crayfish, rectifies markedly. In general, however, the rule of symmetrical bidirectionality holds, and, in fact, it is an important criterion in identifying electrical synapses. The second important functional consequence of this mechanism is that electrical synapses are fast. There is no delay analogous to that seen with chemical synaptic transmission.

The extent of electrical synaptic connectivity in the central nervous system remains unclear. One functional role for electrical synapses that is widely accepted is in the synchronization of the electrical activity of large populations of neurons. For example, in both vertebrates and invertebrates it has been demonstrated that populations of neurosecretory neurons that synthesize and release biologically active peptide neurotransmitters and hormones are connected extensively by electrical synapses. Simultaneous recording from several neurons within such populations reveals that they all are electrically active at the same time, probably resulting in concerted release of their neurotransmitter. Synchronization via electrical synapses may also be important in various aspects of neuronal development, including the formation of chemical synapses. Large numbers of electrical synapses are also found in the retina, where they may influence and coordinate the processing of visual information.

It has been suggested that electrical synapses are less subject to alter-

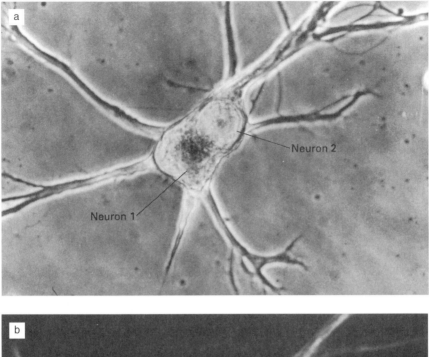

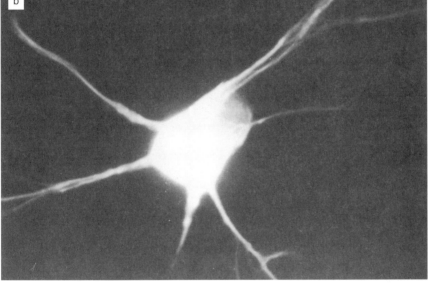

Figure 1–11. Dye coupling via an electrical synapse. *a*: Photograph of two adjoining neurons isolated in a culture dish. The lower cell (neuron 1) was injected with the fluorescent dye Lucifer yellow by one of the authors (Kaczmarek et al., 1979). *b*: The fluorescent image shows that dye has passed into neuron 2.

ation of their properties than chemical synapses and thus might provide an invariant mode of intercellular communication. However, it is becoming evident that the efficacy of electrical synaptic transmission can be regulated, perhaps as extensively as that of chemical synapses. Furthermore, as we shall see in Chapter 19, an examination of the properties of small networks of neurons reveals that many neuronal pairs in such networks are connected by *both* chemical and electrical synapses, and that the efficacy of one of the synaptic types may be modulated by the other. Thus there is no question that more detailed information about electrical synaptic transmission will be necessary as we extend our understanding of intercellular communication in the nervous system.

Summary

The neurons are the cells of the brain that are responsible for intracellular and intercellular information transfer, or signaling. Neurons are asymmetric cells with morphologically and functionally distinct regions that specialize them for signaling. In this chapter we have focused on the unique structural elements characteristic of neurons throughout the animal kingdom. These include the dendrite, among whose functions is the receipt of information from other neurons. The axon, in contrast, is specialized for the intracellular transfer of information over long distances. Finally, we have discussed the synapse, the highly specialized structure that mediates the transfer of information from one neuron to another. It is this intracellular and intercellular communication that is the essence of nervous system function, and that makes the brain on the one hand so complex and difficult to study and yet at the same time so fascinating for the student of cell and molecular biology.

2

Form and Function in
Cells of the Brain

*I*n the first chapter we focused exclusively on neurons, and particularly on those aspects of neuronal structure that specialize them for intra- and intercellular signaling. We will now consider some features of the structure and function of the various classes of *glial cells* that comprise by far the majority of cells in the brain. We will then emphasize that neurons share many structural features with other kinds of cells, including the glial cells. Finally, we will conclude with a discussion of the *cytoskeleton*, and its role in the formation and maintenance of the structure of neurons.

The Brain Consists of Neurons and Glia

In the middle of the nineteenth century the German anatomist Rudolf Virchow recognized that cells in the brain could be divided into two distinct groups: (*1*) neurons, and (*2*) a far more numerous group of cells that appear to surround the neurons and fill the spaces between them. Virchow called this second category of cell the *neuroglia*, or nerve glue, the implication being that one of its functions is to hold the neurons in place. It now appears that this is, indeed, one of the many functions of glia, and certainly the name itself has stuck!

Glial cells can themselves be divided into several subclasses based on their appearance in the microscope. In the central nervous system the two main types of glial cells are the *astrocytes* and the *oligodendrocytes*. As their name implies, the astrocytes have a star-like appearance, with numerous long arms radiating out from a central cell body (Fig. 2–1). The

25

oligodendrocytes also have a central cell body, with radial arms that tend to be shorter and more branched than those of the astrocytes (Fig. 2–1). As will be discussed below, the oligodendrocytes play an essential role in the functioning of neurons by forming the *myelin sheath* around axons in the central nervous system (see Fig. 2–3). In the peripheral nervous system the *Schwann cell*, another class of glial cell, is responsible for forming the myelin sheath.

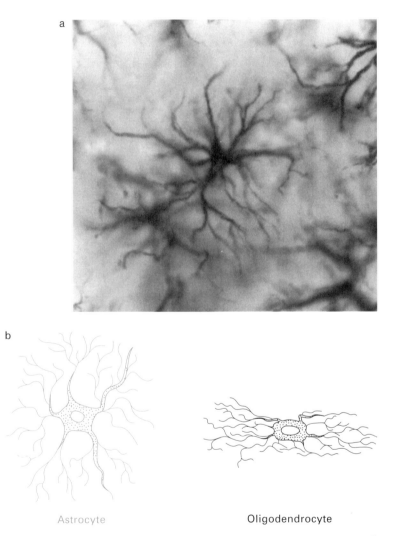

Astrocyte   Oligodendrocyte

Figure 2–1. Morphology of astrocytes and oligodendrocytes. *a*: An astrocyte seen with the light microscope. *b*: Drawings to illustrate the different morphologies of astrocytes and oligodendrocytes. (Micrograph courtesy of Theresa Jones and Bill Greenough.)

In addition to myelination, a number of functional roles have been ascribed to glia. For example, glia are known to

1. act as a scaffolding for neuronal migration and axon outgrowth;
2. participate in the uptake and metabolism of the neurotransmitters that neurons use for intercellular communication;
3. take up and buffer ions from the extracellular environment;
4. act as scavengers to remove debris produced by dying neurons;
5. segregate groups of neurons one from another, and act as electrical insulators between neurons;
6. provide structural support for neurons, fulfilling a role played by connective tissue cells in other organs;
7. play a nurturing role, supplying metabolic components and even proteins necessary for neuronal function; and
8. participate in intercellular signaling, and thereby play a role in information handling and memory storage.

Thus it appears that glia have evolved multiple functional roles.

Glial signaling. In the past, neurobiologists relegated glia to a role secondary to that of neurons because they thought that neurons are uniquely capable of intracellular and intercellular signaling. More recent evidence, however, suggests that glia may in fact be active participants in brain signaling, and it is conceivable that neurons even form functional synapses with glial cells as their partners. Much better established is the fact that astrocytes possess on their cell surfaces the protein receptors for certain neurotransmitters that mediate synaptic signaling between neurons. Astrocytes are also capable of releasing these neurotransmitters, which may then influence nearby neurons or other glia. It is also known that astrocytes can respond to neurotransmitters by producing oscillations in their cytosolic calcium concentration that can spread from one astrocyte to another (Fig. 2–2; see also Plate 3), also producing changes in calcium concentrations in neighboring neurons. Such communication among glial cells, and between glia and neurons, implies that our picture of glia as staid and stodgy cells that play only a supporting role in the drama of brain function is inadequate and in need of revision.

The myelin sheath. Myelination is one role of glia that is well understood. The myelin sheath surrounds many, but not all, axons in the vertebrate nervous system. Although it is formed by glial cells and is not strictly a part of the axon, it is fundamental for axonal function. The sheath is formed by oligodendrocytes on central nervous system axons and by Schwann cells in the peripheral nervous system. When a myelinated axon

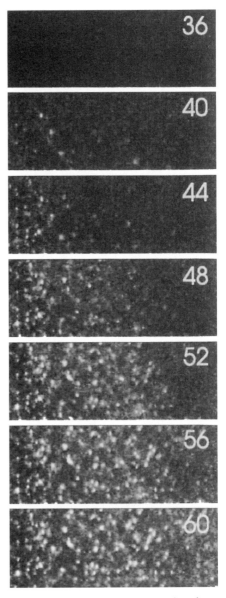

Figure 2–2. Spread of a calcium wave through astrocytes. Astrocytes in a slice from the hippocampus were loaded with Fluo-3, a dye that emits a fluorescent signal when it binds calcium, and were imaged by confocal microscopy (for a more detailed discussion of calcium imaging, see Chapter 9). The numbers on each picture refer to the time (in seconds) when the picture was taken, after a stimulus excited cells in the slice. From an experiment by Stephen J Smith and colleagues (Dani et al., 1992). See also Plate 3.

is examined in cross section with an electron microscope, the axon is found to be surrounded by concentric circles of alternating dark and light bands (Fig. 2–3a). This structure arises by the tight wrapping of the membrane of the oligodendrocyte or Schwann cell around the axon during development (Fig. 2–3b). The cytoplasm of the glial cell is gradually squeezed out of this region as the cell wraps around the axon, so that the concentric circles represent layers of closely apposed glial plasma membrane. One can get a feel for the structure of myelinated axons by examining a roll of paper towels end-on: the central cardboard tube represents the axon, and the layers of paper, the wrapping of glial plasma membrane.

A single Schwann cell may occupy up to about 1 mm of the length of a peripheral nervous system axon. Since some axons may be up to 1 meter or more in length, the myelin sheath consists of a large number of Schwann cells, each occupying its small portion of the axon. Between adjacent Schwann cells are gaps of several micrometers, known as *nodes of Ranvier* (Fig. 2–4). The Schwann cell–covered region between the nodes of Ranvier is known as the *internode*. To carry our analogy further, the myelinated axon can be compared with a large number of rolls of paper towels lined up end-to-end, with small gaps in the paper layer (but, of course, not in the cardboard tubes) representing the nodes of Ranvier.

This multiple-membrane layer, which also happens to be unusually rich in lipid, insulates the axonal cytoplasm (the *axoplasm*) from the extracellular fluid. This means that electrical current can flow across the axonal plasma membrane only at the nodes, and, as we shall see in Part II, this has profound implications for the speed of transmission of electrical signals along the axon. For example, in those species in which birth occurs before myelination, the newborns are extremely limited in motor performance and, in fact, are quite helpless until myelination is complete. The functional importance of myelin is also underscored by the severe impairments in motor function observed in the *demyelinating diseases*, such as multiple sclerosis, which are associated with extensive degeneration of the myelin sheath.

In addition to this critical role in the transmission of electrical signals, other interactions between Schwann cells and neurons have been documented. For example, neurons produce certain molecules, such as growth factors, that are necessary for Schwann cell proliferation. Schwann cells in turn produce molecules that influence the expression of neuronal proteins important for neuronal survival and differentiation. Thus the traditional picture of a purely mechanical interaction between Schwann cells and neurons must be revised to include reciprocal chemical influences as well.

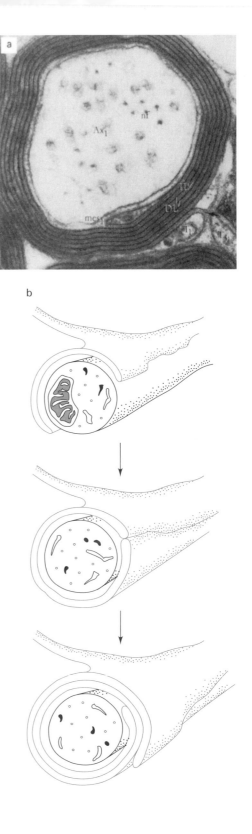

The Nerve Cell Body: Neurons Are the Same as Other Cells

As Ramón y Cajal recognized, the nerve cells, or *neurons*, are the individual signaling elements of the brain. Although we will argue that the intercellular communication that is the hallmark of brain function makes the brain a unique organ, in many respects neurons (and glia) closely resemble other types of cells. Figure 2–5 is a diagram of the archetypal neuron; it is similar to that in Figure 1–3 but with additional organelles included. Note that this neuron consists of processes of different size and shape emanating from a cell body. It is this neuronal cell body, or *soma*, an electron micrograph of which is shown in Figure 2–6a, that most resembles cells in other organs. The most prominent organelle in the cell body is the *nucleus*, which contains the genetic material, DNA. The genomic DNA in neurons is identical to that in other cells in the organism (although in the so-called giant neurons in some invertebrates the genome divides many times without corresponding cell divisions, resulting in as many as 50,000 copies of the genome in the nucleus of some of these cells; the functional consequences of this are not understood). Even though the genome is no different from that in other cells, genes are regulated in specific ways that result in the synthesis of a pattern of proteins specific to neurons. Of course, specific gene expression also occurs in all other tissues and accounts for the existence of specific cell types in liver, muscle, heart, and other organs, in addition to the many different types of neurons and glia found in the brain.

The entire neuron, like all other cells, is enclosed by a *plasma membrane*—a double layer (or *bilayer*) of phospholipid molecules, which acts as a barrier preventing the contents of the cell from mixing with those of the extracellular space. The plasma membrane is also an effective electrical insulator, hindering the diffusion of charged ions in and out of the cell. This is important, because signaling in nerve cells requires the controlled movement of ions across the plasma membrane, a process mediated by specialized proteins located in the membrane.

What other common organelles are found in neuronal cell bodies (Figs. 2–5 and 2–6)? The cell body (as well as the neuronal processes) contains

---

Figure 2–3. The myelin sheath. *a:* Electron micrograph of a cross section through a myelinated axon (modified from Peters et al., 1976). Ax_1, center of axon; *b:* Formation of the myelin sheath. In the first stage (*top*), an axon (*black*) is enclosed by the process of the oligodendrocyte (*blue*). The oligodendrocyte then completely envelops the axon, but has not yet lost its cytoplasm (*middle and bottom*). The mature myelin sheath has cytoplasm only in the inner and outer ends of the spiraled process. (Modified from Peters et al., 1976.)

mitochondria to supply the cell's energy needs. In fact, because a great deal of energy is required to maintain the transmembrane ionic gradients that are essential for neuronal signaling, neurons tend to be particularly rich in mitochondria. The cell body also contains *ribosomes*, which are responsible for the synthesis of proteins destined for insertion into membranes or for secretion; they are located on the membranous sacs of the *rough endoplasmic reticulum*, which is often unusually dense adjacent to the nucleus of neurons, giving rise to the structural feature called the *Nissl substance* (named after its discoverer). Other membranous components include the *smooth endoplasmic reticulum* and the *Golgi complex*, which are involved in the processing of proteins for membrane insertion or se-

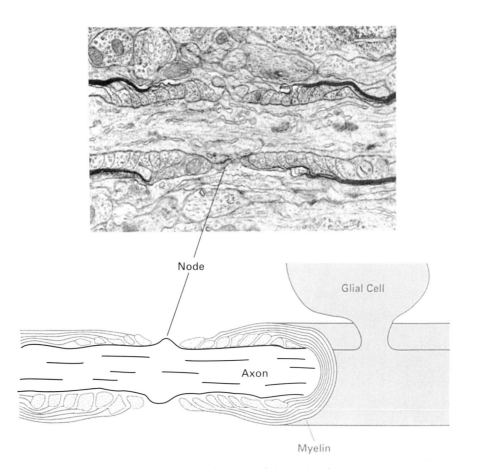

Figure 2–4. Electron micrograph and diagram of the node of Ranvier. At this region, the myelin sheath is interrupted for a short distance between adjacent glial cells, exposing the axonal plasma membrane to the extracellular space. (Micrograph courtesy of Dennis Landis.)

cretion (see Chapter 8), and *lysosomes* and other granules involved in the breakdown and disposal of cellular components.

We have been listing these organelles of the cell body at a rapid pace simply because the reader with a background in cell biology will already be familiar with their structures and functions. Although some features may be particularly characteristic of neurons, such as the presence of the Nissl substance or the density of mitochondria, these are relatively minor quantitative differences, rather than qualitative ones, between neurons and other cells. Only a trained observer would readily identify an electron micrograph such as that in Figure 2–6a as a picture of a neuron rather than of some other kind of cell.

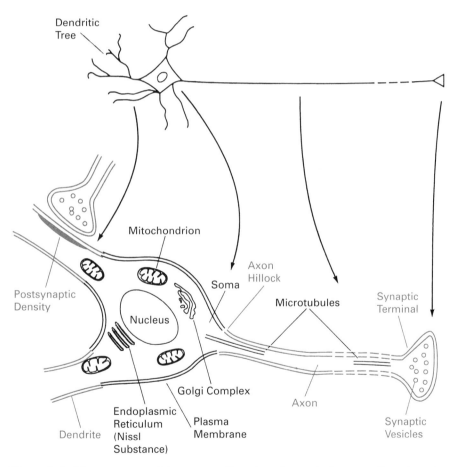

Figure 2–5. Ultrastructure of the neuron. Drawing of a typical nerve cell to show its overall shape and characteristic organelles. Structures and organelles that are common to all types of cells are shown in black (compare with Fig. 1–3).

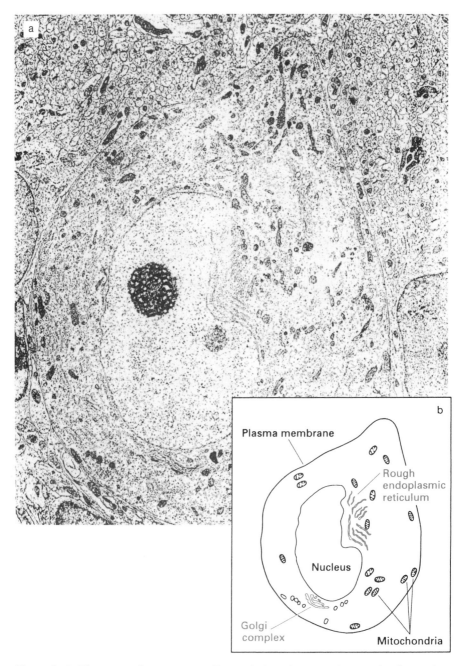

Figure 2–6. The soma of a neuron. *a*: Transmission electron micrograph of a section through the cell body of a typical neuron, a Purkinje cell of the cerebellum (courtesy of Dennis Landis). *b*: Diagram identifying some of the intracellular organelles.

Perhaps the most striking example of the conservation of structures and their functions among different cell types relates to molecular mechanisms of secretion. We will discuss this topic in detail in Chapter 8, but it is worth noting here that almost identical proteins and molecular mechanisms are involved in vesicle trafficking and secretion processes in organisms ranging from yeast to humans. Nothing emphasizes better the unity of cellular biological mechanisms, or that neuronal cell biology is fundamentally the same as that of other cell types.

Formation and Maintenance of Neuronal Form

When one examines a picture of a neuron with its remarkably asymmetric structure (Figs. 1–3 and 2–5), an obvious question comes to mind concerning the mechanisms by which such neuronal polarity arises during development: how do structures such as axons and dendrites originate? In the rest of this chapter we will introduce some of the important molecules and processes that contribute to the formation and maintenance of neuronal structure.

The cytoskeleton. The neuron, like all cells, contains a heterogeneous network of filamentous structures known collectively as the *cytoskeleton*. The major components of this network are the *microfilaments*, the *neurofilaments*, and the *microtubules*.

The function of microfilaments is best understood in skeletal muscle, where they are made up of the proteins actin and myosin. These filaments are present in highly ordered structures and interact to produce muscle contraction. Actin is also found in axons and, as we shall see in Chapter 17, is particularly prominent in the growing tips of axons, the *growth cones*, where it may contribute to the regulation of membrane movement. Actin is also thought to play a critical role in dynamic changes in dendritic spine morphology, of the sort illustrated in Figure 1–5. In many cell types, including neurons, actin accounts for an extremely high proportion of the total protein in the cell.

The neurofilaments are probably the least well understood of the cytoskeletal components. They are long filaments approximately 10 nm in diameter, intermediate in size between actin filaments (about 5 nm) and microtubules (about 20 nm). For this reason they fall into the general class of cytoskeletal components known as *intermediate* filaments in nonneural cells. Certain pathological conditions, including Alzheimer's disease, are associated with a profound disorganization of neurofilaments, but it remains unclear whether the chaotic tangles of neurofilaments seen in the brains of Alzheimer's patients actually cause the progressive senility characteristic of this disease.

Microtubules carry out a variety of functions in different cells. They play an important role in cell movement and are the major component of the *mitotic spindle*, an organelle that participates in cell division. Microtubules are also prominent inhabitants of axons and dendrites. Like the other filaments, they are polymeric structures, made up of large numbers of repeating units of two similar 50 kDa proteins known as α- and β-*tubulin* (Fig. 2–7). The polymerization of tubulin into microtubules depends on the nucleotide GTP and is promoted by *microtubule-associated proteins* (MAPs), which may also help anchor microtubules to membranes or to other cytoskeletal components (Fig. 2–7). A number of different MAPs exist and these are often differentially associated with axons and dendrites. In addition, the amounts of the various MAPs change in characteristically different ways during neuronal development. Figure 2–8 shows a micrograph of a section through the rat cerebellum, stained with an antibody that recognizes one particular MAP, MAP1. The staining is particularly prominent in the dendrites of the large cerebellar Purkinje neu-

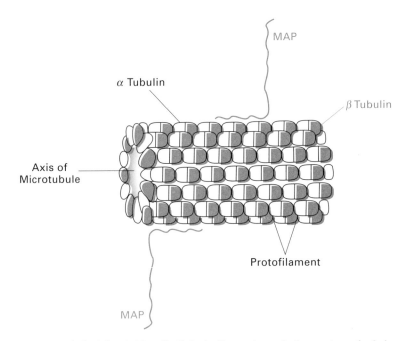

Figure 2–7. A microtubule. The rigid wall of the hollow microtubule consists of a helical array of protofilaments, each of which is a dimer formed from α- and β-tubulin. Microtubule-associated proteins (MAPs) bind to the microtubule.

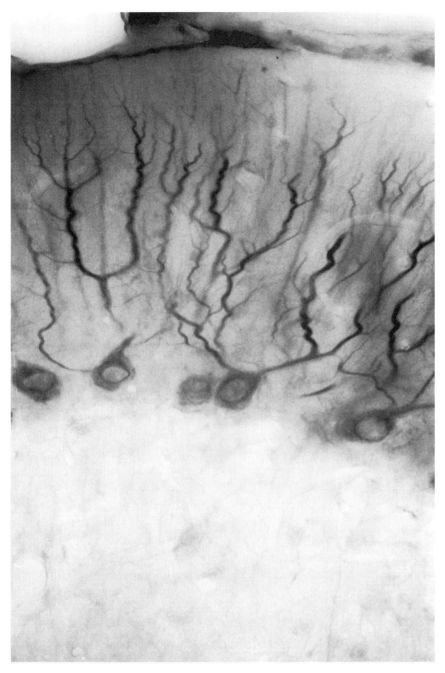

Figure 2–8. Localization of microtubule-associated proteins (MAPs) in axons and dendrites. In this experiment carried out by Andrew Matus and colleagues, a section through a rat cerebellum was stained with an antibody that specifically recognizes one particular microtubule-associated protein, MAP1. The dendrites of the large Purkinje cell neurons stain prominently with this antibody.

rons. Earlier in development, however, MAP1 is restricted to the axons of these cells. Findings such as these suggest that the MAPs play a crucial role in the generation of structural differences between axons and dendrites.

Axonal transport. Another fundamental question that arises from an examination of neuronal structure is how it is maintained during the normal everyday life of the neuron. Since portions of the cell may be as far as 1 meter or more from the cell body, the neuron must have mechanisms for providing proteins and other necessary metabolic materials to its distal regions. It has long been thought that protein synthesis is restricted to the cell body, although there is now compelling evidence for the existence of ribosomes that actively support protein synthesis in some dendrites. Protein synthesis is not known, however, to occur in axons or their terminals. How then do proteins required for normal membrane turnover, and enzymes necessary for metabolic functions such as neurotransmitter synthesis and degradation, reach their appropriate sites in these regions of the neuron? What is the mechanism for providing energy to sites so far removed from the soma?

To carry out these functions, the neuron has evolved a series of elegant transport systems known collectively as *axonal transport*. Of course, all cells are faced with the problem of moving cellular components from one part of the cell to another, but as pointed out above, this problem is particularly acute for neurons. Hence, their transport systems are highly specialized. Such systems are necessary because in the absence of an active process, a typical protein would require approximately 10 days to diffuse passively down a 1 cm axon from soma to terminal.

Axonal transport was first studied in detail as long ago as the 1930s. Through axonal ligation and microscopic examination, a variety of vesicular structures could be seen to accumulate in the proximal portion of the axon immediately behind the ligature (Fig. 2–9). It was inferred from such experiments that vesicles are transported down the axon in a proximal-to-distal (soma-to-terminal) direction. Other early studies of axonal transport used parts of the brain in which the cell bodies are remote from the axons and their terminals. The visual system is particularly useful in this regard since the cell bodies of the retinal ganglion neurons are confined to the retina, and their axons travel to the brain in the optic nerve. Accordingly, a number of investigators applied radioactively or fluorescently labeled materials to the eye and asked whether and how these materials are transported along the optic nerve into the brain. The most extensive of these studies used radioactive amino acids that are incorporated into proteins and provide a marker for following protein transport. It has become evident from such experiments that proteins are transported down the axon at different rates and that each rate probably corresponds to a different form of transport. There is a rapid form of axonal transport that is characterized by transport rates of the order of several hundred millimeters per day, and one or more slow processes that transport proteins at a rate of 1–10 mm per day.

It had long been suspected that components of the cytoskeleton such as microtubules, which run the length of the axon, might play a fundamental role in axonal transport. This has been confirmed by experiments with the microtubule-disrupting drug *colchicine*, which blocks axonal transport. In addition, a technique known as *enhanced-contrast video microscopy* allows the movement of vesicles and organelles along microtubules to be observed in real time. Among the transported organelles that can be seen are mitochondria, which suggests an answer to the question posed above concerning the energy requirements of axons and nerve terminals. The various vesicles carry proteins and other materials to be inserted into membranes or to be released at the nerve terminal.

Molecular motors. How is it that mitochondria and other large vesicular organelles are able to move long distances along microtubules to distal portions of the neuron? Recent experiments have disclosed the existence of

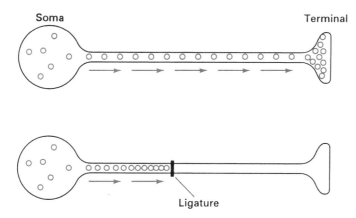

Figure 2–9. Vesicles are transported from soma to axon terminal. Vesicles and organelles are synthesized in the cell body and transported (arrows) by an active process down the axon toward its terminal. When the axon is tied off (ligated), vesicles are seen to accumulate in the axon on the side of the ligature proximal to the cell body. Experiments of this type were first done by Paul Weiss and colleagues in the 1930s.

the molecular machinery, the so-called molecular motors, that drive axonal transport and other cell movements. The best understood of the molecular motors is *myosin*, which interacts with actin to form the basic contractile unit of muscle. In fact, it is now known that a large family of
myosin molecules exists, the members of which participate in such fundamental processes as cell division, cell motility, and changes in cell shape
during development and differentiation. Myosin and other molecular mo-

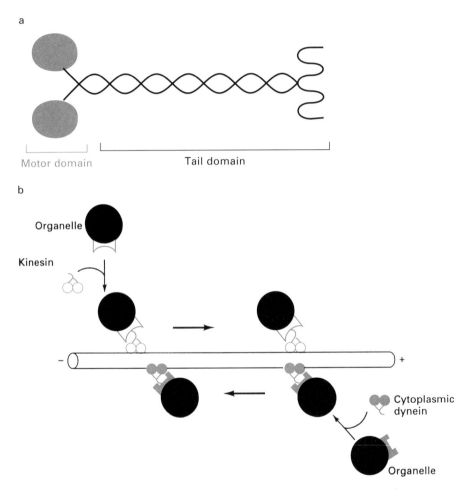

Figure 2–10. Vesicles and organelles are transported by an active process along microtubules. *a*: Molecular architecture of kinesin, a molecular motor. The functional unit
is a kinesin dimer, consisting of a conserved motor domain and a divergent tail. *b*: The
binding and movement of organelles such as vesicles along microtubules are mediated
by kinesin and another molecular motor, cytoplasmic dynein (Sheetz et al., 1989).

tors use the energy derived from ATP hydrolysis to drive movement, by mechanisms that have been studied for a long time but are still not fully understood.

It is not myosin, however, that drives axonal transport. That task falls to *kinesin*, another kind of motor protein. Studies in yeast, nematodes, and fruit flies have identified a large family of kinesin genes, the roles of most of which remain to be determined. The various kinesin proteins are approximately 120 kDa in molecular mass and share a common overall molecular architecture (Fig. 2–10a). The 350 or so amino acids at the amino terminal are highly conserved and constitute the *motor domain*, which contains the enzymatic machinery responsible for the hydrolysis of ATP (the ATPase activity). The remainder of the molecule is divergent in sequence (Fig. 2–10a) and is responsible for targeting the kinesin to a particular kind of organelle or region of the cell. Hence, this divergent tail determines the biological role of a particular kinesin, while the motor domain simply drives the required movement. This modular structure of the kinesins is emphasized by the use of recombinant DNA techniques to make fragments of kinesin molecules that contain only the motor domain. Such purified motor domain fragments alone can produce ATP-dependent movement of microtubules along nonbiological surfaces such as glass.

How does kinesin drive axonal transport of vesicles, mitochondria, and other organelles? Kinesin interacts with both microtubules and vesicles and uses the energy of hydrolysis of ATP to drive the movement of one relative to that of the other (Fig. 2–10b). The central role of kinesin in axonal transport is emphasized by the experiment shown in Figure 2–11. Enhanced-contrast video microscopy reveals that plastic beads coated with pure kinesin can be transported along microtubules in an ATP-dependent manner. The fact that an inert bead can behave like an organelle implies that no proteins on the organelles themselves are necessary for transport (other than those that bind kinesin to the organelle), and that kinesin itself is sufficient to drive this process.

Since in real axons the microtubules are effectively fixed in place by other cytoskeletal components and cell membranes, the net effect of kinesin's action is to move vesicles in a proximal-to-distal (*orthograde*) direction along the axon. Organelles can also be transported in a distal-to-proximal direction—that is, toward the cell body (*retrograde* transport). This is mediated, at least in part, by another molecular motor, a microtubule-associated protein (MAP1c) also called cytoplasmic *dynein*, that is distinct from kinesin. A single microtubule can serve as a track for transport in both the orthograde and retrograde directions, the direction of transport being determined by the nature of the motor that binds to the organelle (Fig. 2–10b).

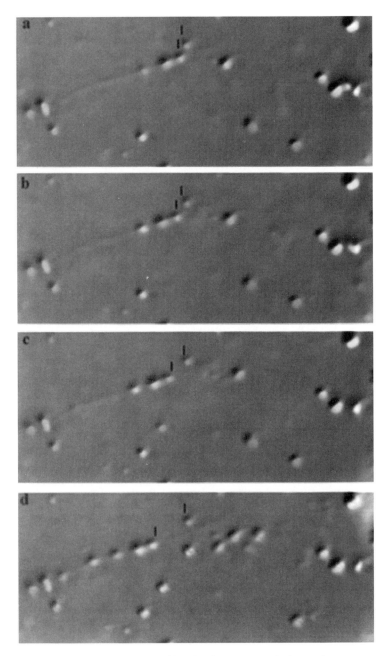

Figure 2–11. Kinesin-dependent movement of beads along microtubules. Video images of kinesin-coated plastic beads moving along a microtubule (raised line running diagonally across the left side of these images) on a glass slide. The two solid markers point to two beads, one of which is on the glass (and hence not moving), and the other of which is on the microtubule. Note the increased distance between the two beads in these successive video images (2 seconds apart). (Video images were provided by Michael Sheetz.)

Summary

The brain, like all other organs, is made up of vast numbers of cells. Unlike some other organs, however, the brain contains a wide variety of cell types. In addition to many different kinds of neurons, which are the main characters of our story, there are several classes of *glial cells*. The glia outnumber the neurons by a factor of 10 or more, but with the notable exception of myelination, their functions are only beginning to be understood. In addition to playing a critical role in the formation of the myelin sheath around axons, glia may be involved in synaptic transmission and in long-distance calcium signaling in the brain.

Neurons share many features in common with other cells (including glia), but they are distinguished by their highly asymmetric shapes. The neuronal *cytoskeleton* is essential for establishing this cell shape during development and for maintaining it in the adult. The neuron utilizes a process known as *axonal transport* for moving vesicles and other organelles to regions remote from the neuronal cell body. Proteins called *molecular motors* make use of the energy released by hydrolysis of ATP to drive axonal transport. Thus the neuron has evolved unique mechanisms to establish and maintain the form required for its specialized signaling functions.

II

ELECTRICAL PROPERTIES
OF NEURONS

We have emphasized in the introductory section that information transfer, within and between nerve cells, is an essential element of nervous system function. We have seen also that neurons are highly asymmetric cells, with processes that often extend a considerable distance from the cell body. The basic question addressed in the next five chapters is how information is transferred intracellularly, from one part of the neuron to another. Chapter 3 deals with the basic phenomenology of electrical signaling. Neurons, like other cells, exhibit a voltage difference across their plasma membranes. Rapid changes in this transmembrane voltage, called *action potentials*, can be propagated from one part of the cell to another and are used by neurons (but not by most other cells) to encode information. Chapter 4 introduces *membrane ion channels*, a ubiquitous class of highly specialized membrane proteins that have evolved to provide exquisite control over the movement of ions across the plasma membrane. We discuss the biophysical and molecular properties of ion channels in considerable detail in this and the next three chapters, because an appreciation of how channels work is essential for understanding electrical signaling. Chapter 5 covers the molecular structure of ion channels and the methods that have been used to investigate these proteins. Molecular cloning and X-ray crystallographic methods now enable us to identify the structural features of an ion channel protein that are responsible for a particular aspect of its function. The goal of such approaches is ultimately to understand electrical signaling in terms of its underlying molecular mechanisms. Chapter 6 examines the ways in which the combined activities of different ion channels give rise to action potentials. Neurons differ from most other cells in their particular ensemble of membrane ion channels, which allow the generation and propagation of action potentials in complex temporal patterns. Finally, Chapter 7 describes the *diversity* of voltage-gated ion channels, with particular focus on calcium and potassium channels. This diversity of channel types allows the electrical behavior of any neuron to be adapted very precisely to its function in the brain.

Electrical Signaling
in Neurons

*A*lthough neurons have many features in common with other cells, they are unique because their primary functions are to receive, modify, and transmit messages. This includes information transfer from one cell to the next, as well as between different parts of the same cell. In this and the following four chapters we will focus on the nature and mechanisms of the electrical signals that neurons use both for intracellular communication and as stimuli for the generation of intercellular messages.

Intracellular Transfer of Information: The Axon

In Chapters 1 and 2 we showed that neurons are highly asymmetric cells and that different parts of the neuron exhibit structural features that enable them to carry out specialized tasks. We will concentrate first on the *axon*, the part of the neuron responsible for transmitting information from one part of the cell to another.

Axons are thin tube-like structures that arise from the neuronal cell body. They vary widely in size, shape, and other characteristics (see Fig. 1–3). Some axons within the central nervous system are only a few micrometers in length, not much greater than the diameter of the neuronal cell bodies from which they arise. In contrast, axons that run from the central nervous system to other parts of the body can be as long as 1 meter in humans and even longer in larger animals. It is immediately apparent that whatever the mechanism of axonal information transfer, it must be able to operate over long distances without garbling or losing messages.

Axon diameter also varies, from less than 1 μm to almost 1 mm, and the diameter of any single axon may be different at different distances from the cell body. Axon diameter is an important factor in determining the speed at which information moves along the axon. Moreover, we shall see that whether or not an axon is myelinated also influences speed of transmission.

We begin here with a descriptive treatment of how information is passed along an axon, and then discuss the diverse patterns of electrical activity exhibited by different kinds of neurons. In subsequent chapters we will describe the mechanisms of these phenomena in detail. To summarize the descriptive message: there is a voltage difference across the axonal membrane, and information is carried in the axon in the form of rapid changes in this voltage difference. These voltage changes, which are generally referred to as *nerve impulses*, *spikes*, or (most commonly) *action potentials*, travel rapidly along the axon from the cell body toward the distal portion of the axon.

Ion Channels Underlie Electrical Signaling in Neurons

Neurons, like all other cells, exhibit a voltage difference known as the *membrane potential* across their plasma membranes. It will become evident in the next chapter that the membrane potential results from the unequal distribution of electrical charge, carried by *ions*, on the two sides of the membrane. Some ions can move across the plasma membrane more readily than others, and the movement of ions may be different under different circumstances (for example, when at rest as compared to during the action potential). Such differential permeability arises because of the presence in the plasma membrane of specialized proteins known as *ion channels*. These

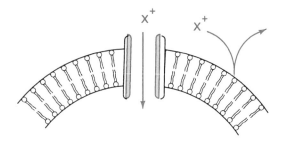

Figure 3–1. Our concept of an ion channel, drawn as a hydrophilic pore (*blue*) that spans the hydrophobic plasma membrane (*black*). Ions (X^+) can cross the membrane only through the aqueous pore provided by the ion channel.

proteins, which will be described in detail in Chapter 4 and will reappear throughout this book, form aqueous pores across the membrane through which specific ions can flow (Fig. 3–1). It is the flow of ions through ion channels that is responsible for electrical signaling in neurons.

Resting Potential and the Passive Membrane Response

When the axon is at rest, that is, when it is not conducting nerve impulses, the value of the membrane potential is called the *resting potential*. In neurons the resting potential is usually in the range −40 to −90 mV. By convention, membrane potentials are expressed relative to the extracellular fluid—that is, negative membrane potentials indicate that the inside of the cell membrane is more negative than the outside. When the membrane potential is less negative than the resting potential the cell is said to be *depolarized*; when it is more negative, the cell is *hyperpolarized*.

It is possible to measure the membrane potential (V_m) by inserting a measuring electrode, connected to an electrometer, into the cell (Fig. 3–2).

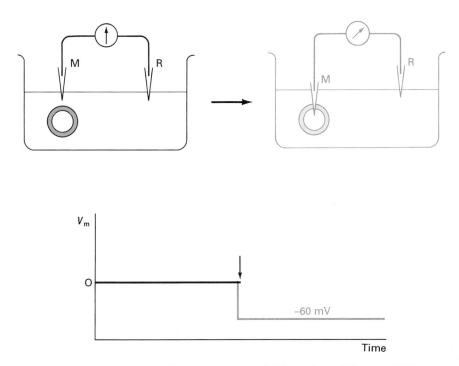

Figure 3–2. Measurement of the resting potential. The voltage difference (V_m) across the cell membrane can be determined as the voltage difference between a measuring electrode (M) inside the cell and a reference electrode (R) in the extracellular fluid.

The electrode can be either a silver wire or a fine-tipped glass pipette filled with a conducting salt solution. When the tip of the measuring electrode is in the extracellular fluid, there is no voltage difference between it and the reference electrode, which is also in the extracellular fluid (left side of Fig. 3–2). When the measuring electrode tip is passed through the plasma membrane, there is a sudden negative voltage deflection of some 40–90 mV relative to the extracellular reference electrode (right side and bottom of Fig. 3–2), reflecting the negative resting potential (V_r).

With appropriate (and very simple) electronics, one can also inject negative (hyperpolarizing) or positive (depolarizing) current into the cell via the same electrode. With negative currents, the membrane potential changes in a hyperpolarizing direction, and the size of the change simply mirrors the amount of applied current stimulus (Fig. 3–3). Such voltage shifts in response to hyperpolarizing current injection reflect *passive* membrane properties. Similar passive responses are seen in response to small depolarizing stimuli (Fig. 3–3). This injection of current through use of electronic instrumentation is a useful experimental manipulation, because it mimics what happens in the nervous system. We shall see that in the real world, neurons are constantly bombarded with physiologically relevant current "injections" that result from synaptic activity or sensory input.

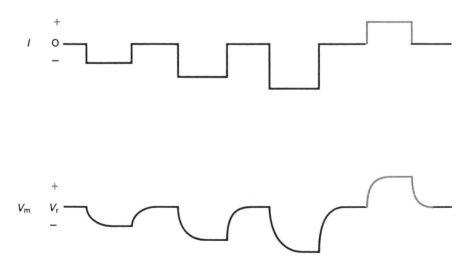

Figure 3–3. Passive response of the membrane. Current (I) can be injected into the cell via an electrode, and the resulting change in membrane potential (V_m) from that at rest (V_r) can be measured with the same or another electrode.

The Plasma Membrane Is a Capacitor
and a Resistor Connected in Parallel

The plasma membrane of a nerve cell or, indeed, of any cell provides a resistance to the flow of ions between the intracellular and extracellular compartments. Accordingly, it can be thought of as an electrical *resistor*, with
the membrane resistance, R_m, being measured in ohms (Ω). In addition,
the lipid bilayer provides an extremely thin insulating layer between two
conducting solutions. This allows the membrane to act as an electrical *capacitor*, a device that is capable of separating and storing electrical charge.
The membrane capacitance, C_m, is measured in farads (F). These considerations allow us to describe the electrical properties of the lipid bilayer
membrane simply in terms of an *equivalent electrical circuit*, as shown in
Figure 3–4a. This description is introduced not to torment the student of
cell and molecular biology, but rather because it is extremely useful in un-

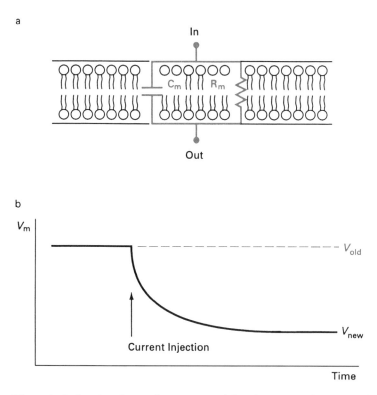

Figure 3–4. Passive electrical properties of the plasma membrane. *a*: The plasma membrane can be depicted as a resistor (R_m) and a capacitor (C_m) connected in parallel.
b: Voltage changes do not occur instantaneously. V_m, membrane potential.

derstanding the electrical behavior of biological membranes under a variety of physiological conditions.

What does all this mean for changes in the voltage difference across the neuronal plasma membrane? Figure 3–3 illustrates that the time course of the change in membrane voltage does not mirror precisely that of the injected current. In fact, the rate of change of the voltage is a function of *both* the injected current (I) and the membrane capacitance (C_m) and is given by:

$$dV/dt = I/C_m$$

This is because the membrane capacitance must be charged (or discharged) before the voltage can change, and this cannot occur instantaneously; rather, it takes some time determined by the membrane *time constant*, τ, which is equal to the product of the membrane resistance and capacitance:

$$\tau = R_m C_m$$

As can be seen in Figure 3–4b, the voltage changes exponentially with time (t), according to the equation:

$$V_t = V_{new} - (V_{new} - V_{old})e^{-t/\tau}$$

In other words, the voltage falls to $1/e$ of its initial value in a time equal to one time constant. Time constants in biological membranes vary over a wide range, even though C_m per unit of membrane surface area is remarkably constant at about 1 μF/cm^2 in all membranes examined. Accordingly, the dissimilar time constants must reflect large differences in R_m from one neuron to another, and even between separate membrane regions of the same neuron. It will become evident in subsequent chapters that such differences in R_m reflect differences in the type, density, and regulation of membrane ion channels. We shall see also that different neurons exhibit distinct and often highly complex patterns of endogenous electrical activity in the absence of external stimulation. The membrane time constant, determined by the complement of ion channels, plays an important role in determining just what a neuron's endogenous activity is, and how the cell reacts to external stimuli.

The Action Potential

All characteristics of the passive membrane response described above apply to hyperpolarizing stimuli of any size and to small depolarizing stimuli (Fig. 3–3). The situation is very different, however, with larger depolarizing stimuli. As the strength of the depolarizing stimulus is increased, a critical stimulus strength, or *threshold*, is reached, below which only a passive response is seen and above which the response looks very different (Fig. 3–5). The actual level of the threshold will vary from neuron to neuron, and at different times within a single neuron (again depending on the complement and regulation of ion channels), but it tends to be in the range 10–20 mV depolarized from V_r. Beyond the threshold, one observes a large change in V_m several milliseconds in duration, superimposed on the passive response (Fig. 3–5). The membrane potential depolarizes very rapidly, and then there is a slightly less rapid return to the resting level. Note that V_m does not go to 0 but actually becomes some 50 mV positive—that is, the inside of the neuronal membrane is briefly positive relative to the extracellular side.

This active response of the membrane when the depolarization exceeds threshold is the nerve impulse, or *action potential*. It is this signal that is responsible for the transfer of information from one part of a neuron to another. The threshold is essential to ensure that small, random depolarizations of the membrane do not generate action potentials. Only stimuli of sufficient importance (reflected by their larger amplitude) result in information transfer via action potentials in the axon. Another important property of action potentials is that they are all-or-none events; this *all-or-none law*, as it is called, is an essential feature of axonal signal transmission. The all-or-none law is illustrated in the right side of Figure 3–5, which demonstrates that any stimulus large enough to produce an action

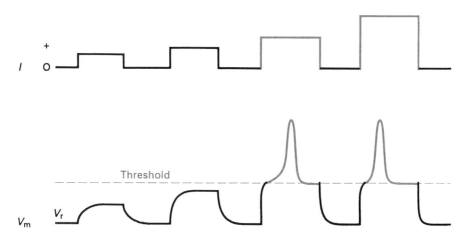

Figure 3–5. Active responses to large depolarizing stimuli. Although small depolarizing responses produce a passive membrane response, as in Figure 3–3, the voltage response to larger depolarizing currents is very different. *I*, current; V_m, membrane potential.

potential produces the same size action potential, regardless of stimulus strength. In other words, once the stimulus is above threshold, the amplitude of the response no longer reflects the amplitude of the stimulus. This is very important; it means that information about stimulus strength must be represented—*encoded*—in the axon in some way other than action potential amplitude.

Although the amplitude of the action potential is generally independent of stimulus intensity, many of its other properties are not. In particular, the *latency*, the time delay from the onset of the stimulus to the peak of the action potential, is a function of stimulus strength. As shown by a careful examination of the two action potentials in Figure 3–5, the stronger the stimulus, the shorter the delay between stimulus and action potential. We shall see that this *strength–latency relationship*, together with another phenomenon known as the *refractory period*, allows the encoding of stimulus strength in terms of the *frequency* of action potentials in the axon.

For several milliseconds after the firing of an action potential, it is impossible to evoke another action potential, no matter how large the depolarizing stimulus; in other words, the axon is *refractory* to stimuli during this time. This *absolute* refractory period is followed by a *relative* refractory period, during which the stimulus must be larger than normal to evoke an action potential. One useful way of thinking about the refractory period is in terms of the threshold (Fig. 3–6). During the absolute refractory period the threshold is essentially infinite, and no stimulus, no

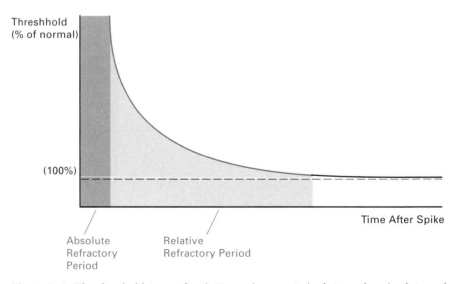

Figure 3–6. The threshold is not fixed. For a short period of time after the firing of an action potential, the threshold is much greater than normal.

matter how large, can exceed it. During the relative refractory period the threshold is larger than normal, that is, it requires a larger than normal stimulus to exceed it. The threshold returns to the normal level with a time course shown in Figure 3–6. Because only an above-threshold stimulus will evoke an action potential, this curve describes the stimulus strength required to generate a second action potential, as a function of time after the first action potential. We shall see in subsequent chapters that the mechanism of the refractory period can be understood in terms of the properties of the membrane ion channels that are responsible for the generation of the action potential. Let us now examine the way the refractory period contributes to neuronal information coding.

Frequency Coding

Consider the response of the axon to a sustained stimulus in the light of these concepts. If the stimulus depolarizes the axon above the normal resting threshold, an action potential results. However, even if the depolarizing stimulus is maintained, a second action potential will be evoked only after the threshold has dropped back below the level of the sustained stimulus (Fig. 3–7a). This will take some time, as described in Figure 3–6. The

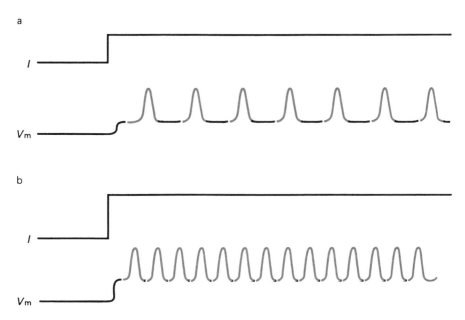

Figure 3–7. Frequency coding in axons. *a*: An above-threshold sustained depolarizing stimulus (*I*) produces action potentials at a certain frequency. *b*: When the depolarizing stimulus is larger, the frequency of action potential firing is greater. V_m, membrane potential.

same will be true for all subsequent action potentials during the stimulus. Thus the axon will fire action potentials as long as the above-threshold stimulus is maintained, but they will be spaced apart in time. Now consider the response of the same axon to a larger depolarizing stimulus (Fig. 3–7b). Again, the second action potential will fire only after the threshold drops back below the stimulus level, but this happens more quickly because the stimulus is larger (and consequently the threshold does not have to drop quite as far). Accordingly, the second and subsequent action potentials occur with less delay. It can be seen from a comparison of Figures 3–7a and 3–7b that the larger stimulus is reflected in a higher frequency of action potentials in the axon. Thus, even though action potential amplitude obeys the all-or-none law and does not reflect stimulus intensity, the phenomena of threshold, latency, and refractory period do indeed allow the encoding of stimulus intensity as a *frequency code* in the axon.

Passive Spread and Action Potential Propagation

Everything we have discussed thus far refers to local changes in the membrane potential at a single point in the axon. However, we have also emphasized that the axon is specialized to move information from one part of the neuron to another. Thus it is time to ask how nerve impulses spread along the axon from the point of a stimulus.

Although it may seem to be a contradiction in terms, a phenomenon known as *passive spread* plays an essential role in the propagation of the active response. Let us look first at passive spread in terms of hyperpolarization of the membrane potential. Suppose an axon is penetrated by several microelectrodes some distance apart, and a hyperpolarizing current is injected through one. As can be seen in Figure 3–8a, a voltage change is observed at all the electrodes, but it is largest at the stimulating electrode and decreases in amplitude with distance away from this electrode. When the amplitude of the voltage response is plotted as a function of distance from the stimulating electrode, it can be seen to fall exponentially with distance (Fig. 3–8b). In other words, the voltage change does spread from one point to another, but it is attenuated with distance, until it eventually becomes so small that it is essentially undetectable. This phenomenon is known as *passive spread* because it can be seen in a dead axon or even in an electric cable with similar properties.

The extent of attenuation of the voltage change is determined by the membrane *space constant*, λ, defined as the distance at which a voltage change has fallen to $1/e$ of its initial value. The voltage V_d at some distance d can be described in terms of V_0, the voltage at distance 0, and the space constant:

$$V_d = V_0 e^{-d/\lambda}$$

The space constant can vary markedly from axon to axon, depending in particular on axon diameter and the molecular characteristics of the axon membrane—again, most notably its complement of ion channels.

   These considerations for hyperpolarizations also serve to describe well the passive spread of a small (subthreshold) depolarizing voltage change. When the local depolarization exceeds threshold, however, the picture changes dramatically. The above-threshold depolarization of course evokes

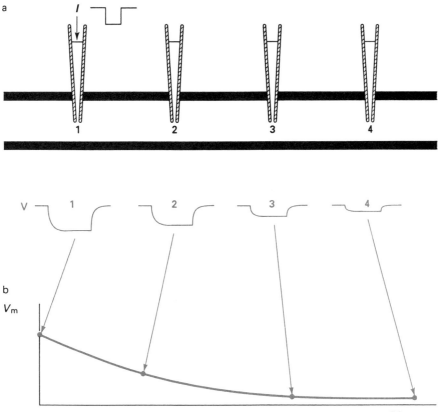

Figure 3–8. Passive spread. a: When current (I) is injected at one point (1) in the axon, a voltage change (V) can be measured at that point. Electrodes in other parts of the axon some distance away (2, 3, 4) measure smaller voltage changes. b: Plot of the decrement in voltage (V_m) over distance.

a very large voltage change, the action potential. There is decrement of this large voltage change as it spreads along the axon, just as there is for smaller depolarizations or hyperpolarizations. However, because the local depolarization is so large, the passive spread is still sufficient (in spite of the attenuation with distance) to depolarize neighboring regions of the axon above threshold, and a full-size action potential is generated at a point adjacent to the original one (Fig. 3–9). This is repeated for each small region of axon until the action potential has swept over its entire length. An often-used and highly appropriate analogy is the lighting of a firecracker fuse: ignition of one point on the fuse brings the neighboring segment above its ignition temperature, and this process continues until the fuse has burned down to its end.

To summarize this descriptive treatment of axonal information transfer, several important characteristics of axonal membranes enable action potentials to carry information faithfully from one part of the neuron to another:

1. There is a *threshold* for generation of action potentials that guarantees that small, random variations in the membrane potential are not misinterpreted as meaningful information.

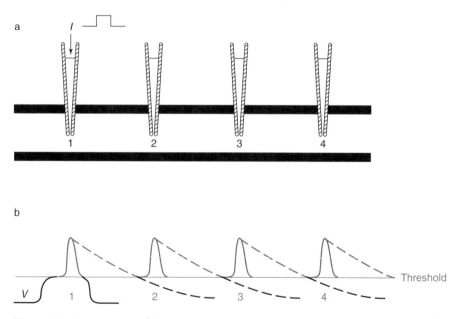

Figure 3–9. Propagation of the action potential. Although the large voltage change (*V*) due to an action potential at one point decreases with distance (dashed lines), the depolarization that spreads to the adjacent region of the axon is still above threshold. Thus a full-size action potential is generated at each point in the axon. *I*, current.

2. The *all-or-none law* guarantees that once an action potential is generated, it is always full size, minimizing the possibility that information will be lost along the way.
3. The *strength–latency relationship* and the *refractory period*, together with the threshold, allow the encoding of information in the form of a *frequency code*.
4. The phenomenon of *passive spread*, which arises simply from the cable-like properties of the axonal membrane, allows the propagation of action potentials along the axon and the transfer of information over long distances within the neuron.

Action Potentials Jump Along Myelinated Axons

We mentioned in Chapter 2 that the speed of action potential propagation along the axon is determined in part by myelination. This comes about because the myelin sheath, which consists of a large number of layers of glial plasma membrane wrapped about the axon, acts as an excellent electrical insulator. The space between the axon and the myelin is not an ion-containing extracellular solution, and no current can flow across the axonal membrane in the regions of myelination. Remember, however, that the myelin sheath is interrupted periodically at the nodes of Ranvier (Fig. 2–4), and at these nodes the ionic conduction pathways that we have been discussing are indeed present. Thus action potentials can be generated only at the nodes. The passive spread of the action potential depolarization along the myelinated portion can bring the adjacent node above threshold, allowing the action potential to "jump" along the axon from node to node. The nodes in the myelinated axon are spaced some 1–2 mm apart, so that the depolarization produced at one node is still well above threshold by the time it reaches the next node. To put this another way, the space constant of the axonal membrane and the spacing between nodes are coordinated to ensure that the action potential is propagated. The high resistance of myelin forces the current to move down the axon rather than leak out across the axonal membrane, and thus the myelin sheath itself contributes to the space constant.

We shall see later that the *voltage-dependent sodium channel* is a particular kind of ion channel that plays a fundamental role in action potential generation and propagation in axons. The sodium channels are not spread evenly throughout the axonal plasma membrane, but are packed together at a very high density at the nodes and are sparse in the intervening membrane under the myelin (Fig. 3–10 and Plate 4). In contrast, *voltage-dependent potassium channels* are present in high density in the *juxtaparanodal region* adjacent to the nodes and help to limit the excitability of the axonal membrane in the Schwann cell–covered internodal region (Fig. 3–10 and Plate 4). Together these factors allow the action potential to jump from node to node, achieving conduction with the minimum use of ion channels or energy-consuming pumps.

This *saltatory conduction* (from the Latin *saltare*, meaning to "leap" or "dance") permits conduction at speeds many times faster than in nonmyelinated axons of the same diameter. Certain diseases of the nervous system, the best known of which is multiple sclerosis, are characterized by loss of myelin from some myelinated axons. Associated with the loss of myelin is a redistribution of the axonal sodium and potassium channels, so that they are spread more evenly throughout the axon and no longer contribute to focusing conduction at the nodes. These demyelinating diseases can have severe consequences, because they result in the slowing (and sometimes the complete blockage) of axonal conduction, with devastating effects on the neuronal pathways in which the demyelinated axons participate.

Having discussed the axonal characteristics that are essential for the generation and propagation of action potentials, we will see now that neurons generally do not fire only single action potentials, or trains of action potentials at constant frequency. Rather, they may exhibit complex temporal patterns of firing that are appropriate for the particular tasks the neurons must carry out.

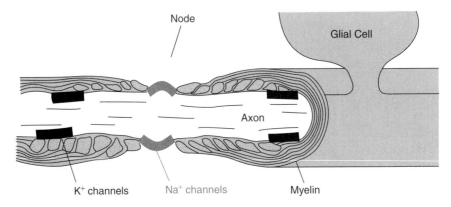

Figure 3–10. Ion channels are differentially distributed in myelinated axons. Voltage-dependent sodium channels (*blue*) are concentrated in the node of Ranvier, while voltage-dependent potassium channels (*black*) are in the juxtaparanodal region. Compare with Figure 2–4 and Plate 4. See Rasband et al. (1999) and Rasband and Trimmer (2001).

Different Patterns of Neuronal Electrical Activity

Cells in different regions of the nervous system are remarkably diverse in their morphology and in their electrical and biochemical properties. In the first part of this chapter we gave a description of action potential generation and propagation in a typical axon. However, even so fundamental a phenomenon as the action potential can vary in shape and size in different neurons (Fig. 3–11). In addition, the pattern of action potential firing exhibits great diversity in different neurons (Figs. 3–12 and 3–13). Again, this diversity reflects differences in membrane ion channels. Diversity in electrical and other properties should come as no surprise when one considers the wide variety of different behaviors and physiological functions that neurons have to control. For example, the neuronal path-

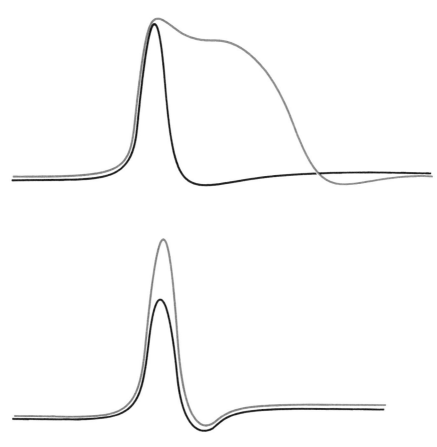

Figure 3–11. Different shapes for action potentials in different neurons. When the electrical activity of different neurons is recorded, action potentials of different amplitudes and durations are seen.

ways and individual neurons that control fast visual reflexes or rapid escape behaviors are very different from those that control slow behaviors including breathing, feeding, and reproduction. In this section we will describe some of the different types of firing patterns that are encountered in nerve cells. In addition, we will provide some examples of how a change in its electrical properties allows a neuron to regulate different types of behavior.

It is important to note that the relatively simple picture we have painted of axonal information transfer becomes more complicated when one moves to the neuronal cell body or dendrites. Dendrites, long thought of as passive elements that do little more than receive information from other neurons, are now known to be capable of generating action potentials and participating in complex ways in neuronal signaling. Furthermore, some

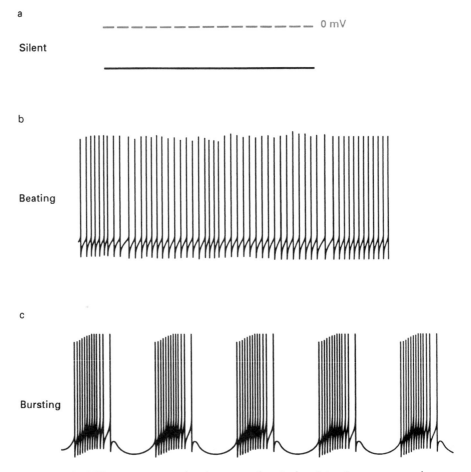

Figure 3–12. Different patterns of endogenous electrical activity. Some neurons do not fire spontaneously at all (*a*). Others may beat (*b*) or burst (*c*) in a regular manner.

cell bodies do not fire action potentials at all—they are said to be *electrically inexcitable*—and they carry out electrical signaling in more subtle ways. Even in those cell bodies that do fire action potentials, the more subtle mechanisms may still be present, leading to far more complex patterns of electrical activity than are usually observed in axons.

Silent, Beating, and Bursting Neurons

Although the generation of an action potential is fundamental to a neuron's ability to transmit information, there are many other aspects of its electrical properties that play important roles in shaping neuronal input and output. Some neurons have a steady, unchanging resting potential in the absence of external stimulation—that is, they are *silent* (Fig. 3–12a). Other neurons, however, generate a variety of endogenous electrical patterns. For example, some cells fire repetitively at constant frequency—that is, they *beat* (Fig. 3–12b). Although external stimulation can change the

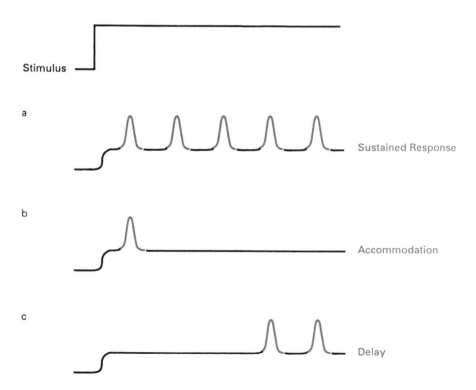

Figure 3–13. Different responses to a sustained stimulus. Some neurons respond to a sustained depolarizing stimulus with a sustained response (*a*), as shown also in Figure 3–7. Other neurons may fire one or a few action potentials and then stop responding (*b*), or may fire action potentials only after a delay (*c*).

firing rate of the cell or inhibit it altogether, the mechanisms that drive repetitive firing are often intrinsic to the neuron itself and do not require continual synaptic activation or other external stimuli.

Some neurons that fire spontaneously in the absence of external stimulation do not fire at fixed regular intervals but instead generate regular bursts of action potentials that are separated by hyperpolarizations of the membrane, as shown in Figure 3–12c. Such cells are termed *bursting neurons*. This ability of a neuron to burst repetitively is used by the nervous system in at least two different ways:

1. Bursting neurons generate rhythmic behaviors. Many fundamental behaviors, such as breathing, walking, swimming, and the chewing of food, require the continual rhythmic stimulation of a group of muscles. Numerous examples of electrical bursting can be found in neuronal circuits that generate such rhythmic motor outputs. Although in many cases the exact form and timing of the bursts, and even their generation, may be regulated by interactions among several different neurons (see Chapter 19), the ability to generate bursts can also be intrinsic to specific neurons that continue to burst in the absence of external inputs.

2. Bursting neurons are used to secrete neurohormones. Neurons, in addition to acting directly on other neurons or on muscle cells, may secrete hormones into the circulation. Figure 3–12c shows the bursting activity of a nerve cell that secretes peptide hormones in the marine mollusc *Aplysia* (a sea hare). This neuron, like many other molluscan neurons, is large and readily identifiable on the basis of morphological, biochemical, and electrical criteria. Accordingly, these cells can be given names; this one, called *neuron R15*, has been studied extensively as a model bursting neuron. Another example of such bursting activity is found in neurons that are located in the hypothalamic region of the mammalian brain and have been termed *magnocellular neurons* (see Chapter 10). Individual magnocellular neurons contain either vasopressin or oxytocin, peptide hormones that are used in the control of water retention and lactation, respectively. For reasons that are not yet fully understood, it appears that a bursting pattern of electrical activity, such as that in the magnocellular neurons and in *Aplysia* neuron R15, is more effective than a steady pacing pattern of firing as a stimulus to the intracellular machinery that causes peptide release (see Chapter 8).

The Response to Sustained Stimulation of a Neuron

Thus far we have been discussing patterns of neuronal activity that are intrinsic to the neuron under study. However, under physiological conditions, neurons are often subjected to external stimuli, for example, a continual barrage of synaptic stimuli from other neurons. Experimentally, such continual stimulation may be mimicked by a sustained depolarization or hyperpolarization from an intracellular microelectrode. Three different ways that a neuron may respond to a depolarizing stimulus are illustrated in Figure 3–13. The cell may generate action potentials repeatedly throughout the period of stimulation, as described in the first part of this chapter, with a constant frequency that reflects the strength of the stimulus (Fig. 3–13a; see also Fig. 3–7). Alternatively, a neuron may fire only one or a few action potentials at the onset of the stimulus and remain silent thereafter (Fig. 3–13b). This response is sometimes termed *accommodation* to the stimulus. Finally, a neuron may not fire at the onset of stimulation but may generate action potentials only after a delay (Fig. 3–13c). In this case, short periods of stimulation fail to trigger any action potentials in the cell.

The first two modes of response may be found in a variety of cells, for example, those that relay sensory information from the environment to the central nervous system. Accommodation in such sensory neurons would result in *behavioral habituation*, the commonly observed decrement in response during a sustained sensory stimulus (see Chapter 20). The third mode, in contrast, would be expected in cells that respond only to excess stimulation. A clear example of this is provided in motor neurons of the ink gland in *Aplysia*. Inking in *Aplysia* is a defensive response to a strong noxious stimulus, such as a mechanical stimulus that punctures the skin. It is believed that the ink that is extruded makes the surrounding water murky and provides camouflage for the animal, allowing it to hide from the predator generating the stimulus. The neurons that control the ink gland are normally not active, and they do not respond to small or transient stimuli; they begin to fire only when they receive the sustained synaptic input that is generated by a large and prolonged noxious stimulus. The mechanism of this delay can be understood in terms of the properties of the particular ion channels in the membrane of these neurons.

Stimulation May Change Neuronal Electrical Properties

There may also be long-term modulation of neuronal properties in response to more subtle external stimuli than the sustained excitation described above. Few behaviors that are controlled by the nervous system remain fixed throughout the life of an animal. For example, feeding and reproductive behaviors have to be turned on and off at appropriate times. A defensive or escape response to a tactile stimulus may be appropriate at one time and not at another. Even the characteristics of essential physiological functions such as breathing may be altered in response to external

stimuli. To a large extent, such changes in the behavior of an animal occur because of changes in the electrical properties of neurons that control
those behaviors. Synaptic or hormonal stimulation may produce either
short- or long-term changes in the shape of action potentials, in the endogenous pattern of firing of a neuron, or in the way the cell responds to
other external stimuli. In Chapter 13 we shall discuss in considerable detail the mechanisms by which such modulations of neuronal electrical properties are brought about.

Summary

The language of intracellular signaling in nerve cells is electrical. There is
a voltage difference known as the membrane potential across the plasma
membrane of all cells. In neurons, information is carried from one part of
the cell to another in the form of action potentials, large and rapidly reversible fluctuations in the membrane potential, that propagate along the
axon. Since action potentials are all-or-none events, their amplitude carries little information about the stimulus that triggered them; instead, several fundamental membrane properties associated with the generation and
propagation of action potentials allow information about stimulus strength
to be encoded in the frequency of action potential firing.

Different neurons exhibit different patterns of action potential firing.
Some neurons are normally silent. That is, their membrane potential remains at the resting potential unless the firing of action potentials is triggered by some external stimulus, and they return to their nonfiring state
when the stimulus is no longer present. However, many neurons exhibit
more complex endogenous electrical activity, often firing action potentials
in a regular pattern without an external stimulus. In some cases it is possible to interpret the pattern of endogenous activity in terms of the particular function that the neuron is assigned in the nervous system.

Finally, the electrical properties of a neuron are not fixed but are subject to modulation by input from the environment. This includes sensory
information from the outside world, hormones released from other parts
of the organism, and chemical and electrical signals from other neurons to
which the neuron is functionally connected. Such modulation of neuronal
properties is of fundamental significance, because it allows the animal to
respond and adapt its behavior in a continually changing environment.

4

Membrane Ion Channels and Ion Currents

The electrical activity of nerve cells—indeed of all cells—depends on the movement of charge, carried by small inorganic ions, across the plasma membrane. The phenomena described in Chapter 3, the membrane potential, the firing of action potentials, and the grouping of action potentials in complex temporal patterns, all arise from such transmembrane ion flow. In addition, modulation of the endogenous electrical activity by external stimuli involves changes in transmembrane ion flow. But how is it that ions can move across the plasma membrane at all? The lipid bilayer of the plasma membrane is an excellent electrical insulator and is largely impermeable to charged species (Fig. 3–1). It requires an enormous amount of energy to move an ion through the hydrophobic interior of the bilayer, and accordingly the cell must make special provision to allow transmembrane *ion current* to flow.

One way for ions to cross the plasma membrane is via energy-driven pumps or transporters, which use the energy from ATP to overcome the energy barrier imposed by the plasma membrane. Such pumps or transporters are proteins that pick up an ion on one side of the membrane, physically transport it across the bilayer, and release it on the other side. Because energy is expended in this process in the form of ATP hydrolysis, it is possible for such active transport processes to move ions against a concentration gradient.

Pumps and transporters are essential for many cell functions, including the establishment and maintenance of concentration gradients of various inorganic ions (most notably sodium, potassium, and calcium ions) across the plasma membrane. Some of them are also *electrogenic*—that is, their activity results in a *net* flow of ions across the membrane; hence they can influence the membrane potential. Nevertheless, pumps and transporters play only a supporting role in electrical signaling in most nerve cells. The stars of this show are the *ion channels*, a ubiquitous class of specialized membrane proteins that span the plasma membrane. These form hydrophilic pores through which ions simply flow from one side of the membrane to the other down their electrochemical gradients (see Fig. 3–1). We will now discuss in considerable detail ways of measuring the activity of ion channels and describe some of their fundamental properties that have been deduced from such measurements. In subsequent chapters we will go on to consider what is known about the molecular structures of ion channel proteins and how their function can be related to their structures.

Single Ion Channels

The possibility that ion currents might flow through hydrophilic pores in the membrane was first suggested in the mid-1950s. Although this idea became widely accepted, more than 20 years passed before the activity of ion channels could be measured directly. The breakthrough came with the advent of *single channel recordings*, methods for measuring the activity of individual ion channels either in their native membrane or after their insertion into artificial bilayer membranes constructed from phospholipids. The most important development was *patch clamp recording* (Fig. 4–1). This technique, developed by Erwin Neher, Bert Sakmann, and co-workers, allows the current passing through single ion channels in the membrane of a cell to be measured directly. The information derived from this revolutionary approach, for which Neher and Sakmann were awarded the Nobel Prize, has dramatically advanced our understanding of ion channel properties in neurons (and other cells).

To carry out a patch clamp recording, a glass pipette, with an internal diameter of the order of a micrometer or so at its tip, is placed against the membrane of a cell. The application of suction to the inside of the pipette can lead to an electrical seal between the glass and the membrane. This seal becomes so tight that ions effectively are prevented from leaking out through it. Depending on the exact size of the patch of membrane under the pipette and the density of ion channels in the membrane, one or more ion channel proteins may be isolated under the pipette. Current carried by ions flowing into or out of the cell through these channels can be detected by a sensitive current-to-voltage converter that is connected to the inside of the electrode (Fig. 4–1a).

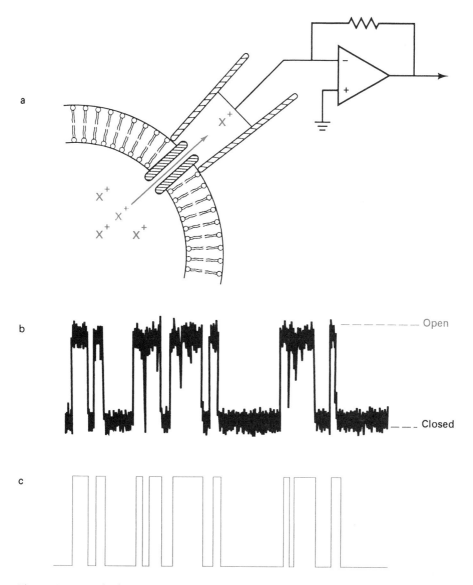

Figure 4–1. Patch clamp recording of single ion channel activity. *a*: Illustration of the cell-attached mode of patch clamp recording, with a current-to-voltage converter that is connected to the electrode (Hamill et al., 1981) to measure the flow of ion X^+ across the membrane. *b*: An example of recordings of single ion channel activity obtained with this method. *c*: Simple computer programs can be used to produce idealized single channel records, which reproduce faithfully the openings and closings seen in the real record.

When a single ion channel is isolated under the pipette, the patch clamp technique can be used to reveal abrupt transitions between an open state, during which a detectable amount of current flows through the channel, and a closed state, during which no current flows. These *functional states*, measured electrophysiologically, must be the manifestation of stable *structural conformations* of the ion channel proteins. Figure 4–1 shows an example of a real channel recording (Fig. 4–1b) together with an idealized description of its opening and closing (Fig. 4–1c). The upward transitions are openings and the downward transitions are closings of the single ion channel. The computer-generated idealized record is free of noise and hence suitable for computer-aided quantitative analysis of channel activity.

For some purposes it may be desirable to have access to both the intracellular and extracellular sides of the patch membrane. In the cell-attached patch recording technique it is possible to alter the composition of the extracellular medium in the pipette, but there is no direct access to the inside of the patch. Fortunately, other configurations of single channel patch recording have been invented that do provide for manipulations of both the inside and the outside of the patch. Two such variants of patch clamping are termed *inside-out* and *outside-out* cell-free patch recording, illustrated in Figure 4–2. Both techniques rely on the fact that the seal between the glass pipette and the cell membrane is tight not only electrically but also mechanically. Accordingly, when a cell-attached patch pipette is pulled away rapidly from a cell, the patch of membrane frequently comes away with it. In the inside-out configuration the cytoplasmic membrane surface is exposed to the bathing medium, whereas in the outside-out patch the external membrane surface is accessible. Many ion channels can survive for a long time in such cell-free patches of membrane, and a full characterization of the properties of the channels can be carried out readily.

Ion Flow Through Ion Channels Is Fast

That such measurements of single channel currents can be made at all should not be taken for granted—it really is rather astonishing. Ion channels are proteins, and when we measure the activity, the opening and closing, of a single ion channel, we are observing the activity of a single protein molecule! Compare this with the standard enzyme assay in a test tube, where typically one is measuring the sum of the activities of some 10^{10} or more protein molecules. The ability to measure single channel activity is due in part to advances in modern electronics; current-to-voltage converters capable of measuring as little as 10^{-13} A (0.1 pA) of current are available. In other words, there is a highly sensitive assay for ion channel activity. However, this assay would not be sufficiently sensitive to measure single channel currents if the rate of ion transport through channels were not remarkably fast.

The current flowing through a single ion channel, such as that illustrated in Figure 4–1, is typically in the 1–20 pA range. This corresponds to the movement of some $0.6–12 \times 10^7$ ions per second through the chan-

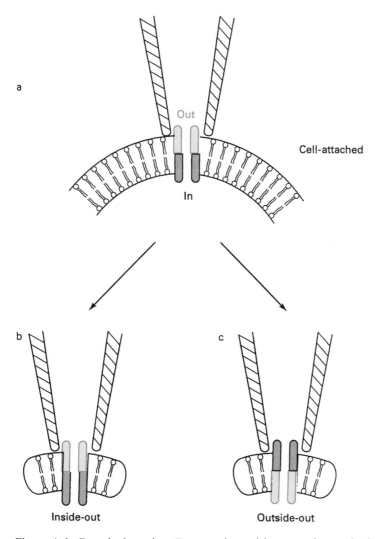

Figure 4–2. Detached patches. Because the seal between the patch electrode and the plasma membrane is mechanically stable (*a*), it is possible to pull the electrode off the cell with the patch remaining attached to the electrode. Depending on the conditions under which this is done, one can obtain either an inside-out patch (*b*), in which the former cytoplasmic portion of the channel (*black*) is exposed to the bathing medium, or an outside-out patch (*c*), in which the former extracellular portion of the channel (*blue*) is exposed to the bathing medium (see Hamill et al., 1981).

nel. If we think of an ion channel as an enzyme whose job is to catalyze ion transport, then the turnover rate for this enzyme is of the order of 10^7–10^8 reactions per second. Turnover rates for most enzymes tend to be of the order of 10^2 per second, with the fastest being in the range of 10^5 per second. Active transport systems also have turnover rates in the 10^2–10^4 per second range; indeed it can be shown that they have a theoretical limit of about 10^5 reactions per second because of the time it must take them to physically carry the ion across the membrane.

These uniquely high turnover rates for ion channels lead to the fundamental conclusion that the ion transport that they mediate *must* be via diffusion through a pore. The fact that we can measure single channel events at all makes this conclusion inevitable; single carrier currents could be no larger than about 10^{-3} pA and would not be detectable with presently available techniques. This in turn has enabled us to draw a picture of an ion channel (see Fig. 3–1) as a membrane-spanning hydrophilic pore, which must be accurate in general outline if not in detail. The astonishing thing is that this could be done years ago, well before high-resolution protein structural information became available for any ion channel. The landmark determination, by X-ray crystallography, of the three-dimensional structure of a voltage-dependent potassium channel in the late 1990s confirmed in remarkable detail many predictions that had been made on the basis of functional measurements more than 20 years earlier (see Chapter 5).

Different Kinds of Ion Channels

There are many different types of single ion channel activities, even in the membrane of a single neuron. These may be classified according to several different criteria:

1. *single channel conductance*, a measure of the rate at which ions pass through the open channel;
2. *ion selectivity*, the nature of the ions that are allowed to pass through the open channel;
3. *gating*, the opening and closing of the channel under the influence of such factors as the transmembrane voltage, the binding of neurotransmitters, hormones, and other agents to sites on the outside of the channel, and the actions of certain intracellular metabolites and enzymes; and
4. *pharmacology*, the susceptibility of the channel to various compounds that may block the pore or otherwise influence channel properties.

Single channel conductance. The voltage across the patch of membrane may be set to different levels, and the size of the current that flows through the open channels (Fig. 4–3a) can then be plotted against the voltage, as has been done in Figure 4–3b. For many channels, a straight line is obtained over a wide range of voltages. Such a plot provides two pieces of information: the *unitary* or *single channel conductance* of the channel and the

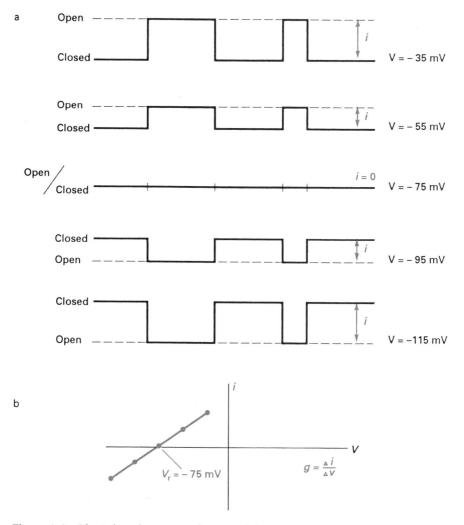

Figure 4–3. Ohm's law determines the size of the single channel current. *a*: The amplitude of the current (*i*) passing through a single ion channel varies as the voltage across the membrane is changed. *b*: Plot of the single channel current amplitude as a function of voltage (*V*). The current is zero at the reversal potential (V_r), equivalent to the equilibrium potential for the ion that passes through the channel. The equilibrium potential will be discussed in the next chapter. *g*, single channel conductance.

reversal potential for the current that flows through the channel. Knowledge of the latter allows conclusions to be drawn about the ion(s) that can permeate the channel.

The conductance of a channel is a measure of the ease of flow of current through the channel. Recall that the electrical conductance G is the inverse of electrical resistance R. Conductance is closely related to *permeability*, which is the term we have been using to describe the ease with which an ion moves across the plasma membrane. The unitary or single channel conductance (g) is the slope of the open channel current versus voltage plot (Fig. 4–3b). It is given by the equation:

$$g = \Delta i / \Delta V$$

This equation is simply Ohm's law, a fundamental law of physics that we will discuss in more detail in Chapter 6. When i is given in amperes and V is in volts, the unit of conductance is siemens (S) or reciprocal ohms (note that i is used to denote the current passing through a single channel, and I the *macroscopic* or total membrane current that passes through the many channels in the cell membrane; similarly, g is the single channel conductance and G the macroscopic membrane conductance). Single channel conductances are usually given in picosiemens (pS, 10^{-12} S). The conductances of channels in biological membranes that have been measured to date are generally in the range of 5–400 pS.

Ion selectivity. Another critical piece of information about an ion channel is the nature of the ions that normally flow through the channel when it is open. Channels are able to *select* for one kind of ion over another. For example, channels in biological membranes will allow either cations or anions to flow, but not both. Within these broad classes of cation and anion channels, most channels are also selective for one particular cation or anion. For example, we shall see that the action potential is dependent on the presence in axons of two distinct cation channels, one highly selective for sodium ions and the other for potassium ions. Selectivity is so fundamental a property of an ion channel that channels are often named according to the ions they prefer (e.g., *sodium* channels, *potassium* channels, *calcium* channels, *chloride* channels).

How do ion channels exhibit selectivity, often exquisite selectivity, for one ion over another? They do so because they are far more than simple holes in the membrane. Although a detailed discussion of channel selectivity mechanisms is well beyond the scope of this book, the X-ray determination of the structure of a potassium channel has demonstrated strikingly that an ion, together with its strongly bound shell of water molecules, must make a tight fit with the narrowest region of the channel protein, the *selectivity filter*, to pass through it (although there is more to selectivity than this). This will be discussed at more length when we consider ion channel structure and function in Chapter 5.

Gating. By now it will be evident that ion channels are not simply inert pores in the membrane. Rather, they are dynamic entities that can undergo extremely rapid transitions between an open state, in which they conduct ions, and a closed state, in which they do not allow ions to pass. These open/closed transitions, which are readily apparent in single channel recordings such as that in Figure 4–1, must reflect conformational changes in the channel protein.

The opening and closing of a channel is often termed *gating*, because it is convenient and instructive to modify our simple picture of the ion channel as a pore (Fig. 3–1) to include a hinged gate, presumably an integral part of the channel protein, that can swing open to allow ion flow or shut to prevent it (Fig. 4–4a). These two states of the protein are in dynamic equilibrium, and the amount of time the channel spends in each state will depend on the relative values of the free energies of the two states. These free energies in turn will be reflected by easily measured quantities, the *rate constants*, for channel opening and closing (Fig. 4–4a).

Ion channel gating may be influenced by a variety of external conditions. We often say that such conditions cause channels to "open" or "close," but what we really mean that the relative free energies of the open and closed states have been changed, so that the channel is more likely to be open or closed than it was previously. This will be seen in the single channel records as a change in the rate constant for opening or closing, or sometimes for both (Fig. 4–4b).

Voltage-dependent gating. Many channels, particularly those that shape the ongoing electrical behavior of a neuron, are *voltage-dependent* channels. The frequency with which such channels open and close depends on the membrane potential. As we shall see in the next chapter, different types of channels may either increase or decrease the amount of time that they spend in the open state as the voltage across the membrane is made more positive. Figure 4–5a shows the behavior of a voltage-dependent ion channel at different membrane potentials. At negative potentials, such as the resting potential of the cell, the channel opens infrequently or not at all and closes again quickly. As the potential is made positive, the channel begins to open more frequently and stay open longer until, at potentials more positive than about +20 mV, the channel is fully activated. The important point here is the amount of *time* that the channel spends in the open and closed states. The amplitude of the open channel current also changes with voltage, in the manner described in Figure 4–3, but this is not important in the present context (it will be discussed in detail in Chapter 6). Figure 4–5b is a graph of the probability of the channel being open (open probability, P_o), as a function of voltage. The data points fall on a sigmoid curve, the steepness of which reflects the channel's sensitivity to voltage.

What is the structural basis for this sensitivity of channel opening and closing to voltage? The hypothetical gate depicted in Figure 4–4 must act as a *voltage sensor*, detecting the strength of the electric field across the membrane. It is presumed that this part of the channel protein possesses some net charge and can move under the influence of the electric field to

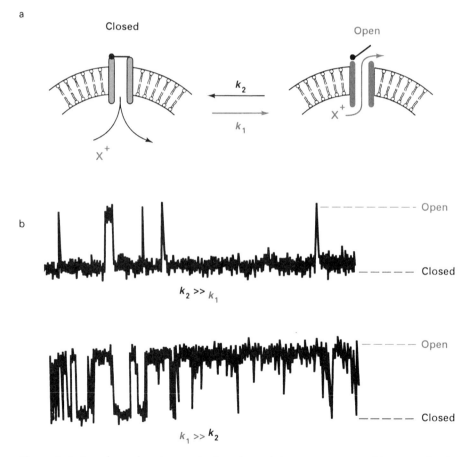

Figure 4–4. Ion channel gating. *a*: An ion channel drawn as a pore with a gate (bar). There is a dynamic equilibrium between the closed and open states, determined by the opening (k_1) and closing (k_2) rate constants. *b*: The proportion of time that the channel spends open depends on the relative values of k_1 and k_2.

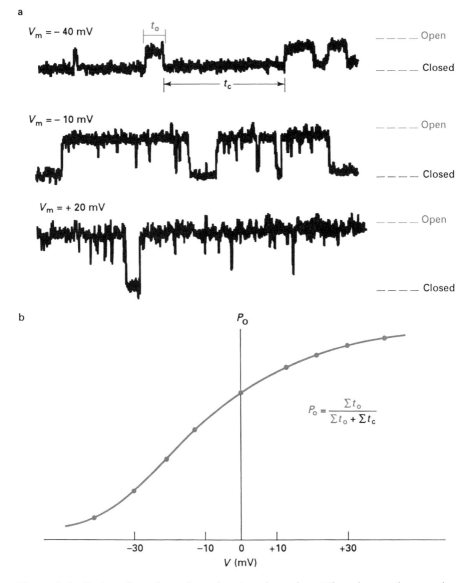

Figure 4–5. Gating of a voltage-dependent ion channel. *a:* When the membrane voltage (V_m) is varied, the amount of time that the channel spends open (t_o) and closed (t_c) changes. *b:* The channel open probability (P_o) can be plotted as a function of voltage (V). The data fit a sigmoid curve, with the open probability being highest at the most depolarized voltages.

open or close the channel pore and hence allow or prevent ion flow. In Chapter 5 we will consider the progress that has been made in identifying the voltage sensor in different kinds of voltage-dependent ion channels.

Gating controlled by neurotransmitters or intracellular messengers. The activity of many ion channels is tightly linked to the action of *neurotransmitters*, chemicals released from one neuron that influence the activity of other neurons. The gating of other channels may be influenced by intracellular *messenger* molecules or ions—for example, calcium ions. The way neurotransmitter binding or intracellular messengers influence the opening and closing of the channel gate will be discussed in detail in Chapters 11 and 12.

Single channel kinetics. Further characterization of an ion channel can be carried out by measuring the mean open time and mean closed time for a large number of transitions between the open and closed states. For a voltage-dependent channel, these measurements must be made at several different voltages (as in Fig. 4–5), and the voltage at which they were measured must be stated. Histograms of the number of openings or closings of a given duration can also be plotted. Such information enables simple models of the behavior of the channel to be made. Here we will provide one example of the use of such information.

Some channels show "bursty" kinetic behavior (Fig. 4–6) that cannot be interpreted simply in terms of transitions between a single open and a single closed state. Measurement of the closed times of this channel will show that periods during which the channel is closed fall into two groups: "short" closed times, which represent the brief closings of the channel *during* one burst of openings, and "long" closed times, which represent the

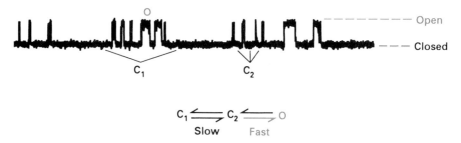

Figure 4–6. Single channel kinetics. The activity of channels cannot always be described in terms of a simple transition between one open and one closed state. Some channels exhibit bursty kinetic behavior. The behavior of the channel shown here can be explained if the channel has one open state (O) and two distinct closed states (C_1 and C_2).

times *between* the bursts of openings. A simple model for such bursty behavior consists of two closed states, C_1 and C_2. During a burst itself, the channel flips between the open state (O) and one of the closed states (C_2). Occasionally, however, the channel enters the other closed state (C_1). Return from this closed state is slow, accounting for the long periods between the bursts. A simple model of this type allows the calculation of rate constants for the transitions between each of the three states of the channel. The way that these rates are affected by membrane voltage, neurotransmitters, drugs, and other parameters can then be analyzed, to provide a mechanistic description of the regulation of channel gating.

Pharmacology. Since physiologically relevant chemicals such as neurotransmitters and intracellular messengers can bind to ion channels, it will come as no surprise that nonphysiological chemicals, both naturally occurring and synthetic, can also bind to channels and influence their properties. As we will emphasize throughout this book, ion channels are proteins, and small molecules often can bind selectively and with high affinity to specific proteins. Although small-molecule pharmacological probes are available for many different kinds of ion channels, let us take as an example the sodium channels that are essential for axonal action potentials. As summarized in Table 4–1, a number of creatures that use toxins either for self-defense or to subdue their prey have evolved toxins targeted against axonal sodium channels. Among the most useful of these naturally occurring toxins for neuroscientists is *tetrodotoxin* (TTX), which is found in the Japanese puffer fish *fugu*, and which, at nanomolar concentrations in the extracellular medium, can bind to sodium channels and block the

Table 4–1 Agents That Bind to Sodium Channels and Alter Their Properties

Agents	Actions
Tetrodotoxin (TTX) Saxitoxin (STX) μ-Conotoxins	Block channel from outside
Batrachotoxin Aconitine Grayanotoxin	Alkaloid neurotoxins that activate the channel
α-Scorpion toxins Sea anemone toxins	Slow the rate of inactivation
β-Scorpion toxins	Shift voltage dependence of inactivation to more negative potentials
Local anesthetics	Block channel, mostly from inside

flow of sodium through the channels. It is thought that TTX enters the external mouth of the sodium channel and physically occludes the pore. This block is seen in single channel records as long periods without channel activity (Fig. 4–7a). Although these records are reminiscent of those for the channel with multiple closed states in Figure 4–6, in this case there is an additional state, a *blocked* state, that represents a channel bound with TTX, rather than a separate stable closed conformation of the channel protein itself (Fig. 4–7b).

Activation and inactivation. One important characteristic of the kinetic behavior of a voltage-dependent ion channel is its rate of *activation*. When the membrane potential is changed abruptly, the channel open probability (P_o) may change rapidly, until a new steady-state open probability is attained for the new voltage. This increase in the channel's open probability is its activation. The rate of activation of some voltage-dependent ion channels—for example, sodium channels—is very fast, reaching a maximum within a few milliseconds after the change in membrane voltage (Fig. 4–8). However, other channels—some potassium channels for example—exhibit slower rates of activation (Fig. 4–8).

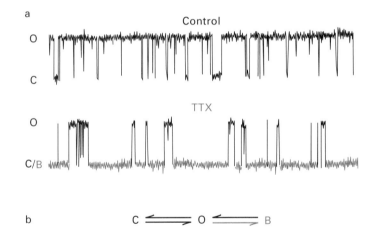

Figure 4–7. Block of sodium channels by tetrodotoxin (TTX). *a*: The control trace shows the activity of a sodium channel under conditions that it is open (O) most of the time and does not exhibit inactivation. Note the occasional brief closings (C). The bottom trace shows the same channel in the presence of nanomolar concentrations of TTX. There are long nonconducting periods, during which TTX is bound to the channel and occludes the pore. Note that when the channel is not blocked, brief closings can still occur. *b*: Kinetic scheme that can account for the gating observed in the presence of TTX. The open channel can enter a blocked state (B), from which it recovers only when TTX exits the channel.

As important for the electrical behavior of a neuron as the rate of activation of its different channels is their rate of *inactivation*. Some channels, once they have been induced to open by a change in voltage, maintain their new rate of opening for a prolonged period. This is the case for the slowly activating potassium channel illustrated in Figure 4–8. Other channels, however, following their activation, undergo a progressive decrease in openings. This is illustrated in Figure 4–8 for our voltage-dependent sodium channel. The rate of loss of channel activity is termed the *rate of inactivation*. Most potassium channels also undergo inactivation, although it is generally slower than that of sodium channels. Thus channel activity can be not only *voltage* dependent but also *time* dependent. At early times, voltage-dependent activation causes sodium channels to open, but at later times inactivation begins to dominate and eventually the channels are never open, even though the depolarization is maintained. As we shall see in Chapter 6, inactivation of various ion channels plays an essential role in shaping action potentials and in determining the electrical characteristics of many neurons.

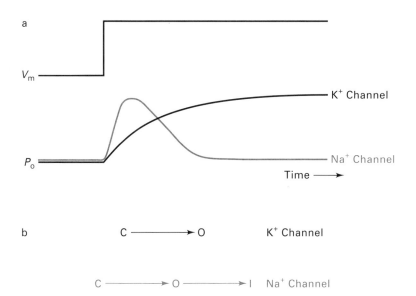

Figure 4–8. Activation and inactivation of ion channels. *a*: In response to an abrupt depolarization of the membrane voltage (V_m), the open probability (P_o) of sodium channels increases rapidly and then decreases again, even though the depolarization is maintained. In contrast, the P_o of potassium channels increases more slowly and remains increased throughout the depolarization. *b*: Kinetic schemes that can account for the gating behavior shown in a. A nonconducting inactivated state (I), from which the channel recovers only very slowly, is necessary to explain the gating of the sodium channel. C, closed state; O, open state.

Macroscopic Ion Currents Result from the Activity of Populations of Ion Channels

Let us now examine how the microscopic currents flowing through a population of ion channels combine to generate the much larger macroscopic current recorded from the whole cell. The voltage-dependent axonal sodium channels that open rapidly in response to a change from a negative to a more positive membrane voltage provide an excellent example (Fig. 4–9). When one channel is present in a patch (Fig. 4–9a), the response to depolarization is an increase in channel open probability, followed by a decrease again as the channel inactivates (see also Fig. 4–8). When several sodium channels are present in the patch (Fig. 4–9b,c), the current record begins to resemble the whole-cell sodium current (Fig. 4–9d), measured by the techniques we will describe below. In other words, the whole cell sodium current is the sum of the currents passing through all of the sodium channels in the plasma membrane. In the whole cell, the rapid change in the probability of opening of the individual sodium channels (Fig. 4–8a) is manifest as a rapid increase in the total sodium current (Fig. 4–9d). Note also in Figure 4–9 that the total current returns to zero even though the depolarization is maintained, as a consequence of the inactivation of the individual ion channels (again, compare with the channel open probability depicted in Fig. 4–8a). These current traces emphasize once again the fundamental fact that the activity of many ion channels is both voltage and time dependent.

These considerations can be expressed in a more quantitative way by means of a simple yet useful equation. The macroscopic current I carried by one type of ion channel is given by:

$$I = NP_o i$$

where N is the number of functional channels of that type present in the membrane, i is the current carried through a single channel when it is open, and P_o is the probability of a channel being open. As we have seen, i depends on the voltage across the membrane, and we shall see that P_o (and sometimes N) may be a function of voltage and time, and may be modulated by neurotransmitters and/or intracellular metabolic events.

A *dilemma in measuring voltage-dependent ion currents.* From these considerations it will be evident that I is an important parameter to measure, in order to understand channel gating and the electrical behavior of a neuron. Recall from Figure 4–5, however, that channel opening is often voltage dependent. At the same time, channel opening itself will generally result in a change in voltage, and this in turn will influence channel gating. How, then, in the face of this positive feedback loop, is one to measure I

and study effectively the voltage-dependent regulation of channel gating? The answer is to devise a method to hold the membrane voltage constant, even though ion channels are opening and closing. To do this, in the 1930s K. C. Cole and colleagues invented an electronic feedback system called the *voltage clamp* to hold the membrane potential constant at a voltage chosen by the investigator. In its simplest form (Fig. 4–10a) the voltage

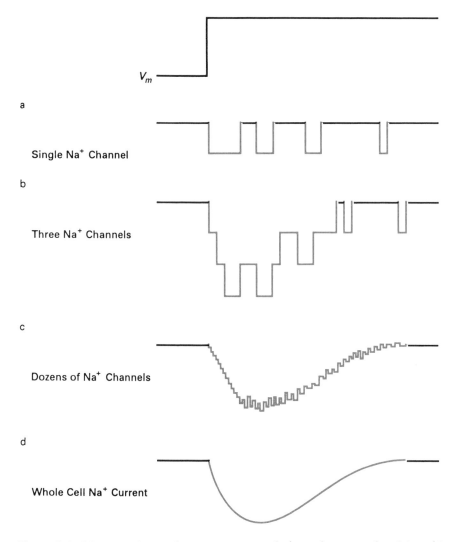

V_m

a

Single Na$^+$ Channel

b

Three Na$^+$ Channels

c

Dozens of Na$^+$ Channels

d

Whole Cell Na$^+$ Current

Figure 4–9. Macroscopic membrane currents result from the summed activity of individual ion channels. *a*: During a sustained depolarizing voltage pulse (V_m) single sodium channels open and then inactivate. The inward currents carried by sodium rushing into the cell through the open sodium channels are shown as downward deflections. The more channels there are in the patch (*b* and *c*), the more closely the patch current resembles the sodium current recorded from the whole cell (*d*).

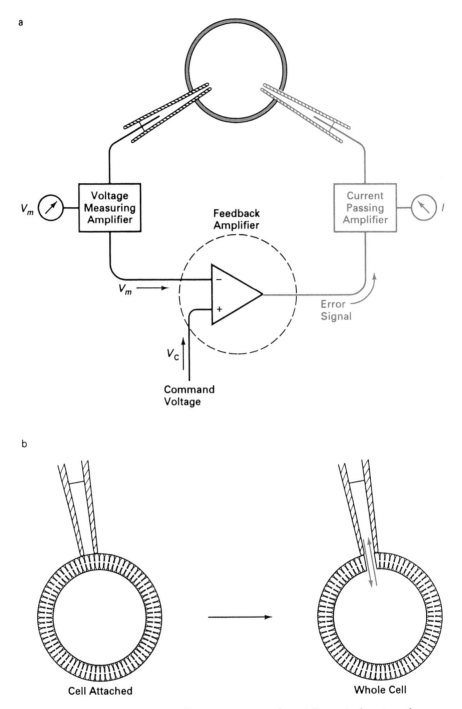

a

V_m

Voltage
Measuring
Amplifier

Feedback
Amplifier

Current
Passing
Amplifier

I

V_m

−

+

Error
Signal

V_c

Command
Voltage

b

Cell Attached

Whole Cell

Figure 4–10. How is the whole cell current measured? *a*: Schematic drawing of a two-electrode voltage clamp, which uses three separate amplifiers to control the membrane voltage. *b*: Whole-cell mode of the patch recording technique (see Hamill et al., 1981).

clamp consists of two separate electrodes, one connected to a voltage-measuring amplifier to measure the transmembrane voltage and the other connected to a current-passing amplifier. A negative feedback loop is created by adding a feedback amplifier, which compares a voltage set by the experimenter ($V_{command}$) with the measured membrane voltage (V_m). The difference between these two voltages is known as the *error signal*, and the feedback system injects current through the current-passing electrode to maintain the error signal as close as possible to 0. By this means, V_m is forced to be equal to $V_{command}$; in other words, the membrane voltage is controlled by the experimenter, and the signal that is measured is the amount of current required to maintain that particular voltage. This current is, in fact, equal to the macroscopic current I flowing across the membrane at that voltage.

Other ways to measure the macroscopic membrane current. A more recent method that has been developed to measure currents in whole cells is a variant of the patch clamp technique, known as *whole-cell patch recording* (Fig. 4–10b). In this method, a conventional patch electrode is sealed to a cell as described in Figure 4–1, and the membrane under the patch is then destroyed by either a pulse of suction or a large abrupt change in voltage. The solution in the pipette can then exchange freely with the cytoplasm of the cell, and the cell can be voltage clamped with appropriate electronics connected to the inside of the pipette. This configuration can be considered analogous to a very large outside-out patch (Fig. 4–2c), consisting of most of the cell's plasma membrane, with a very large number of ion channels contributing to the current flow across the membrane.

   One problem that sometimes arises with the whole-cell patch clamp technique is that the exchange of molecules and ions between the pipette solution and the cell's cytoplasm (Fig. 4–10b) can prove disruptive to the normal function of the cell. Although this exchange may also be an asset for some types of experiments, many interesting regulatory phenomena may simply disappear during whole-cell patch recordings, and under these circumstances the less invasive intracellular microelectrode voltage clamp is the method of choice. For cells that are too small to tolerate the insertion of two independent microelectrodes, a single microelectrode can be used to measure voltage and inject current. The electrode is "switched" electronically between voltage measuring and current injection modes to clamp the voltage of the cell. To provide an effective clamp, the switching must occur at a rapid rate so that membrane voltage does not change significantly during the brief periods of voltage measurement (when no current is being injected and the cell is briefly out of clamp). For technical reasons, this technique is less effective for recording rapid and large changes in membrane currents, but it is extremely useful with small cells or cells within intact areas of the nervous system that cannot be visualized easily for penetration with two microelectrodes.

We have emphasized these techniques for measuring membrane currents under voltage clamp because of their critical importance for our understanding of neuronal membrane properties. Keep in mind that of the three parameters involved in regulating the transmembrane ion current—the ionic gradients, the voltage, and the gating of ion channels—the first two can be manipulated by the experimenter and, accordingly, the regulation of channel gating can be investigated in a rigorous way.

Ion Channels, Ion Currents, and Neuronal Electrical Activity

Why should we go to these lengths to measure ion currents and to investigate the regulation of ion channel gating in a rigorous way? Recall that when ion currents flow across the plasma membrane through ion channels, the distribution of charge and hence the membrane voltage will change; this can result in action potentials, either in isolation or grouped in complex patterns, as we saw in Chapter 3. Let us re-examine the action potentials in Figure 3–11, in the context of the ion channels that are important for their generation. As shown in Figure 4–11, the depolarizing upstroke of the action potential is associated with the opening of sodium channels and the entry of positively charged sodium ions into the cell (*inward current*, which is *depolarizing*). The repolarization, in contrast, is associated with the opening of potassium channels and the exit of positively charged potassium ions from the cell (*outward* or *hyperpolar-*

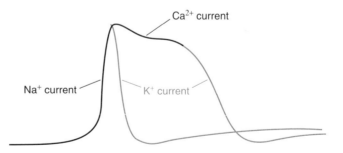

Figure 4–11. Different ion channels contribute to the action potential. Inward depolarizing currents carried through sodium and/or calcium channels are responsible for the upstroke and plateau of the action potential (*black*). Outward potassium current mediates repolarization (*blue*). The relative proportion of these currents determines the different shapes of action potentials such as those in Figure 3–11.

izing current). Some cells fire longer action potentials, often associated with calcium channels that stay open longer and produce a longer-lasting inward *calcium current* (Fig. 4–11). The important points here are *(a)* multiple classes of ion channel exist; and *(b)* the combined activities of different kinds of inward and outward current channels with different kinetic properties determine the precise form of neuronal electrical activity, including the size and shape of action potentials (Fig. 3–11) and their grouping in characteristic temporal patterns (Fig. 3–12). In Chapter 6 we shall expand on this rather superficial summary and describe in more detail how voltage clamp analysis of ion currents has provided profound insights into the mechanisms of generation of action potentials and complex patterns of neuronal electrical activity. First, however, we shall discuss ion channels as membrane proteins, whose properties can be studied not only electrophysiologically but also by techniques of protein biochemistry and molecular and structural biology.

Summary

Electrical activity in neurons (and other kinds of cells) results from the movement of ions across the plasma membrane through specialized membrane proteins known as ion channels. Exquisitely sensitive techniques are available to measure the current passing through single ion channels, as well as the macroscopic membrane current carried by a population of ion channels. These techniques have enabled the detailed characterization of various essential properties of ion channels, including their selectivity for particular ions, their pharmacology, and the way their activity is regulated by membrane voltage and other factors. There are many different kinds of ion channels in the neuronal plasma membrane, and their activities sum to generate action potentials and complex patterns of action potential firing.

5

Ion Channels Are
Membrane Proteins

*I*n the last chapter we described methods of measuring the activity of single ion channels and the macroscopic membrane currents resulting from the activity of populations of ion channels, and discussed some of the key functional properties of channels that can be deduced from such measurements. Let us now consider ion channels as protein molecules, the amino acid sequences of which are known from molecular cloning techniques. The powerful combination of electrophysiological, molecular biological, and direct structural approaches has provided novel insights into ion channel structure and function in recent years.

Cloning Strategies for Ion Channels

We shall now digress briefly to discuss some standard methods in molecular biology that can be used to determine the complete amino acid sequence of a protein such as an ion channel. Methods that have been extremely important historically include cloning by *protein purification*, *positional* cloning, and cloning by *sequence homology*. We will describe each of these here in the context of the ion channels for which they have been most useful. The discussion of methodology will be brief, however, in part because these techniques are in routine use for many different kinds of proteins and will be very familiar to the student of cell and molecular biology. In addition, these techniques are rapidly being supplanted by the astonishing progress in sequencing whole genomes from a variety of creatures, including humans.

Cloning by protein purification. The sodium channel whose functional properties we have already introduced was the first voltage-dependent ion channel to yield its biochemical structure to scientists. This occurred in large
part because of the relatively large number of pharmacological agents that
interact specifically with the sodium channel protein (Table 4–1). These
include tetrodotoxin (TTX; see Fig. 4–7) and a related toxin from marine
dinoflagellates, saxitoxin (STX), both of which block the channel when
applied to the outside of the membrane. Such agents have been of use to
biochemists as well as physiologists. Using these specific toxins to label
sodium channel proteins, several groups in the early 1980s were able to
extract and purify the channel from membranes of mammalian skeletal
muscle and brain and from the electric organ of electric eels. The latter is
a particularly rich source of the channel, which the eel uses to generate
sufficient current to stun its prey. In all cases a very large glycoprotein
(about 260 kDa) was purified, termed the α *subunit*. In addition, two
smaller proteins that copurify with the α subunit, the $\beta 1$ (39 kDa) and $\beta 2$
(33 kDa) *subunits*, were found in rat brain.

With purified sodium channel (or other) protein available, it is possible to use routine techniques of protein chemistry to identify the amino
acid sequences of short stretches of the protein. This sequence information can then be used to obtain a DNA clone that encodes the α subunit
of the sodium channel protein (Fig. 5–1). First, messenger RNA from a
tissue that expresses the protein is purified and used as a template by the
enzyme *reverse transcriptase* for the synthesis of DNA that is *complementary* (cDNA) to the messenger RNA template. The resulting *cDNA library* is a collection of DNA sequences, representative of the various messenger RNA species that are present in the tissue of choice.

The next task is to select from this large collection of cDNA molecules
the one that encodes the sodium channel α subunit. This is where the limited amino acid sequence information, derived from the purified protein,
comes into play. It is possible to chemically synthesize short pieces of DNA
(*oligonucleotides*) whose nucleotide sequences encode the identified amino
acid sequences. These oligonucleotide probes can then be used in several
different ways to purify from the cDNA library specific cDNA species that
encode all or part of the protein of interest. One of these ways is by the
hybridization of complementary nucleotide sequences. Under appropriate
conditions, the oligonucleotide corresponding to the desired sequence can
be made to bind tightly—that is, to hybridize—to complementary sequences in the cDNA library. If the oligonucleotide has been labeled with
a radioactive or fluorescent tag, the tag can be used to identify and purify
cDNA species that encode the sodium channel (Fig. 5–1). The nucleotide
sequence of the cDNA can then be obtained using standard methods, and

the complete amino acid sequence can be deduced from it. This procedure is far faster and less tedious than using protein chemistry techniques to attempt to obtain the entire amino acid sequence.

This approach has been made even easier by the widespread use of the *polymerase chain reaction* (PCR) to produce large amounts of cDNA. Two separate oligonucleotides (the *primers* for the PCR), each corresponding in sequence to a different part of the protein amino acid sequence, are allowed to hybridize to complementary sequences in the cDNA library (the *template* for the PCR). An enzyme called *DNA polymerase* is then used to fill in the nucleotide sequence, corresponding to that of the template, between the two oligonucleotides. Thus a copy has been made of that portion of the template, between the sequences at which the primers bind. By carrying out multiple copying cycles, this sequence in the cDNA template can be amplified manyfold. The amplified cDNA can then be used in hy-

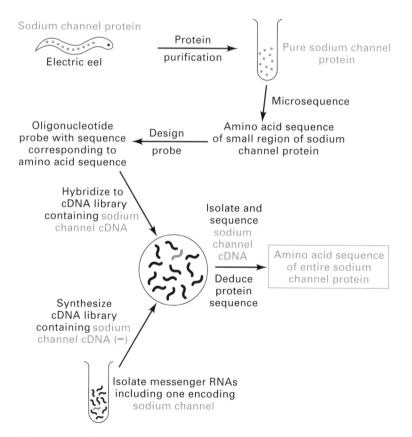

Figure 5–1. Cloning via protein purification. See text for details.

bridization experiments to isolate longer cDNA clones from the library, until eventually a cDNA that encodes the entire sodium channel is obtained.

Positional cloning. In contrast to the situation for sodium channels, the lack of a rich source of protein has made it extremely difficult to purify potassium channels. In the absence of sequence information from purified protein, it is not possible to carry out molecular cloning based on sequence, and an alternative approach is required. For potassium channels, the critical alternative approach was provided by the study of mutant fruit flies.

The fruit fly *Drosophila melanogaster* was an invaluable resource for genetic studies throughout the twentieth century, and the sequencing of its entire genome has opened new horizons as we enter the twenty-first century. Later in this book, we shall see examples of how *Drosophila* continues to provide novel insights into neuronal development and mechanisms of learning. To examine one of these creatures closely, it must be anesthetized with ether (otherwise it just flies away). Occasionally, instead of simply going to sleep as a good fly should, a fruit fly will shake its legs, wings, and abdomen when exposed to the anesthetic (Fig. 5–2a). This reaction is due to mutations in specific genes, and a number of strains of mutant flies that exhibit this behavior have now been bred. Among these strains of mutant flies are several that have defects in one particular gene, a piece of DNA that has been termed the *Shaker* locus.

A number of studies have indicated that the *Shaker* locus encodes voltage-dependent potassium channels. Abnormally long action potentials are recorded in axons of *Shaker* flies (Fig. 5–2b). When these prolonged action potentials in the giant fibers arrive at the neuromuscular junction, they cause unusually prolonged transmitter release, prolonged muscular contraction, and shaking. As we shall discuss in detail in the next chapter, potassium channels are responsible for the repolarization of action potentials in axons, and the defect in some of the *Shaker* flies was found to result from the total loss of a particular kind of inactivating potassium current (Fig. 5–2c). Not all mutations within the *Shaker* locus cause the entire loss of this current; some mutations alter only its amplitude or kinetics. Such findings suggest that the *Shaker* locus might contain a gene encoding a potassium channel.

For many years an important advantage of using *Drosophila* in research was the availability of a precise genetic map of densely spaced markers on each of its four chromosomes. Such a genetic map is even more valuable now in conjunction with the complete genome sequence that became available in 2000. The genetic markers make it possible to define the relative position of a mutation (such as *Shaker*) and to identify cloned segments of DNA that include the mutant locus. Such positional cloning provides an alternative to cloning by protein sequence when purified protein is not available. Identifying through positional cloning the sequence of the protein encoded by the *Shaker* locus proved to be a difficult task, which took several years of characterization of the DNA around the locus. As we shall see below, the effort was well worthwhile.

Cloning by sequence homology. Once the cDNA encoding a protein is in hand and its sequence is available, it is a simple matter to search for cDNAs for related, or *homologous*, proteins, using the fundamental oligonucleotide hybridization strategy outlined in Figure 5–1. The only difference is that the sequence on which the cloning is based comes not from purified protein but rather from the already isolated cDNA. More recently, with the availability of whole genome sequences from an increasing number of organisms, the sequence is used to search computer databases containing genome sequence information. As we shall see in Chapter 7, the widespread

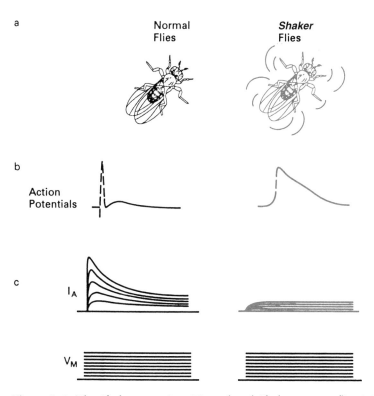

Figure 5–2. The *Shaker* mutation. Normal and *Shaker* mutant flies (*a*) differ in their action potentials (*b*) and potassium currents (*c*) (from the work of Mark Tanouye, Larry Salkoff, Bob Wyman, and colleagues). I_A, current; V_m, voltage.

use of these approaches has uncovered a quite remarkable diversity of ion channel proteins in many creatures, from bacteria to humans.

Ion Channel Structure Inferred from Sequence

Structure of sodium channels. A cDNA encoding the full amino acid sequence of the α subunit of the eel sodium channel was isolated in the mid-1980s by means of the cloning strategy described in Figure 5–1. The protein predicted from the cDNA sequence contains about 2000 amino acids and accounts for 208 kDa of the total 260 kDa molecular weight, the remainder apparently being accounted for by carbohydrates attached to the channel protein.

What can an unwieldy string of 2000 amino acids tell us about the structure of the channel? Luckily there are a few general rules relating amino acid sequence to protein structure that can be used to provide clues as to which regions of the protein may lie within the lipid membrane itself. One of the more important of these rules is that a string of 23 or so hydrophobic amino acids can span a normal cell membrane and is likely to be organized in the form of an α helix of amino acids. Such strings of hydrophobic amino acids in a protein can readily be picked out from a *hydrophobicity plot.* Each amino acid is assigned a *hydrophobicity value,* which reflects its ability to interact with water. Amino acids with nonpolar side chains interact poorly with water—they are strongly hydrophobic—and are given a high positive value. In contrast, polar amino acids are given a negative value. A running average of these values over several amino acids is then calculated around each amino acid in the protein sequence and plotted as a function of position along the protein chain. A hydrophobicity plot for the α subunit of the sodium channel is shown in Figure 5–3a. Twenty-four possible transmembrane stretches of amino acids can be found.

The apparent complexity of the structure of the sodium channel can be substantially reduced—its sequence contains four internal domains, each of which strongly resembles the others. These are marked I, II, III, and IV in Figure 5–3. Within each of these homologous regions there are six possible transmembrane segments labeled S1–S6. With this information it is possible to construct a model for the arrangement of different parts of the protein across the plasma membrane (Fig. 5–3b). It should be emphasized that such a structure remains only a hypothetical model until direct structural determinations are made on the channel protein itself. As we shall see later, many features of the predicted structure of voltage-dependent potassium channels have been confirmed quite spectacularly by such a direct structural determination.

Structure of potassium channels. When the long-sought sequence of the *Shaker* locus finally became known, it was found to possess some quite remarkable features. The first arresting feature of the proteins encoded by the *Shaker* locus is that they are only about one-quarter the size of the sodium channel protein we described above. Only a single domain consisting of six putative transmembrane regions, S1–S6, is found in the protein (Fig. 5–4). The second remarkable feature is that more than one type of channel can be made from the RNA produced from the *Shaker* locus (Fig. 5–4). The DNA coding for the channel does not run continuously through

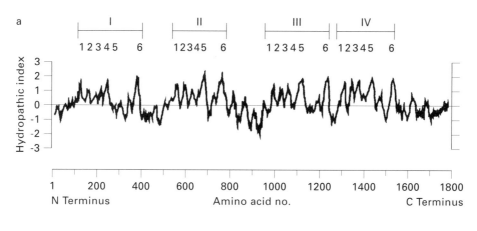

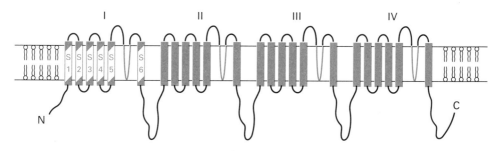

Figure 5–3. The α subunit of the sodium channel. *a*: Hydrophobicity plot for the α subunit of the sodium channel. *b*: Model for the arrangement of the sodium channel α subunit in the plasma membrane. There are six membrane-spanning segments (*blue*, S1–S6) in each of the four homologous domains (I–IV).

the locus. Rather, regions coding for the protein (termed *exons*) are separated by stretches of noncoding DNA (termed *introns*). Because RNA is synthesized from this DNA, it initially includes these noncoding introns. During the production of the mature messenger RNA that encodes the protein, the introns are removed and the exons are *spliced* together. In the *Shaker* locus there are several different regions that can code for alternative carboxyl-terminal and amino-terminal regions of the channel protein (Fig. 5–4). Different patterns of cutting and splicing of RNA can therefore produce channels that possess the same sequence in the central region, which contains most of the hydrophobic segments, but that have different sequences at their carboxyl or amino termini. Figure 5–4 demonstrates the production of two Shaker proteins, ShA and ShB. These

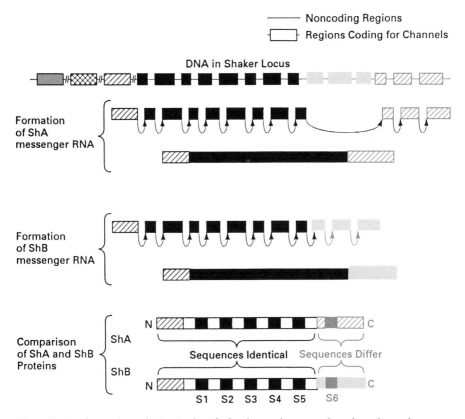

Figure 5–4. Alternative splicing in the *Shaker* locus that was cloned at about the same time by several different laboratories. Lily and Yuh Nung Jan and co-workers showed that RNA transcribed from this locus can be processed to encode one of several different Shaker proteins, including Shaker A (ShA) and Shaker B (ShB) (Schwarz et al., 1988).

two proteins are identical throughout much of their sequences, but differ after the fifth hydrophobic segment.

The Use of Heterologous Expression Systems

How do we know that the DNA molecules isolated by these cloning strategies actually encode ion channels? Does the sodium channel α subunit alone constitute a complete functional sodium channel or are other proteins, such as the associated subunits that copurify with the α subunit, required for conduction, gating, and selectivity? Does the protein product encoded by the *Shaker* locus indeed exhibit potassium channel activity? These kinds of questions can be addressed by heterologous expression of the ion channel in a cell that contains few endogenous ion channels. Oocytes of the South African toad *Xenopus laevis*, and certain mammalian cells in tissue culture, have been particularly useful for this purpose.

Xenopus oocytes. To an electrophysiologist, the *Xenopus* oocyte is a dull cell. It bears few of the interesting channels that give neurons and other excitable cells their distinctive electrical characteristics. On the other hand, oocytes are very large and their electrical properties can be measured easily using standard techniques. In the early 1970s it was found that when messenger RNA encoding a protein from some other cell type is injected into the oocyte, the RNA is translated faithfully into protein. Moreover, the oocytes can carry out many of the normal post-translational modifications of the foreign protein, including the addition of carbohydrate or phosphate groups, and are able to insert the protein into the appropriate compartment of the cell. So it is with ion channels. When messenger RNA prepared from an excitable tissue is injected into the oocyte and several days are allowed to elapse so that the synthesis of proteins can occur, new ion channels appear in the oocyte membrane. The exact pattern of channels expressed depends on the source of the messenger RNA.

It is also possible to express in oocytes a particular channel in isolation, by injecting messenger RNA derived from a cDNA clone encoding only that channel. This technique is shown in Figure 5–5 for the sodium channel. When purified messenger RNA that codes only for the α-subunit of a rat brain sodium channel is injected into an oocyte, functional sodium channels are expressed (Fig. 5–5). These results indicate that the α subunit is sufficient to produce a functional channel. However, the rate of inactivation of the sodium channels expressed from pure α-subunit messenger RNA differs from that observed when total messenger RNA from rat brain is used (Fig. 5–5), because other associated subunits are also expressed when total brain messenger RNA is used, and these modify the functional properties of the expressed sodium channels.

Heterologous expression in oocytes can also be used to study whether the *Shaker* locus does indeed encode a potassium channel and whether the different proteins that can be constructed from the *Shaker* locus by alternative splicing give rise to channels with different electrical properties. Figure 5–6 shows currents, recorded in oocytes, after injection of messenger RNA coding for ShA or ShB. In response to depolarization of the membrane, both the ShA and ShB channels activate and then inactivate as the depolarization is maintained. The rate at which ShB inactivates, however, is more rapid than for ShA (Fig. 5–6). In addition to ShA and ShB, several other Shaker splice variants exist with different amino- or carboxyl-terminal regions. Although all of these give rise to inactivating potassium

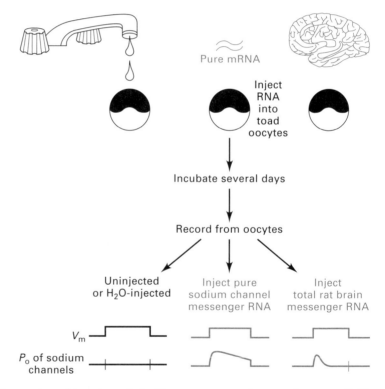

Figure 5–5. Expression of ion channels in *Xenopus* oocytes. In control oocytes (*left*), few channels are present in the membrane to respond to a depolarizing voltage pulse. In contrast, injection of messenger RNA encoding the sodium channel α subunit leads to expression of sodium channels whose open probability (P_o) can be increased by depolarization (*center*). The properties of the sodium channels expressed from total brain messenger RNA (*right*) are different. V_m, membrane voltage.

currents, their rates of activation and inactivation vary substantially. As we shall see below, the molecular structures responsible for one type of inactivation process are now understood.

Roughly 100 other genes encoding voltage-dependent potassium channels have now been identified, through techniques such as positional cloning and sequence homology, in organisms ranging from bacteria to nematode worms to flies to humans (see Chapter 7). Some of these closely related proteins give rise to non-inactivating or slowly inactivating potassium currents rather than rapidly inactivating currents in heterologous expression systems. In fact it appears that there is a spectrum of types of voltage-dependent potassium channels, with different functional properties, all of which fall within this family of proteins that are related structurally. Although not all of the potassium channel genes give rise to multiple protein products in the way the *Shaker* locus does, it is quite evident that the diversity of potassium channels is far greater than had been suggested from electrophysiological studies.

Mammalian cell expression systems. Certain kinds of mammalian cell lines that express very few endogenous ion channels have also been exploited for the heterologous expression of ion channels. Cells in a tissue culture dish are mixed with the cDNA encoding the ion channel under conditions that permit many of the cells to take up the cDNA (Fig. 5–7a). Such *transfection* with cDNA avoids the necessity of transcribing messenger RNA, which is fragile and difficult to manipulate in vitro. In addition, mam-

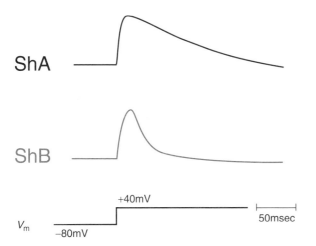

Figure 5–6. The Shaker A (ShA) and Shaker B (ShB) splice variants (see Fig. 5–4) expressed in *Xenopus* oocytes exhibit different inactivation kinetics. V_m, membrane voltage.

malian cell transfection can lead to a high level of expression of the ion channel, often in amounts sufficient for biochemical analysis. Of course, standard patch clamp techniques can be used to characterize the functional properties of the expressed channel.

Expression of mutant channels. Heterologous expression of ion channels can also be used to systematically investigate the relation between sequence and function in the channel protein. Pieces of cDNA can be constructed in which the sequence encoding the protein is modified, or *mutated*, at specific sites, using molecular biological techniques that are in standard use in many laboratories. The mutated cDNA can then be used to either transfect mammalian cells or to produce messenger RNA that can be injected into *Xenopus* oocytes as described above. Such *site-directed mutagenesis* experiments can be used to ask what role particular amino acids

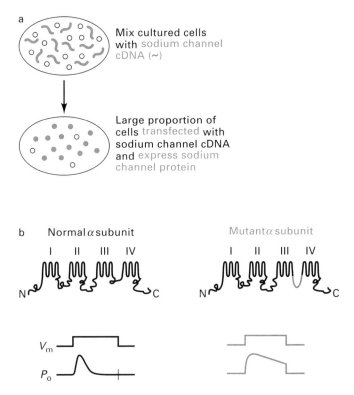

Figure 5–7. Transfection and site-directed mutagenesis. *a*: Many of the cells in a tissue culture dish will take up cDNA added to the medium and express the protein that it encodes. *b*: Site-directed mutagenesis provides information about portions of a channel sequence that contribute to its functional properties. P_o, open probability; V_m, membrane voltage.

or structural features play in the functioning of the protein. In the case of sodium channels, mutations in the intracellular loop between homologous domains III and IV cause changes in channel inactivation rate (Fig. 5–7b), thereby implicating this region of the channel molecule in the inactivation process. We shall be providing numerous additional examples of this approach, for ion channels as well as for other important neuronal proteins, throughout this book. For example, it is clear from clever mutagenesis and heterologous expression experiments that four Shaker subunits come together in the membrane to form a structure that resembles the sodium channel α subunit. In other words, potassium channels are functional *tetramers* (Fig. 5–8), and heterotetramers exist in which different subunits such as ShA and ShB interact to form a mixed complex with functional properties different from those of the homotetrameric channels.

The Relation of Structure to Function in the Voltage-Dependent Ion Channels

A large number of such mutagenesis experiments have now been carried out on the voltage-dependent sodium and potassium channels, and many of the results from one kind of channel are generally applicable to the other. As examples of this general approach, we shall focus on three sets of studies that have characterized channel sequences involved in voltage-dependent activation, ion conduction and selectivity, and rapid inactivation in the voltage-dependent ion channels. We shall then go on to examine the high-resolution three-dimensional structure of a potassium channel and discuss the insights from and implications of this structure for aspects of channel function.

Gating currents and the voltage sensor. It is evident that for a channel to respond to changes in voltage across the cell membrane, it must contain some charged structure that can act as a voltage sensor and actually move when the voltage across the membrane is changed. This in turn may trigger the rearrangement of the protein that allows the opening or closing of the ion channel pore. The charge on the voltage sensor is known as the *gating charge*.

Immediately after a change in voltage, the movement of a gating charge within an ion channel protein should itself register as a flow of current across the membrane. This gating current is very much smaller than that due to the flow of ions through the channel, and it is also very brief. Gating current flows only while the channel protein is undergoing the movement to a new conformation and this can occur very rapidly. The ionic

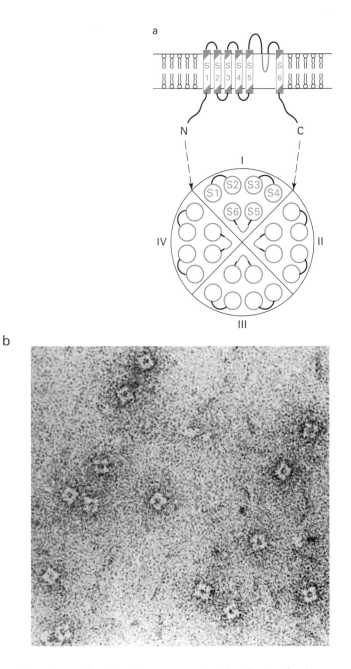

Figure 5–8. Potassium channels are functional tetramers. *a*: Each subunit of voltage-gated potassium channels is thought to have six membrane-spanning segments (S1–S6), as in each domain of sodium channels (see Fig. 5–3). Four subunits (I–IV) come together to form the functional channel. (Modified from Ranganathan, 1994.) *b*: Purified Shaker protein viewed with the electron microscope. Note the apparent four-fold symmetry. (Micrograph courtesy of Nigel Unwin [see Li et al., 1994].)

102

current, by contrast, starts to flow only after the new conformation of the protein is achieved (Fig. 5–9a). The gating currents for sodium and potassium channels in the squid giant axon and some other preparations have been measured (Fig. 5–9b). To do this it is first necessary to eliminate, either through the use of drugs or electronic wizardry, the very much larger ionic currents flowing across the lipid membrane through the ion channels. The movements of charge that can be recorded under these conditions generally match those expected for the movement of a physical "gate" that controls the entry and exit of ions through the channel. A perfect match, however, is not obtained because not all of the charge movements within an ion channel protein lead directly to the opening or closing of the channel (Fig. 5–9c).

A leading contender for the voltage sensor is found in the S4 segments of the voltage-dependent ion channels. Figure 5–10a shows that this stretch of amino acids contains repeated basic residues, either arginines or lysines, in every third position. If the S4 region were to form an α-helix within the membrane, these positively charged residues would come to be arranged in a spiral form around the helix, as shown in Figure 5–10b. The positively charged residues are likely to be stabilized by negatively charged amino acids, such as aspartate or glutamate, situated on adjacent helices. It has been proposed that a change in the electric field across the α-helix, such as would occur when the membrane is depolarized, leads to an uncoupling of the positive residues from their partners, followed by a displacement or rotation of the helix. This would result in the movement of charge in the direction of the imposed electric field and the establishment of a new equilibrium conformation.

It is possible to produce mutant channels in which the positively charged amino acids in the S4 region are replaced by neutral or negative charges. This has been done for both sodium and potassium channels. When such mutant channels are expressed heterologously, the voltage dependence of their activation differs from that of wild-type channels in ways that are generally consistent with the idea that segment S4 is a sensor of the membrane voltage. In addition, elegant experiments with reagents that interact chemically with specific amino acids have provided compelling evidence that the S4 segment actually moves in a direction perpendicular to the plasma membrane when the transmembrane voltage is changed.

A *ball-and-chain mechanism for rapid channel inactivation.* What channel structures contribute to inactivation in the voltage-dependent ion channels? A classic experiment performed by Clay Armstrong, Francisco Bezanilla and Eduardo Rojas in the 1970s demonstrated that activation on the one hand, and inactivation on the other hand, must involve different parts of the

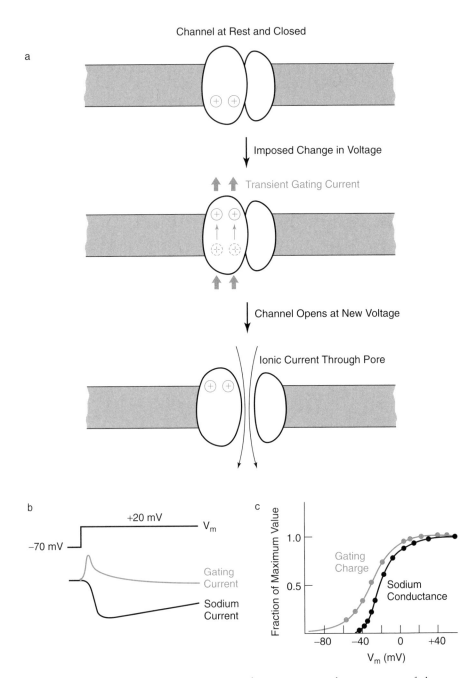

Figure 5–9. Gating currents. *a*: Generation of gating currents by movement of charges in an ion channel protein after a change in voltage. *b*: After a step in voltage, the gating current precedes the ionic current. *c*: Comparison of the voltage dependence of gating charge movement with that of the sodium conductance in an axon (this topic is covered further in a review by Armstrong, 1981). V_m, membrane voltage.

Sodium I

Val-Ser-Ala-Leu-Arg-Thr-Phe-Arg-Val-Leu-Arg-Ala-Leu-Lys-Thr-Ile-Ser-Val-Ile-

Sodium II

Leu-Ser-Val-Leu-Arg-Ser-Phe-Arg-Leu-Leu-Arg-Val-Phe-Lys-Leu-Ala-Lys-Ser-Trp-

Calcium I

Val-Lys-Ala-Leu-Arg-Ala-Phe-Arg-Val-Leu-Arg-Pro-Leu-Arg-Leu-Val-Ser-Gly-Val-

Calcium II

Ile-Ser-Val-Leu-Arg-Cys-Ile-Arg-Leu-Leu-Arg-Leu-Phe-Lys-Ile-Thr-Lys-Tyr-Trp-

Shaker

Leu-Arg-Val-Ile-Arg-Leu-Val-Arg-Val-Phe-Arg-Ile-Phe-Lys-Leu-Ser-Arg-His-Ser-

Rat Kv1.1

Leu-Arg-Val-Ile-Arg-Leu-Val-Arg-Val-Phe-Arg-Ile-Phe-Lys-Leu-Ser-Arg-His-Ser-

b

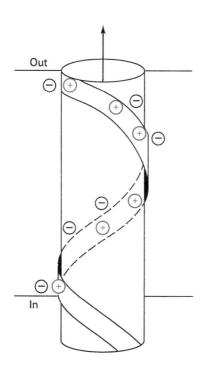

Figure 5–10. The S4 region. *a*: Amino acid sequence of S4 regions in domains I and II of several different kinds of sodium and calcium channels and in two voltage-dependent potassium channels, Shaker A and Kv1.1. *b*: Possible arrangement of basic residues in S4 regions in a helix that spans the membrane (modified from Catterall, 1986).

channel protein. They perfused the inside of an axon (the squid giant axon, which we shall discuss in the next chapter) with pronase, a heterogeneous mixture of proteolytic enzymes, and found that this treatment eliminates inactivation but does not affect activation/deactivation of the axonal sodium current (Fig. 5–11a). This experiment demonstrated unequivocally

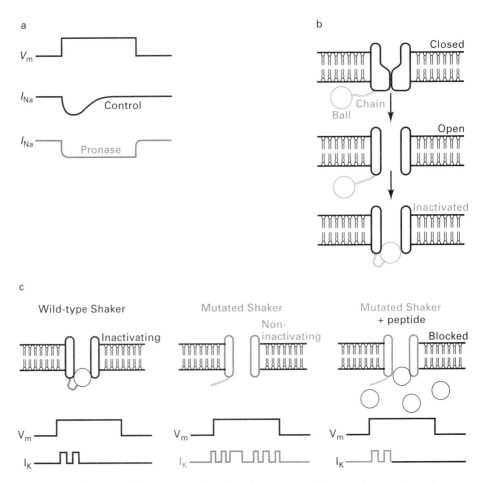

Figure 5–11. Ball-and-chain model for inactivation of sodium and potassium channels. *a*: Sodium channel inactivation before (*black*) and after (*blue*) pronase treatment. I_{Na}, sodium current. *b*: Inactivation results from block of the open channel by a part of the channel protein. *c*: Removal of the amino-terminal 20 amino acids of *Shaker* by mutagenesis eliminates rapid inactivation. Inactivation of the mutated *Shaker* can be restored by application of a synthetic peptide, whose sequence corresponds to the amino-terminal 20 amino acids, to the cytoplasmic side of the channel. I_K, potassium current.

that the channel component responsible for inactivation, the *inactivation gate*, is a protein domain that must be accessible from the cytoplasmic face of the membrane. Armstrong and Bezanilla also demonstrated that the activation gate is not accessible to pronase from the cytoplasmic side and hence must involve a different domain of the protein. This finding, which has been instrumental in shaping our ideas about how sodium channels work, led Armstrong and Bezanilla to propose a *ball-and-chain* model for sodium channel inactivation (Fig. 5–11b). According to this scheme, the inactivation gate (the ball) is a portion of the channel protein, tethered to the remainder of the channel by another stretch of amino acids (the chain). When the channel activates, current flows through the open channel, but only until the ball blocks its internal mouth; thus, according to this scheme, inactivation is a special form of channel block (Fig. 5–11b).

In a series of important experiments carried out in 1990, Richard Aldrich and his colleagues demonstrated that the ball-and-chain model accurately describes the rapid inactivation of Shaker potassium channels expressed in *Xenopus* oocytes. They first applied trypsin, a more specific proteolytic enzyme, to the cytoplasmic face of detached membrane patches containing Shaker channels and found that rapid inactivation was removed, mirroring the earlier pronase experiment with squid axon sodium channels. They then mutated Shaker to remove 20 amino acids from the amino terminal of the protein and found that the resulting channels activated normally but did not inactivate (Fig. 5–11c), suggesting that this amino-terminal region constitutes the ball. Shortening or lengthening that portion of the protein connecting the ball to segment S1 changed the rate at which the channels inactivate, which is consistent with the idea that this portion constitutes the chain. Finally, when the mutated Shaker, lacking the 20 terminal amino acids (and hence non-inactivating), was expressed in oocytes, a synthetic peptide corresponding in sequence to these 20 amino acids was able to block the channel when it was added to the cytoplasmic face of detached membrane patches (Fig. 5–11c). Taken together, these experiments provide strong evidence that the rapid inactivation of potassium channels reflects channel block by a tethered blocking particle that is an integral part of the channel protein. They also emphasize the power of carefully designed molecular mutagenesis experiments in assigning specific channel functions to particular parts of the channel protein. Interestingly, it is *not* the amino terminus that is responsible for the rapid inactivation of cloned sodium channels. Instead, mutagenesis experiments have demonstrated that the intracellular loop between the third and fourth homologous channel domains (see Fig. 5–7) is critical for inactivation, by a mechanism that appears to be more complex than the classic ball-and-chain model.

Two kinds of potassium channel inactivation. This ball-and-chain inactivation of Shaker has been termed *N-type* inactivation, to reflect the fact that it involves the *amino* terminal of the channel protein. However, not all potassium channels undergo the rapid inactivation exhibited by Shaker. It is now evident from cDNA sequence comparisons that while many other potassium channels closely resemble Shaker in most respects, a large proportion of them lack a ball and chain. When a sequence corresponding to the Shaker ball-and-chain is added by mutagenesis to the amino terminal of a nonrapidly inactivating potassium channel, it can exhibit N-type inactivation. In addition, the synthetic ball peptide is capable of blocking many other potassium channels, suggesting that they share with Shaker a sequence in the channel mouth that acts as a ball receptor.

All the voltage-dependent potassium channels exhibit another form of inactivation during a prolonged depolarizing pulse. This has been termed *C-type* inactivation, in part to distinguish it from N-type, and because sequences near the *carboxyl* terminal (as well as others) are involved. N-type and C-type inactivations are mechanistically distinct, and C-type inactivation is usually (but not always) considerably slower than N-type inactivation. It is now clear from mutagenesis experiments that C-type inactivation involves large regions of the channel protein and probably requires a more global change in channel conformation than the simple block characteristic of N-type inactivation. C-type inactivation plays an important role in regulating neuronal firing rates. It is seen in most or all the voltage-dependent potassium channels, including Shaker channels that have had their N-type inactivation removed by mutagenesis. In contrast, N-type inactivation is restricted to Shaker and a few of its cousins.

The channel pore. Another clear example of assigning function to particular channel sequences is the identification of the region that forms the ion-selective conduction pore in voltage-dependent potassium channels. Mutagenesis experiments have demonstrated that the scorpion toxin *charybdotoxin*, a blocker of the external pore of some potassium channels, interacts with amino acids in the region between transmembrane segments S5 and S6 of Shaker (Fig. 5–12a). It could also be inferred that the S5–S6 linker must span the membrane, because some amino acids in this linker are accessible to the potassium channel blocker tetraethylammonium (TEA), applied from the *inside* (Fig. 5–12a). This finding was a surprise, because the S5–S6 linker had originally been modeled as an extracellular loop based on hydrophobicity plots; it serves as a warning that cartoons of channel structure are subject to revision in the face of real data.

Further evidence that the S5–S6 linker (now called the *P domain*) contributes importantly to the channel pore comes from the finding that mutations in this region can change the ion selectivity and conduction properties of Shaker channels. Finally, when the P domains of two different potassium channels with different conduction properties are swapped, the size of the single channel currents of the resulting *chimeric* channels is determined by the small P domain rather than by the remaining approximately 500 amino acids of the channel sequence (Fig. 5–12b–d). This experiment provides an unusually clear demonstration of the critical role of the P domain in potassium channel conduction and selectivity; it has been confirmed quite spectacularly by direct structural determination.

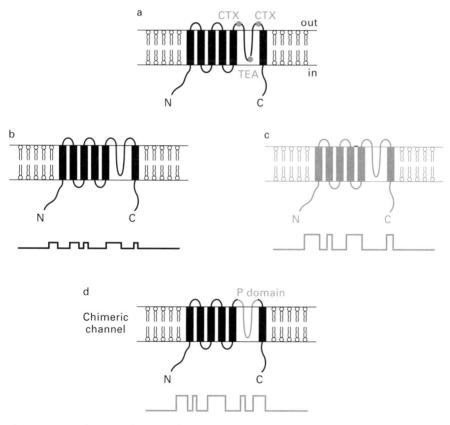

Figure 5–12. The pore domain of potassium channels. *a*: The amino acids marked in blue are critical for binding the pore blockers tetraethylammonium (TEA) from the inside of the channel, and charybdotoxin (CTX) from the outside. *b–d*: The region between membrane-spanning segments S5 and S6 is important for the conduction and selectivity properties of chimeric channels.

The Three-Dimensional Structure of a Potassium Channel

A word of caution is in order concerning all these conclusions from mutational analysis. Site-directed mutagenesis of course demonstrates the relation of *sequence*, rather than *structure*, to channel function. Until recently it has only been possible to infer structure from the sequence information, but now that the real three-dimensional structure of a potassium channel has become available, it is interesting to reflect on how accurate some of our cartoons of channel structure have been. Nevertheless, there have been some surprises that require us to modify our picture of channel structure. We shall see in Chapter 11 that this has also been necessary in the case of the nicotinic acetylcholine receptor/channel, for which structural data also exist.

A prokaryotic potassium channel. The amino acid sequence of the P domain is remarkably invariant among different potassium-selective channels, even those that may differ substantially in their gating or other properties. Mutations within a critical region of the P domain, the so-called potassium channel *signature sequence*, disrupt the ability of the channel to discriminate between potassium and sodium ions, thereby confirming the essential role of this region in channel conduction and selectivity. Thus it came as a surprise to find such a signature sequence in a protein from the bacterium *Streptomyces lividans*. This protein is predicted from its sequence to have two membrane-spanning domains that flank a P domain, which is different from Shaker with its six predicted membrane-spanning domains (Fig. 5–4), but reminiscent of a large family of eukaryotic potassium channels that we shall describe in Chapter 7. This protein, nicknamed KcsA, forms a tetramer that can mediate the flux of potassium (but not sodium) when it is reconstituted in lipid vesicles, confirming that it is indeed a potassium-selective ion channel.

Roderick MacKinnon and colleagues were able to obtain protein crystals of the purified KcsA protein and determine its three-dimensional structure at high resolution (3.2 Å, which allows one to see atomic detail) using standard techniques of *X-ray crystallography*. This was a remarkable tour de force, because although the structures of many cytosolic proteins have been solved by these techniques, membrane proteins tend to lose their ordered structures when they are removed from the lipid bilayer, and have been very difficult to crystallize.

The structure elucidated by MacKinnon's laboratory (Figs. 5-13 and 5-14, and Plate 5) is very beautiful to channel afficionados. The four subunits of the tetramer are arranged to form an "inverted teepee," the apex of which points toward the intracellular side of the membrane (Fig. 5–13a).

The extracellular entry to the pore, at the base of the teepee, is evident from a view looking down on the membrane (Fig. 5–13b). As had been predicted many years earlier from biophysical measurements, the portion of the channel that selects for potassium over other ions (the selectivity filter) is a narrow region toward the extracellular surface of the membrane (Fig. 5–14). Two potassium ions can occupy the selectivity filter simultaneously, with a third in a water-filled cavity deeper in the pore, again in accord with predictions from long ago.

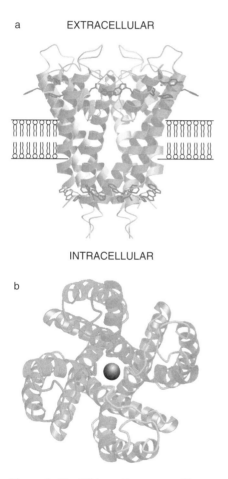

a   EXTRACELLULAR

INTRACELLULAR

b

Figure 5–13. Ribbon diagrams to illustrate the three-dimensional structure of the KcsA potassium channel that was solved by Rod MacKinnon and colleagues. *a*: View from the side. Note the "inverted teepee" shape. *b*: View looking down on the entry to the channel from the extracellular side. A potassium ion (*black*) is shown in the central pore formed by the fourfold symmetrical protein (*blue*). See also Plate 5. (Modified from Doyle et al., 1998.)

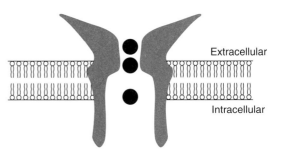

Extracellular

Intracellular

Figure 5–14. Cartoon to illustrate the pore of the KcsA channel (*blue*). The narrow selectivity filter is near the extracellular side of the channel. Three potassium ions (*black*) in single file can occupy the pore simultaneously (modified from Doyle et al., 1998).

Although questions about the structural changes associated with channel gating are not addressed by these studies, the high-resolution three-dimensional structure of KcsA confirms beautifully many of the predictions from mutational analysis about potassium channel conduction and selectivity. Indeed, this structure goes considerably further, providing an elegant and satisfying molecular explanation for the high conduction coupled with exquisite selectivity that is a hallmark of potassium channels.

Summary

Advances in channel molecular biology have made it clear that there are notable similarities in the molecular structures of sodium and potassium channels. Both are predicted to have 24 membrane-spanning segments, in addition to a domain that contributes to the channel pore. In sodium channels this overall structure is achieved with a single primary subunit that contains four homologous domains each with six membrane-spanning segments. In contrast, the primary subunit of potassium channels is much smaller and resembles one of the four homologous domains in the sodium channel; four of these primary subunits come together to form a functional potassium channel. Molecular mutagenesis experiments have revealed channel protein sequences involved in such functions as voltage-dependent activation, inactivation, and ion selectivity. An interesting finding from these experiments is that at least some functions of voltage-dependent channels do not involve global changes in protein conformation, but can be assigned to discrete structural modules in the channel protein. Many of the inferences from mutational analysis, particularly those related to channel conduction and selectivity, have been confirmed and extended by the elucidation of the three-dimensional structure of a bacterial potassium channel.

6

Ion Channels, Membrane
Ion Currents, and the
Action Potential

A great deal of what we know about ion channels, including information about selectivity and gating of different types of channels,
was already understood long before single channel recording and
the application of molecular and structural approaches revolutionized the
field. This understanding developed because, for more than 60 years, the
voltage clamp invented by K. C. Cole allowed us to record the macroscopic membrane current in some cells. As we discussed in Chapter 4, the
macroscopic current is the combined current flowing simultaneously
through all the active ion channels in the cell. In the current chapter, we
shall expand on this topic, to describe in detail just how such voltage clamp
measurements of ion currents have led to a detailed mechanistic understanding of the action potential. Let us begin with a review of the fundamental physicochemical concept of the *equilibrium potential*, which is
essential for understanding all electrical phenomena in biological membranes. We will then go on to consider how voltage- and time-dependent
sodium and potassium currents combine to give rise to the action potential. It is important to keep in mind throughout that there is nothing mys-
terious about the phenomena we are discussing here—they arise logically
from the properties of just a few kinds of membrane proteins, the sodium
and potassium channel proteins that (as we have seen in Chapter 5) are
becoming increasingly understood in molecular detail.

Ionic Equilibria and Nernst Potentials

The rate of flow of an ion across the plasma membrane is determined by

1. the *concentration gradient*, the difference in the concentrations of the ion on the two sides of the plasma membrane;
2. the *voltage difference* across the plasma membrane; and
3. the *conductance* of the ion channels, the ease with which ions move through the ion channels across the plasma membrane.

The simplest example. Consider the case (Fig. 6–1) of a plasma membrane that separates two aqueous solutions, representing the inside and outside of a cell, each solution containing only the generic ions X^+ and Y^- This hypothetical membrane contains ion channels selective for X^+, but none for Y^-, so only X^+ can cross the membrane. Let us suppose further that the concentration of X^+ and Y^- on one side of the membrane (*inside* the cell) is 10 times as high as it is on the other side (*outside* the cell). In other words, $[X^+]_i = 10[X^+]_o$ and $[Y^-]_i = 10[Y^-]_o$. Suppose, in addition, that initially there is no voltage difference across the membrane (that is, $V_m = 0$). Furthermore, there is no net charge on either side of the membrane, because the charges on X^+ and Y^- cancel each other. In the first instant after this condition is set up (left side of Fig. 6–1), there will be a tendency for X^+ to diffuse down its concentration gradient from inside to outside the cell, via its selective ion channel. This will of course cause a redistribution of charge across the membrane; the inside of the membrane has lost some of its positive charge and the outside has gained some, so there will now be a voltage gradient across the membrane with the inside negative relative to the outside. This voltage gradient will tend to slow the diffusion of X^+, since the positive ion does not want to leave the region of negative charge. This continues over time with the flow of X^+ (the *ion current* across the membrane) becoming slower and slower, until eventually the voltage gradient becomes large enough to oppose the concentration gradient. At this point there is no longer any net flow of X^+, and hence the voltage is no longer changing (right side of Fig. 6–1). It is important to note that the number of ions that flows across the membrane to give rise to the voltage difference is very small relative to the total number of ions in the intracellular and extracellular compartments. In other words, the voltage difference across the membrane is established without any significant change in the ion concentration gradient.

   The voltage required to exactly oppose the flow of any given ion X is called the *equilibrium potential* (E_X) for that particular ion (Fig. 6–1). It will at once be evident that E_X is entirely dependent on the transmem-

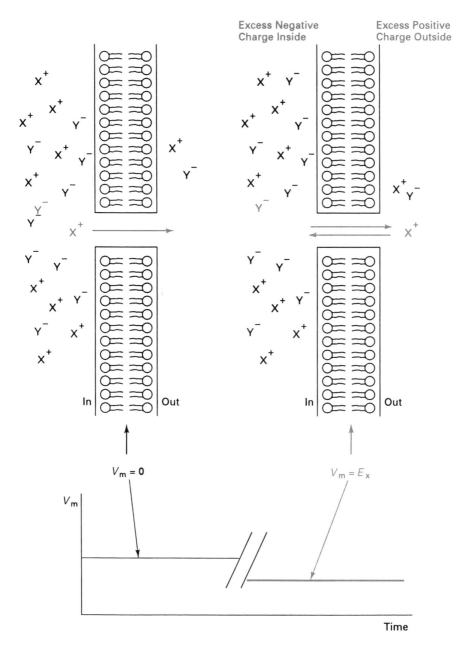

Figure 6–1. The Nernst equilibrium potential. Assume the membrane contains ion channels selective for a single charged ion, X^+, which is asymmetrically distributed on the two sides of the membrane. The counterion, Y^-, cannot cross the membrane. X^+ will flow across the membrane from the side of high concentration to that of low concentration (*left*), until the buildup of charge is sufficient to oppose net ion flow (*right*). The transmembrane voltage (V_m) is 0 before X^+ begins to flow. At equilibrium $V_m = E_x$.

115

brane concentration difference. Near the end of the nineteenth century the physical chemist Walther Nernst described the relationship of E_X to $[X^+]i$ and $[X^+]o$ with the equation that bears his name:

$$E_X = \frac{RT}{zF} \log_e \frac{[X^+]_o}{[X^+]_i}$$

where R is the gas constant, T is the temperature in degrees Kelvin, z is the charge on the ion, and F is the Faraday (the amount of charge in coulombs carried by a mole of monovalent ions). For monovalent ions at room temperature (approximately 20°C), the Nernst equation reduces to:

$$E_X = 58 \log_{10} \frac{[X^+]_o}{[X^+]_i}$$

For the 10-fold inside-to-outside concentration gradient we have been discussing here, it is evident that E_X will be -58 mV; in other words, when the inside of the cell is 58 mV more negative than the outside, the voltage gradient will balance the concentration gradient and there will be no net ion flow. As long as X^+ is the only ion able to cross the membrane, the voltage across the membrane, V_m, will be equal to E_X. A change in the concentration gradient will of course lead to a shift in E_X and a corresponding shift in V_m.

A *real membrane.* Let us now return to the real world and consider what happens when there are several ions with different concentration gradients across the membrane, and several kinds of ion channels selective for these different ions. The example we shall use is the membrane of the giant axon of a marine mollusc, the squid *Loligo*, which has been of enormous value in elucidating the physicochemical mechanisms underlying action potential generation and propagation. The extracellular medium for the squid giant axon contains ions at concentrations very similar to those in seawater, and the following relationships are *approximately* true for the ionic gradients across this membrane:

1. $[K^+]_i = 20[K^+]_o$
2. $[Na^+]_o = 10[Na^+]_i$
3. $[Cl^-]_o = [Cl^-]_i$ (This is not strictly correct since chloride ion concentration is somewhat higher outside than in; however, negative charges on intracellular organic macromolecules balance out the excess extracellular chloride.)

There are of course other ions both in seawater and inside the cell, but these are either present at low concentrations or do not have ion channels that permit them to cross the membrane. Accordingly, they contribute very little to the transmembrane flow of ion current, and we may restrict our discussion to the major charge carriers, potassium, sodium, and chloride.

The axonal membrane also contains sodium-, potassium-, and chloride-selective ion channels, and for the squid axon (and most other axons) *at rest* the following relationships also hold:

4. The permeability of the membrane to chloride (P_{Cl}) is essentially 0 (that is, $P_{Cl} = 0$). In other words, the chloride channels are always closed.
5. The permeability to sodium (P_{Na}) is very low. In other words, the sodium channels are mostly closed.
6. The permeability to potassium (P_K) is relatively high. In other words, the potassium channels are often open.

How then can we determine the membrane potential given these relationships? The Nernst equation can describe the membrane potential when only a single ion X^+ can flow, since under these conditions $V_m = E_X$. Many years ago David Goldman, and independently Alan Hodgkin and Bernard Katz, derived the following equation to describe the membrane potential in terms of the concentration gradient and permeation properties of several different permeant ions:

$$V_m = \frac{RT}{zF} \log_e \frac{K_o + [P_{Na}/P_K]Na_o + [P_{Cl}/P_K]Cl_i}{K_i + [P_{Na}/P_K]Na_i + [P_{Cl}/P_K]Cl_o}$$

When the chloride and sodium channels are closed (that is, when P_{Cl} and P_{Na} are zero) and the membrane is permeable only to potassium, the permeability terms in both the top and bottom of the Goldman-Hodgkin-Katz equation are zero. Under these conditions the equation reduces to the Nernst equation and the membrane potential is determined only by the single permeant ion, potassium. When V_m is measured experimentally in the squid axon (and in many other nerve cells), it is usually found to be very close to, but slightly less negative than, the equilibrium potential for potassium. In the particular case of the squid axon, for example, V_m is usually about -70 mV, whereas the E_K calculated from the potassium concentration gradient by the Nernst equation is -75 mV. The fact that the measured V_m is usually slightly less negative than E_K reflects the fact that the resting sodium permeability, although small, is not zero. That is, the sodium channels may be open occasionally at rest, although much less so than the potassium channels. Thus, to a limited extent, sodium also contributes to setting the resting membrane potential.

This resting potential, then, is exactly large enough to balance the ion flow caused by the various permeant ions with their different concentration gradients and membrane permeabilities. At this voltage the net charge movement is zero. It is important to note that when only a single type of ion can cross the membrane, the system comes to *equilibrium* and there is no net flow of that ion (Fig. 6–1). In the squid axon and other real cells, however, V_m is not exactly equal to the equilibrium potential for any of the permeant ions. No individual ion is at equilibrium, and each will continually flow down its own concentration gradient. Thus there will be some current (I) carried by each ion. In this case the membrane is at a *steady state* rather than equilibrium. The total membrane current (I_m), which must be zero because the voltage is not changing, is the sum of the currents carried by the individual ions. In other words, I_m is given by the following:

$$I_m = I_1 + I_2 + I_3 + \cdots + I_n = 0$$

where I_1, I_2, and so on are the currents carried by n different ions. It can be seen that for this sum to be equal to zero, different currents must have different signs. By convention, as we have mentioned in Chapter 4, the flow of positive ions across the membrane into the cell (inward current) is considered to be negative, and the flow of positive ions out of the cell (outward current) is positive. The opposite holds for the flow of negative ions.

If the total I_m is zero, and only sodium and potassium can flow, the currents carried by sodium and potassium (I_{Na} and I_K, respectively) must be equal and opposite. That is, $I_{Na} = -I_K$. How can this be when P_K is so much greater than P_{Na} (that is, the potassium channels are open so much more than the sodium channels)? The answer is that I for any given ion is dependent on more than just whether its channels are open or closed. From Ohm's law, which we introduced briefly in Chapter 4, we know that the current flow between two points depends on the voltage difference (V) and resistance to current flow (R) between those points:

$$I = \frac{V}{R}$$

For the flow of an ion X^+ across a membrane, the relevant voltage difference is ($V_m - E_X$) and is called its *driving force*. We can consider that R is equivalent to the *inverse* of the permeability for that ion (intuitively we can see that *permeability*, a measure of the *ease* of ion flow, is inversely related to the *resistance* to ion flow). In reality, R is actually the inverse of the *electrical conductance* (G), a measure of the ease of ion flow that is similar to, but not identical with, permeability. For our purposes, however, the terms conductance and permeability both reflect the extent to which ion channels are open and may be used interchangeably. Accordingly, we can rewrite Ohm's law to describe the current carried by any ion as follows:

$$I_X = (V_m - E_X)G_X$$

Since $I_{Na} = -I_K$ at rest, it must follow that

$$(V_m - E_{Na})G_{Na} = -(V_m - E_K)G_K$$

Now remember that V_m is very close to E_K, so the driving force for potassium flow $(V_m - E_K)$ is very small. By contrast, the driving force for sodium $(V_m - E_{Na})$ is large enough to generate an inward sodium current equal to the outward current carried by potassium, in spite of the very much lower sodium conductance. This point, that the current carried by a given ion is dependent on *both* the membrane conductance and the driving force for that ion, is fundamental. We will return to it later in the context of the currents that flow during the action potential.

Let us now suppose that G_{Na} suddenly becomes much higher than G_K and is maintained at this high level (Fig. 6–2a). Initially sodium ions will rush into the cell down their concentration gradient and the ion current carried by sodium (I_{Na}) will increase (Fig. 6–2b). At this time there is a net current, and the system is no longer at a steady state. As positively charged sodium ions build up inside the cell, the membrane depolarizes (Fig. 6–2c). This depolarization brings the membrane potential, V_m, closer to E_{Na}, thereby decreasing the driving force for sodium, and so I_{Na} will begin to decrease again (Fig. 6–2b). At the same time the V_m is farther from E_K, so I_K increases as a result of the increased driving force for potassium. These changes in the sodium and potassium currents combine to slow the rate of change of V_m (Fig. 6–2c). Eventually a new steady state is reached at a different voltage. I_K and I_{Na} are again equal and opposite, but are larger than they were before, reflecting the increase in total membrane conductance.

From these considerations we can see intuitively what the Goldman-Hodgkin-Katz equation tells us mathematically. When the ion concentrations are kept constant, V_m depends on the relative values of G_K and G_{Na}. Figure 6–3 is a simple graph that describes the V_m when G_K is fixed and G_{Na} is varied from much smaller than to much greater than G_K. The two extremes are the limiting cases of the Goldman-Hodgkin-Katz equation, where it reduces to the Nernst equation and V_m is equal to either E_K or E_{Na}; intermediate conductance ratios lead to intermediate values for V_m.

Since V_m is a function only of ion conductance and concentration gradient, in theory a change in either or both of these parameters could be used to alter V_m. However, on the one hand, it seems likely that changes in concentration gradients sufficiently large to produce significant changes in V_m would be very slow, and would disrupt many other cellular functions. On the other hand, the opening and closing of ion channels in the plasma membrane can be modulated very rapidly by a variety of mechanisms. We shall see throughout this book that a selective change in the activity of one or another ion channel, with a consequent change in the membrane conductance for the ion that flows through that channel, is used routinely by nerve cells as a means of changing V_m and rapidly producing meaningful electrical signals.

Ion selectivity revisited. Let us return to the question of ion selectivity of channels, which we introduced in Chapter 4, in the context of this concept of the Nernstian equilibrium potential. An important clue to the ion selectivity of a channel is provided by the *reversal potential* (V_r) for the

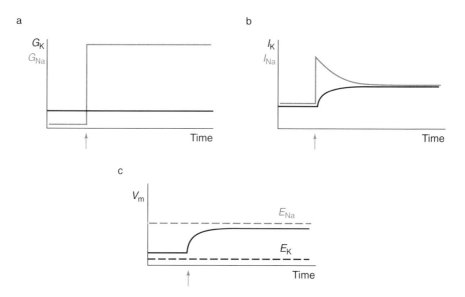

Figure 6–2. Conductance changes lead to voltage changes. Effect of a change in sodium conductance (G_{Na}) (*a*) on membrane currents carried by sodium (I_{Na}) and potassium (I_K) (*b*) and on the membrane voltage (V_M) (*c*). The time at which the sodium conductance is changed is indicated with blue arrows. E_K, potassium equilibrium potential; E_{Na}, sodium equilibrium potential; G_K, potassium conductance.

single channel current, the voltage at which no current flows through the channel even when it is open. Recall that for the hypothetical channel illustrated in Figure 4–3, this occurs at −75 mV. At this potential the channel may still open and close, but no net flow of ions occurs during the openings. From our discussion of Nernstian equilibrium potentials it will be evident that the reversal potential for the current through a channel is equal to the equilibrium potential for the ion that passes through the channel. Thus we may infer that current through the channel in Figure 4–3 is probably carried by potassium ions. Because E_K is very close to −75 mV, there will be no net flow of potassium at this potential *even when the channel is open.* It can be seen that these considerations for single channels are identical to those for total membrane currents, which result from the summed activity of large numbers of single channels.

As with the total membrane current, the Nernst equation provides a ready test for the ion selectivity of a single channel. For example, for a potassium channel, increasing the extracellular concentration of potassium (that in the patch pipette) by a factor of 10 should shift the reversal potential by 58 mV to a more positive potential. Altering potassium concentration, however, should not alter the reversal potential of channels selective for other ions, such as sodium ions, if no change has been made in sodium concentration. Some channels, however, can allow more than one species of ion to cross the membrane. To determine the extent to which a

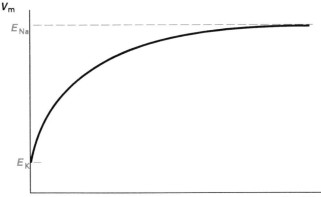

Figure 6–3. The membrane potential depends on the ratio of the membrane conductances for sodium and potassium. When the sodium conductance (G_{Na}) is very low, the membrane potential (V_M) approaches the potassium equilibrium potential (E_K); in contrast, when the sodium conductance is very much higher than the potassium conductance (G_K), the membrane potential approaches the sodium equilibrium potential (E_{Na}).

potassium channel selects for potassium over other ions, these manipulations should be made in the presence of other potential permeant ions, for example, sodium ions. A channel that strongly prefers potassium over sodium will always exhibit a reversal potential at E_K, whatever the sodium concentration on either side of the membrane. If, however, the reversal potential deviates from E_K in the presence of sodium ions, this indicates that the channel is not completely selective and allows some sodium to flow through it.

Again we may compare this with the total membrane current in a neuron at its resting potential. This current is equal to zero (that is, it reverses its sign) near but not precisely at E_K because the membrane is permeable mostly but not exclusively to potassium. One possible interpretation of this finding is that there is one class of ion channels, permeable mostly to potassium and slightly to sodium, that is responsible for the total membrane current. Such channels, called *nonselective cation channels*, do exist. We know, however, that most channels in neurons are selectively permeable to one or another ion. The combination of a high potassium and low sodium permeability comes about because under resting conditions the potassium channels are sometimes open (and allow current to pass), whereas the sodium channels are closed virtually all of the time.

One difficulty in the interpretation of whole-cell macroscopic current recordings is that the membrane of a neuron has many different types of ion channels, which are selective for different ions and whose gating is influenced in different ways by voltage and neurotransmitters. Is it indeed possible to measure *selectively* the whole-cell sodium current, as we have shown in Figure 4–9? One advantage of heterologous expression of sodium (or other) channels in low-background cell types (see Figs. 5–5 to 5–7) is that the expressed channels are generally the dominant channels in the plasma membrane, and can be studied without contamination by other channel types. In real neurons, although it is not always easy, a careful choice of voltages and the use of drugs that block other channels often allow one to record currents that represent the opening and closing of a single class of ion channel. This will become evident below in our discussion of the ion currents responsible for the action potential and for determining patterns of neuronal firing.

Ionic Mechanisms of the Action Potential

Changes in ion channel activity such as those described above are exactly what happens during the nerve impulse. We will begin by summarizing the sequence of changes during an action potential (Fig. 6–4), then we will discuss in depth the experimental evidence for this sequence of events.

When an axon is depolarized beyond the action potential threshold, the depolarization itself causes large numbers of voltage-dependent sodium channels to open. This is seen as a rapid increase in G_{Na} (Fig. 6–4a), which quickly rises to a level very much higher than G_K (as in Fig. 6–2). As a result, inward sodium current increases (Fig. 6–4b), the membrane depolarizes further, and V_m approaches E_{Na} (Fig. 6–4c). In contrast to the situation described in Figure 6–2, however, a further series of changes occurs *as a result of the depolarization*. By the peak of the action potential there is (*1*) sodium channel inactivation, and hence a rapid decrease in

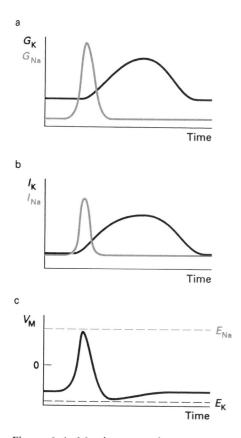

Figure 6–4. Membrane conductances, currents, and voltage during an action potential. *a*: The first change during an action potential is an increase in the sodium conductance (G_{Na}) to a level much greater than at rest. This is followed by a slower and longer lasting increase in the potassium conductance (G_K). *b*: The sodium (I_{Na}) and potassium (I_K) currents change in accordance with the changes in conductance. *c*: The result of these changes is the characteristically shaped action potential. E_K, potassium equilibrium potential; E_{Na}, sodium equilibrium potential; V_M, membrane potential. See Hodgkin and Huxley (1952a,b,c) and Hodgkin et al. (1952). A sophisticated quantitative analysis is presented by Hodgkin and Huxley (1952d).

G_{Na} back to its resting level; and (2) a slower increase in G_K. As a result, the inward I_{Na}, which had been transiently very large, begins to drop and, somewhat more slowly, I_K begins to increase. As the outward I_K becomes larger than the inward I_{Na}, the net current flow is now outward (hyperpolarizing), and it begins to drive V_m back toward the resting level. Notice that the increase in G_K is prolonged compared to that in G_{Na} (Fig. 6–4a), and thus for some period after the spike the V_m may actually be more negative than the normal resting potential (Fig. 6–4c), that is, closer to E_K. This phenomenon is called the *afterhyperpolarization* of the spike. Finally, G_K begins to decrease again, and at some time after the end of the action potential the membrane conductances have returned to their normal resting levels. The time course of these changes (Fig. 6–4) can vary from cell to cell, but in general, axonal action potentials are very fast. In the squid giant axon, for example, the entire sequence of events described above is over in a few milliseconds. In other cells, for example, in certain neurons in the pituitary gland of vertebrates, action potentials may last for tens of milliseconds; in cardiac muscle cells they may be hundreds of milliseconds long.

Voltage clamp studies of the squid giant axon. The sequence of events described in Figure 6–4 is of fundamental importance, and the reader is encouraged to examine this figure carefully before proceeding further. The studies that led to the elucidation of these events represented a partnership between several brilliant investigators on the one hand, and a magnificently well-suited experimental preparation on the other. The work of J. Z. Young, K. C. Cole, Alan Hodgkin, and Andrew Huxley on the squid giant axon ranks among the great success stories of twentieth-century science. Hodgkin and Huxley received the Nobel Prize for their studies, and some have remarked that it is unfortunate that the Atlantic squid *Loligo* cannot be similarly honored.

Young, a British zoologist, found in the mid-1930s that the mantle of the squid is innervated by a giant axon up to 1 mm in diameter. The giant axon arises from the fusion of a large number of smaller neurons. It can be removed from the animal, and the axoplasm can be extruded and replaced by saline solutions of defined ionic composition; in other words, the transmembrane ion gradients can be manipulated by the experimenter. The axonal plasma membrane is surprisingly robust and survives this maltreatment with its electrical properties intact. The large size of the axon makes it easy to place electrodes both inside and outside the membrane to measure (and control) the transmembrane voltage. Recall from Chapter 4 that the importance of controlling as well as measuring the voltage arises from the fact that the sodium and potassium conductances themselves change as a function of voltage, and the membrane is not at steady state during the action potential. It will be evident that depolarization produces an increase in G_{Na}, which then produces further depolarization. This in turn further increases G_{Na}, and an unstable positive feedback loop results that gives rise to the *regenerative* all-or-none action potential. Accordingly, the only way to study the regulation of membrane conductance effectively is to measure the conductance properties at fixed voltages, by means of K. C. Cole's voltage clamp that we described near the end of Chapter 4.

Voltage- and time-dependent ion currents. Hodgkin and Huxley (as well as Cole) immediately recognized the importance of controlling the membrane voltage, and the experimental convenience of working with a large and manipulable axon. They carried out a series of seminal experiments (interrupted by World War II) on voltage-clamped squid giant axons. The results of these studies were published in a classic series of papers by Hodgkin and Huxley (one of them in collaboration with Bernard Katz) in 1952. They are wonderfully insightful papers, not easy reading, but essential for the serious student of neurophysiology and membrane biophysics.

Hodgkin and Huxley asked what happens when one voltage clamps the axon near the resting potential, and either hyperpolarizes it or depolarizes it before returning to the original voltage (the *holding potential*). As shown in Figure 6–5a, small hyperpolarizing or depolarizing pulses of the same size produce small inward or outward currents, respectively. These *leak currents* are not time dependent (they reach their maximum amplitude in a time that is too short to be resolved by the recording instrumentation), and they are the same size in inward and outward directions for equal-amplitude hyperpolarizations and depolarizations. When the current amplitude is plotted against the voltage during the pulse (the *pulse* or *command potential*) for these small hyperpolarizations and depolarizations, the resulting *current-voltage (I–V) relationship* is a straight line (Fig. 6–5b). Such a straight line I–V relationship is also seen for a linear resistor in a nonbiological electrical circuit (Fig. 6–5c). Time- and voltage-independent ion channels contribute to the leak current. It can be seen that the I–V curve intersects the zero current axis at V_r. This is not surprising, since V_r is defined as the voltage at which the net current flow is zero.

This linear leak current is all that is seen for hyperpolarizing voltage clamp pulses, whatever their amplitude. What happens when a larger pulse, one that normally exceeds the threshold for action potential generation, is given in the depolarizing direction? Remember that the membrane voltage is held constant by the voltage clamp, so no action potential is per-

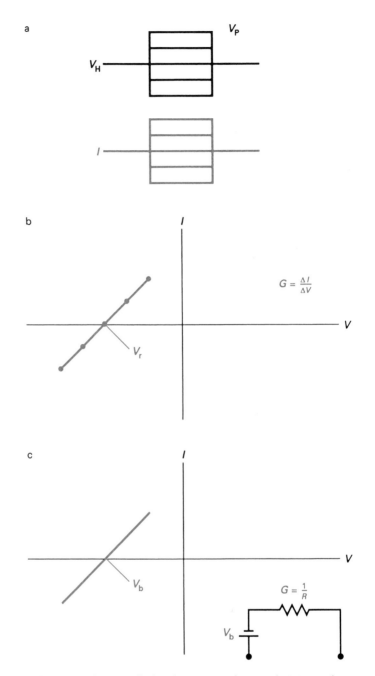

Figure 6–5. Leak currents. *a*: When small depolarizing or hyperpolarizing voltage clamp steps are made from the holding potential (V_H) to the pulse potential (V_p), small time-independent currents (I) are seen. *b*: A plot of these currents as a function of voltage (V). V_r, reversal potential. *c*: A similar current-voltage relationship is seen for a linear resistor in a nonbiological electrical circuit, containing a battery of voltage (V_b).

mitted to occur. It is immediately obvious that the membrane current is *not* at steady state during these larger depolarizing pulses, and time-dependent currents flow (Fig. 6–6a). There is an inward-going (negative by convention) current during the first millisecond or two after the beginning of the depolarizing pulse, and then the current reverses sign and becomes outward or positive during the remainder of the pulse. When a series of such pulses is given to different depolarizing voltages, a family of curves is generated as shown in Figure 6–6b. Note that as the amplitude of the voltage pulse increases, the early inward component of the current (blue) first increases, and then begins to decrease until it reverses sign and becomes outward at very large depolarizations. In contrast, the later outward component of the current (black) remains outward and continues to increase in amplitude with larger depolarizations.

How can one interpret these complex voltage- and time-dependent ionic currents? The relationship between the imposed membrane voltage and the membrane current that flows at that voltage can be investigated in more detail by constructing *I–V* curves. The early and late components of the current can be examined separately by measuring the current at different times. The peak inward current (usually after about 1–2 msec in the squid axon) is taken as a measure of the early component, and the current near the end of the pulse is the late component (also called by Hodgkin and Huxley the *delayed outward current*). As we shall see below, the early and late components can also be separated on the basis of other criteria, confirming that it is appropriate to make this distinction on the basis of their kinetic properties. The *I–V* curves in Figure 6–6c extend the conclusions drawn from an inspection of the current traces themselves. Both components of the current exhibit markedly nonlinear *I–V* curves, the early inward component first increasing and then decreasing in amplitude, then reversing in sign. The late outward component continues to increase (with increasing slope) over the entire voltage range examined. For these large depolarizations, then, the membrane is no longer behaving like a linear resistor; rather it rectifies, and the membrane conductance exhibits voltage dependence in this voltage range. As we know from our consideration of voltage-dependent ion channel gating in Chapter 4, these conductance changes result from voltage-dependent changes in the open probability of the channels responsible for the membrane currents.

Sodium and potassium carry the inward and outward membrane currents. Hodgkin and Huxley noted that the early inward current has the right sign, amplitude, voltage dependence, and kinetics to be responsible for the upstroke of the action potential. For example, the fact that the inward current turns on only at voltages depolarized from rest provides an explanation for the

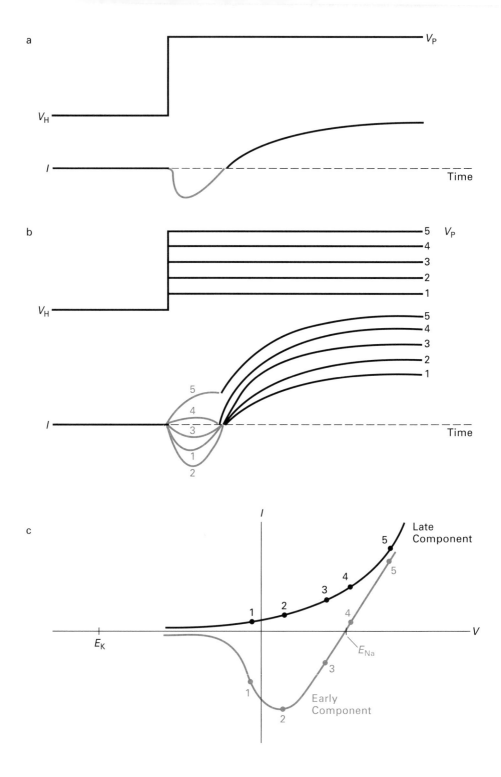

a

V_P

V_H

I

Time

b

5 V_P
4
3
2
1

V_H

5
4
3
2
1

I

5
4
3
1
2

Time

c

I

Late
Component

5

4

3

2

1

E_K

E_{Na}

4

5

V

1

2

3

Early
Component

phenomenon of a threshold for action potential generation. Similarly, the delayed outward current has the right characteristics to be responsible for the repolarization. They subsequently went on to ask which ions are the charge carriers for the inward and outward currents, using a series of *ion substitution* experiments. When the sodium was removed from the extracellular medium and replaced by an equivalent amount of some nonpermeant monovalent cation (for example, choline), the late component of the current was not affected, but the early component was outward over the entire voltage range examined (Fig. 6–7a). This is because the sodium concentration gradient is now reversed, and when the sodium channels open, sodium leaves rather than enters through the channels. When the extracellular sodium concentration is varied over a wide range, so as to systematically vary E_{Na}, it can be seen that the V_r for the early current is always equal to E_{Na} (Fig. 6–7b). This result confirms that this component of the membrane current is carried entirely by sodium and there is no significant contribution by any other ion.

The delayed current is not affected by the extracellular sodium concentration. Hodgkin and Huxley suspected that the delayed current was carried by the outward flow of potassium ions, but were unable to confirm this directly because they had difficulty changing the intracellular potassium concentration without damaging the axons. However, subsequent ion substitution experiments, on squid axon and other cell types, confirmed that V_r for the delayed current is always equal to E_K, demonstrating that potassium, and only potassium, is the charge carrier for this current component. Because of its kinetics, and the voltage-dependent gating that gives rise to rectification in the *I–V* curve, this current is often called the *delayed rectifier potassium current*.

Pharmacological tools have also proven to be extremely useful in separating the two components of axonal current. As discussed in Chapter 4, the Japanese puffer fish toxin tetrodotoxin (TTX) is a potent and selective blocker of sodium channels (Fig. 4–7). In the presence of TTX the

---

Figure 6–6. Nonlinear voltage-dependent currents. *a*: When the depolarizing pulses are made very much larger than those in Figure 6–5, time-dependent currents (*I*) are seen to flow. During a sustained depolarization, there is an early component of the current that is inward (*blue*) and a later component that is outward (*black*). V_H, holding potential; V_p, pulse potential. *b*: When a series of pulses is given to different depolarizing pulse potentials, the currents change with voltage in a characteristic way. *c*: Plot of the early and late peak currents (*I*) as a function of voltage (*V*) (see Hodgkin and Huxley, 1952a,b,c; Hodgkin et al., 1952). E_K, potassium equilibrium potential; E_{Na}, sodium equilibrium potential.

early sodium component of the current is eliminated, and the delayed potassium component can be studied in isolation (Fig. 6–8).

It is interesting that the puffer fish is a delicacy in Japan, and chefs are specially trained to remove the TTX-containing organs for the preparation of this dish; however, these organs are not removed entirely, because the tingle one gets from a small dose of TTX is apparently one of the major reasons this dish is so popular. In spite of the undoubted skill of these highly trained chefs, mistakes are made and there are still several deaths per year in Japan from TTX poisoning.

The story of potassium channel blockers has (until recently) been less colorful. Several organic compounds with quaternary ammonium groups, the most useful of which is tetraethylammonium (TEA; see Fig. 5–12), are selective blockers of the delayed rectifier potassium current in squid axon,

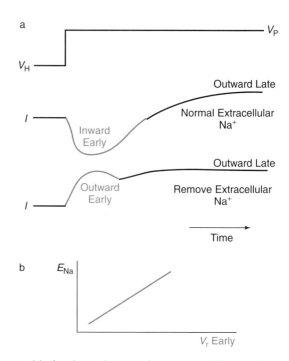

Figure 6–7. Sodium ions are responsible for the early inward current. a: When sodium ions are removed from the extracellular solution, the early phase of the current I $(blue)$ changes from inward to outward because of the change in the sodium equilibrium potential. V_H, holding potential; V_p, pulse potential. b: Plot of the reversal potential (V_r) of the early current as a function of the sodium equilibrium potential (E_{Na}). The relationship is exactly that predicted by the Nernst equation for a current carried exclusively by sodium ions. The late component of the current is not affected by manipulation of the sodium concentration.

allowing the early sodium current to be examined in isolation (Fig. 6–8). As we shall see in the next chapter, there can be many kinds of potassium currents in nerve cells, and these blockers do not affect all potassium currents to the same extent. The pharmacology of potassium channels has also expanded with the discovery that certain toxins, for example, the bee venom toxin *apamin*, the scorpion venom component *charybdotoxin*, and the snake venom toxin *dendrotoxin*, can selectively block certain classes of potassium channels.

Sodium current inactivation. An essential feature of an action potential is the activation of the sodium current by membrane depolarization. But as we

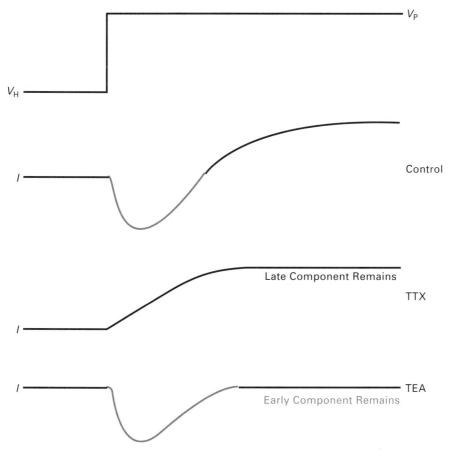

Figure 6–8. Pharmacological agents selectively block the early and late components of the current (I). Tetrodotoxin (TTX) blocks the early component of the current, whereas tetraethylammonium (TEA) blocks only the late component. V_H, holding potential; V_p, pulse potential.

have seen, depolarization not only makes the sodium current turn on, it also causes it to turn off very soon thereafter. This *inactivation* occurs during the depolarizing pulse. It is distinct from *deactivation* (or reversal of activation), which occurs after the end of the pulse as a result of the return of the membrane voltage to the hyperpolarized holding potential. Inactivation of the sodium current of course reflects the inactivation of individual sodium channels (Fig. 4–9). An examination of Figure 6–8 makes it clear that the switch from net inward to net outward current during a depolarizing pulse is due not only to the slow turning on of the delayed outward potassium current but also to the fact that the opposing inward sodium current has inactivated and gone to sleep.

Figure 6–9 summarizes in cartoon form the sequential activation, inactivation, and recovery from inactivation of sodium channels. Under rest-

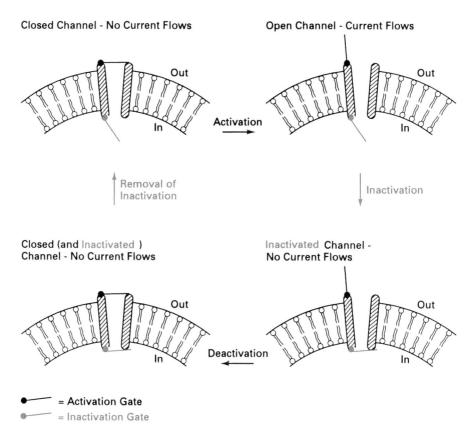

Figure 6–9. Opening, closing, and inactivation transitions in voltage-dependent sodium channels. The gating transitions in sodium channels during and following a depolarizing pulse are summarized. See text for details.

ing conditions (Fig. 6–9, upper left) the black activation gate is closed and no current flows. When the membrane is depolarized (right side of Fig. 6–9), this activation gate undergoes voltage-dependent opening. As shown on the upper right of Figure 6–9, the channel is now open and current can flow. The same depolarization that opens the activation gate also leads to slower closing of the red inactivation gate (Fig. 6–9, lower right). Although the membrane is still depolarized and the activation gate is still open, no current can flow because the inactivation gate is closed. After the end of the depolarizing pulse, deactivation, the reversal of activation, occurs and the activation gate closes. Again, no current can flow (Fig. 6–9, lower left). At this time a depolarization cannot evoke any current, because even though the activation gate will open as a result of the depolarization, the inactivation gate remains closed for some time following the pulse. Only after inactivation is removed is the channel back in its resting state (Fig. 6–9, upper left) and available to be opened by another depolarization.

How do we know that the diagram in Figure 6–9 is a reasonable description of how sodium channel inactivation works? The inactivation of the sodium current can be investigated by using *conditioning prepulses*, prior to the voltage clamp test pulse during which the sodium current is measured. If the membrane is depolarized briefly (prepulsed) immediately before the test pulse, it is found that the amplitude of the sodium current is smaller than in the absence of a prepulse (Fig. 6–10a). This is because the prepulse depolarization has caused inactivation of a portion of the current, and it has not yet recovered from this inactivation by the time the test pulse is given. In contrast, with a *hyperpolarizing prepulse*, the sodium current during the test pulse can be larger than the control (Fig. 6–10b). This shows that at the holding potential, which often is close to the cell's resting potential, the level of depolarization is sufficient to cause some resting or steady-state inactivation, which is removed by the hyperpolarizing prepulse. This is illustrated in a plot of the relationship between membrane voltage and extent of inactivation (Fig. 6–10c).

We have seen that sodium channel inactivation is a time-dependent process that contributes to the switch from inward to outward current during an action potential. The recovery of sodium current from inactivation is also time dependent. The time course of recovery from inactivation can be investigated by varying the time between a depolarizing prepulse and a test pulse. The prepulse produces inactivation, and recovery to the normal amplitude sodium current takes several tens of milliseconds. Typically, recovery is half complete after about 15 msec in the squid axon. This of course means that sodium current inactivation will long outlast the action potential that produces it.

The functional implications of the long time course of recovery from

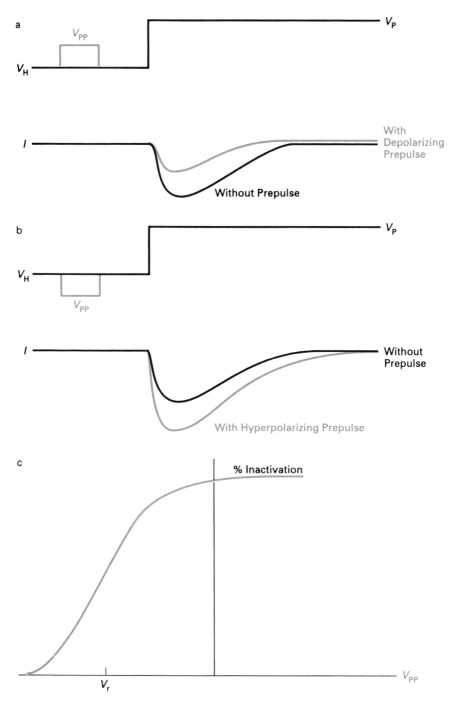

Figure 6–10. Sodium current inactivation. When the late component of the current (I) is blocked, for example, with tetraethylammonium (TEA), it is possible to examine the kinetics of the sodium current in isolation. Effect of a depolarizing (a) or hyperpolarizing (b) prepulse (V_{pp}) on the amplitude of the sodium current during a subsequent depolarizing pulse (V_p). V_H, holding potential. c: Degree of inactivation as a function of voltage. V_r, reversal potential.

sodium channel inactivation are profound. Since the peak of the action potential is a voltage at which inactivation will be complete (Fig. 6–10c), sodium current will be inactivated for some period of time, and the cell will be unable to fire a second action potential until there is sufficient recovery from this inactivation. It will be evident, then, that *sodium channel inactivation is the ionic mechanism underlying the refractory period*. The elevated threshold during the refractory period reflects sodium channel inactivation, and the return of the threshold to normal (Fig. 3–6) corresponds to removal of inactivation. Effectively, sodium channel inactivation sets the upper limit of action potential frequency in an axon. We shall see, however, that a variety of potassium channels also participate in determining the actual rate at which a neuron fires.

It is important to emphasize that there is nothing magic about inactivation gating (or any of the other gating transitions) in ion channels. With our understanding of ion channels as protein molecules, gating can be thought of as a rapid change in the three-dimensional structure of the protein, from a conformation that allows conduction to one that does not, and vice-versa. The closed and inactivated states of the channel reflect different protein conformations, neither of which conducts ions (recall the cartoon of the inactivating Shaker potassium channel in Fig. 5–11b, and compare with Fig. 6–9). Many of the gating transitions (and hence protein conformational changes) that we have described are voltage dependent, implying that they result from the movement of some charged region of the ion channel protein, in the electric field across the plasma membrane.

Ion Pumps Maintain the Ion Concentration Gradients

It is evident that neurons cannot continue to fire action potentials forever. When membrane currents flow, ions are moving down their concentration gradients. The currents are relatively small at steady state, but of course are much larger during action potentials. If action potential firing continues, eventually the sodium and potassium concentrations on the two sides of the membrane will be equal, the membrane potential will be zero, and the state of the cell can be well described by the word "dead". It may take a long time to run down the ionic concentration gradients in an axon as large as the squid giant axon, but in smaller cells significant changes may occur after relatively few action potentials. Fortunately, the energy driven pumps come to the rescue before any damage is done.

A particular active ion transporter, the *sodium-potassium-ATPase* or *sodium-potassium pump*, mediates the pumping of sodium out of and potassium into the cell to maintain the ion concentration gradients. Another way to think of this is to say that the pump is responsible for charging up the membrane battery. The pump is an enzyme that hydrolyzes ATP and uses the energy to move each ion against its concentration gradient (Fig. 6–11). This transport activity may involve some sort of movement or rotation of the pump in the membrane. The stoichiometry of the sodium-potassium-ATPase, the transport ratio for sodium and potassium, is not 1:1, but instead 3:2. In other words, three sodium ions are transported outward for every two potassium ions transported inward and, as a result, the pump produces a net outward current. This kind of pump is said to be *electrogenic*, because its activity causes the cell to hyperpolarize, and it contributes (although usually only to a limited extent) to the setting of the resting potential.

Although we have de-emphasized their contribution to neuronal excitability, we can see that ion pumps do indeed play an essential role. They

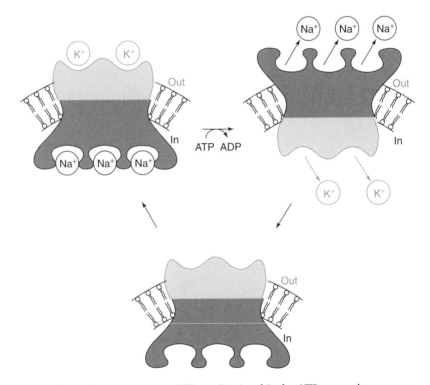

Figure 6–11. The sodium–potassium–ATPase. Depicted is the ATPase, a plasma membrane pump that uses the energy of hydrolysis of ATP to move three sodium ions from the inside of the cell to the outside and, at the same time, move two potassium ions from the outside to the inside.

are not quite as flashy as the channels that allow for such rapid flow of ions, but they are always there in the background, working away quietly to ensure that the ion concentration gradients that are essential for electrical signaling are maintained.

Summary

The flow of ions down their electrochemical gradients, through populations of ion channels in the neuronal plasma membrane, gives rise to transmembrane ion currents. It is the sum of the various currents flowing at any point in time that determines the neuron's membrane potential. Thus the normal firing pattern of a neuron, and its response to different kinds of stimulation, can be seen as a play of interactions among the currents generated by the different kinds of ion channels in its membrane. The activities of the sodium and potassium channels responsible for axonal action potentials are themselves dependent on voltage. Voltage clamp studies, which allow the measurement of the current flowing through these channels at fixed voltage, have provided a detailed understanding of the sequence of changes in sodium and potassium channel activity that give rise to action potentials.

7

Diversity in the Structure and Function of Ion Channels

*T*hus far we have been discussing the axonal membrane as if it had only two kinds of ion currents, a voltage-dependent potassium current that is responsible for the axon's electrical activity (or rather its lack of activity) at rest, and a voltage-dependent sodium current that underlies the large and rapid membrane depolarization during the action potential. Although the work of Hodgkin and Huxley demonstrated that these two currents could provide a reasonably accurate picture of the electrical activity of the squid giant axon, it is now evident that there is a considerable diversity of ion currents in axons, and even greater diversity in neuronal cell bodies and dendrites.

The electrical behavior of cell bodies and dendrites certainly tends to be more varied than that of axons. Some neuronal cell bodies do not fire action potentials, and are said to be *electrically inexcitable* because they lack the rapid voltage-dependent sodium current. Other neurons produce pacing, bursting, and the wide range of responses to external stimuli described in Chapter 3. The cell bodies of such neurons may exhibit many other ion currents in addition to or in place of the classic action potential currents. These other currents, which may be regulated by (*1*) voltage, (*2*) neurotransmitters that bind to receptor sites on the extracellular side of the channel, (*3*) intracellular calcium, (*4*) intracellular metabolic modulators, or (*5*) some combination of these factors interact to generate complex patterns of neuronal electrical activity such as that exhibited by *Aplysia* neuron R15 (see Fig. 3–12c).

Since ion currents reflect the activity of ion channels, the diversity in ion currents must be matched by an equivalent diversity in the ion chan-

139

nel proteins that underlie these currents. Single channel recording and molecular cloning techniques have been used to demonstrate that the diversity is even greater than had been imagined; in many cases these techniques reveal that currents that were thought previously to be carried by a single population of ion channels in fact reflect the activity of several different kinds of ion channels. Only through a knowledge of the molecular basis of this diversity can we begin to understand its contribution to the electrical behavior of the neuron.

This chapter will focus on the diversity of the major classes of *voltage-dependent* ion channels (see Table 7–1). We do not mean to give short shrift to the *neurotransmitter-gated* ion channels, which are essential for chemical synaptic transmission and for the modulation of neuronal electrical properties. This group, including a variety of potassium-, calcium-, and chloride-selective channels, will be considered in detail in later chapters. Some of the neurotransmitter-gated channels are also voltage dependent, making the distinction between these two channel classes somewhat blurred. Thus, the choice of channels to be discussed here rather than in later chapters is by necessity somewhat arbitrary.

Calcium Channels

In axons the most important channels for the generation of inward currents are the voltage-dependent sodium channels whose properties and structure were discussed in the last two chapters. However, there are several other classes of channels that contribute substantially to inward current flow in many neuronal cell bodies (and in some axons and dendrites). Among these are nonselective cation channels that allow the flow of both

Table 7–1 Examples of the Major Classes of Voltage-Dependent Ion Channels

Channel Type	Activation Voltage Range	Physiological Function
Axonal sodium channels	−30 to +20 mV	Upstroke of action potential
Calcium channels	Variable	Calcium action potentials; calcium-mediated intracellular events, including neurotransmitter release
Potassium channels	Extremely variable	Action potential repolarization; spacing of action potentials; regulation of resting potential

sodium and potassium. The molecular properties of these channels have not been investigated thoroughly, and we will not discuss them further. Instead, let us focus on calcium channels, which play a critical role in the lives of neurons (and other cells).

Calcium currents. In most neurons a depolarizing voltage clamp step elicits an inward current with kinetics very different from those seen in the squid axon. The current may rise to its peak more slowly, and inactivate only partially and far more slowly, than in the squid axon (Fig. 7–1a). When pharmacological treatments and/or ion replacement are used to eliminate any sodium current, an inward current that rises slowly to its peak and inactivates only partially (if at all) can still be elicited by the depolarizing pulse (Fig. 7–1a). In fact, when the neuron is released from voltage clamp under these conditions, it is often found that it can still fire action potentials *even in the complete absence of sodium current*, although the shape and duration of these action potentials can be very different from those observed when sodium current is present (Fig. 7–1b; see also Fig. 3–11). Further ion substitution experiments reveal that most neurons exhibit a substantial voltage-dependent calcium current (I_{Ca}). In some cases this is responsible for much or all of the regenerative depolarization during the rising phase of the action potential.

Interestingly, the very brilliance of the studies of Hodgkin and Huxley, which defined the sodium and potassium currents as both necessary and sufficient to account for action potentials in the squid axon, led to skepticism in assessing the work of early pioneers in the calcium current field. Although the calcium current experiments stood up to critical scrutiny, there was a reluctance on the part of many neurophysiologists to complicate with another ion current what had been a satisfying and apparently complete picture of membrane excitability. The neurophysiology community did not suspect in the 1960s just how drastically this simple picture was to be modified in the years to come.

Diversity of calcium channels. In some neurons, a plot of the peak calcium current as a function of voltage (Fig. 7–1c) closely resembles that for the sodium current (Fig. 6–6c), except that the current approaches zero at very depolarized voltages, reflecting the more depolarized value for the calcium reversal potential, E_{Ca}. In other neurons this curve appears more complex, indicating that more than a single population of calcium channels gives rise to the current–voltage (I–V) relationship. In fact, on closer inspection with single channel recordings, even the simpler I–V relationships can turn out to be generated by more than one species of calcium channel. It now appears that there are several distinct categories of calcium channels in

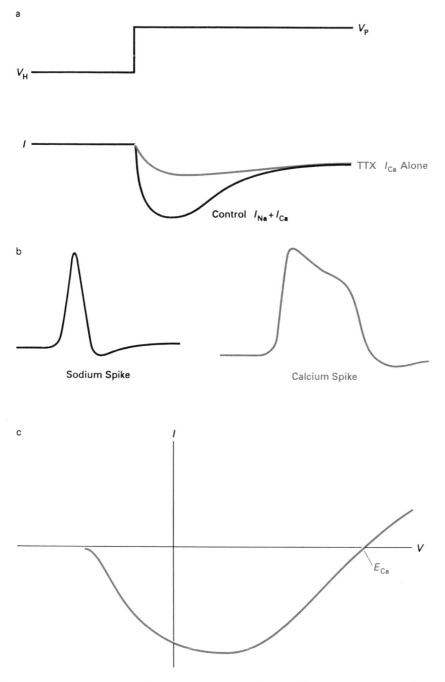

Figure 7–1. Currents carried by calcium ions. *a*: When tetrodotoxin (TTX) is used to block the sodium component (I_{Na}) of inward current (I), a calcium current component (I_{Ca}) remains. V_H, holding potential; V_P, pulse potential. *b*: The sodium action potential is contrasted with the action potential in cells in which the inward current is carried predominantly by calcium. *c*: Current–voltage (I–V) relationship for the calcium current. E_{Ca}, calcium equilibrium potential.

many neurons, which can be distinguished on the basis of their voltage dependence, kinetics, single channel conductance, pharmacology, and molecular structures, as well as by their location in the neuron.

Pharmacological probes confirm calcium channel diversity. As we have seen with sodium channels, selective drugs and toxins have been particularly useful in identifying and discriminating among the different components of calcium current. The *dihydropyridines* are synthetic organic compounds (Fig. 7–2a) that bind to one particular class of calcium channel, the *L-type* channels, which exhibit long-lasting macroscopic currents. Dihydropyridine *antagonists* cause the L-type channels to spend less time in the active state, whereas *agonists* promote a more active mode of channel activity characterized by longer channel openings (Fig. 7–2b). Other classes of calcium channel are resistant to the dihydropyridines but can be identified by their interaction with peptide toxins. For example, the venom of the fish-hunting cone snail, *Conus geographus*, contains a 27 amino acid peptide called *ω-conotoxin GVIA* (Fig. 7–3). This peptide inhibits another type of calcium current, the *N-type* calcium current, in neurons. Another larger peptide toxin, *ω-Agatoxin IVA* (Fig. 7–3), found in the venom of the funnel web spider, *Agelenopsis aperta*, selectively inhibits a calcium channel called the *P-type* calcium channel, which is responsible for most of the calcium

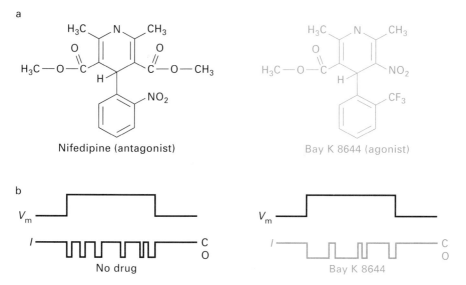

Figure 7–2. Dihydropyridines modulate calcium channel activity. *a:* Structures of a dihydropyridine (DHP) antagonist (*black*) and agonist (*blue*). *b:* L-type calcium channel activity in the absence (*black*) or presence (*blue*) of a DHP agonist. I, current; V_m, membrane voltage.

current in cerebellar Purkinje neurons as well as many other types of neurons. Like many other small bioactive peptides, these toxins contain multiple disulfide bonds (Fig. 7–3) that probably confer upon them the rigid three-dimensional structure necessary for their selective binding to different classes of calcium channels.

Purification and cloning of calcium channel subunits. Through procedures analogous to those described in Chapter 5 for sodium channels, these specific pharmacological agents have been used to purify calcium channels from several different tissues. As in the case of sodium channels, there is a large (175–230 kDa) subunit, termed α_1, that is sufficient to form a functional voltage-dependent calcium channel and one or more smaller subunits (β, γ, α_2, and δ; see Fig. 7–4a). Although the smaller subunits are not *required* for channel activity, they do interact with the α_1 subunits and *modulate* the kinetic properties of the channels. As we shall see later in this chapter, auxiliary subunits also exist for potassium (and sodium) channels, and they influence not only channel functional properties but also channel targeting and localization in the plasma membrane.

Molecular cloning, based on protein sequence as described for sodium channels in Chapter 5, has been used to study the structural basis for the functional and pharmacological diversity of calcium currents. Multiple distinct genes for both the α_1 and β subunits have been identified (Fig. 7–4b). Furthermore, all of the α_1 and most of the β subunit messenger RNA transcripts can undergo alternative splicing, a way of generating several distinct messenger RNAs and hence several different protein products from a single gene as we saw for the Shaker potassium channel. The bottom line is that many calcium channel α_1 subunits can be expressed in the brain (and other tissues), and when their interactions with β and other subunits

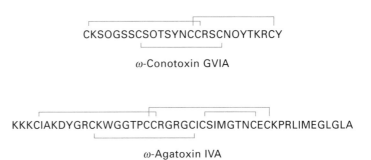

CKSOGSSCSOTSYNCCRSCNOYTKRCY

ω-Conotoxin GVIA

KKKCIAKDYGRCKWGGTPCCRGRGCICSIMGTNCECKPRLIMEGLGLA

ω-Agatoxin IVA

Figure 7–3. Peptide toxins that block calcium channels. The sequences of two useful toxins (single letter amino acid codes; O = hydroxyproline). Note the multiple disulfide bonds (*blue*) between cystine (C) residues.

is considered, the number of combinatorial possibilities is enormous. The diversity hinted at by calcium current kinetics and pharmacology pales in the face of this molecular heterogeneity.

Molecular organization of calcium channels. What have we learned about the structure and function of calcium channels from molecular cloning approaches? First, as emphasized above, heterologous expression tells us that there is a single polypeptide, the α_1 subunit, that is capable of forming a

a

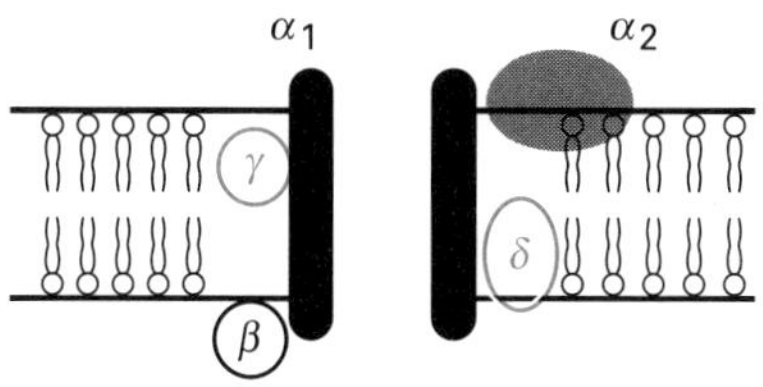

b

Gene	αSubunit Subtype	Functional Channel Subtype
Ca$_v$1.1	α_{1S}	L
1.2	α_{1C}	L
1.3	α_{1D}	L
1.4	α_{1F}	L
Ca$_v$2.1	α_{1A}	P/Q
2.2	α_{1B}	N
2.3	α_{1E}	R
Ca$_v$3.1	α_{1G}	T
3.2	α_{1H}	T
3.3	α_{1H}	T

Figure 7–4. Subunits of calcium channels. *a*: Purified calcium channels consist of as many as five types of subunits. *b*: Multiple genes contribute to calcium channel diversity (modified from Dunlap et al., 1995 and Ertel et al., 2000).

functional channel, reminiscent of the picture of sodium channels described in Chapter 5. Even more strikingly similar to sodium channels is the membrane organization of the calcium channel protein, predicted from the α_1 subunit amino acid sequence. Hydrophobicity plots predict 24 transmembrane segments, which can be divided into four homologous domains, each consisting of six transmembrane segments. This organization is so similar to that of sodium channels that we need not provide a new diagram here, but simply refer the reader to the diagram of sodium channel structure in Figure 5–3. Recall that this overall structural homology is recapitulated for voltage-dependent potassium channels as well (Figs. 5–4 and 5–8).

Calcium channels are special. Calcium channels are of particular interest because calcium is far more than simply a charge carrier across the plasma membrane. As essential as calcium ions are in contributing to action potentials and other aspects of neuronal electrical activity, this role may be secondary to the intracellular messenger actions of calcium. Calcium that enters the cell interacts with calcium-binding proteins to regulate a variety of intracellular enzymes. Furthermore, intracellular calcium ions regulate the gating of several types of ion channel and can even feed back and participate in the inactivation of some of their own channels. In addition, an essential characteristic of neuronal signaling, the release of chemical neurotransmitters at synapses, is controlled directly by intracellular calcium. In this sense, calcium can be thought of as the transducer of an electrical signal, depolarization, into chemical signals inside the cell.

All of these features set calcium apart. It will thus come as no surprise that the activity of calcium channels themselves is subject to intricate modulatory influences, in cardiac and skeletal muscle as well as in neurons. We shall be hearing much more about the regulation and consequences of calcium channel activity throughout this book.

Channels That Carry Outward Current: The Potassium Channels

Even more impressive than the diversity of calcium channels is that exhibited by the potassium channels. Some half dozen or more voltage-dependent potassium currents were first identified on the basis of voltage clamp experiments. This number has expanded dramatically as single channel and molecular biological approaches have been used to study potassium channels (Fig. 7–5). As in the case of other channels, kinetics, voltage dependence, pharmacology, single channel properties, and molecular structure have been used to characterize the various potassium channels. We will summarize here the physiological properties of some of these channels in the context of their cloning and molecular structures. By necessity we can only touch on their diversity in the limited space available.

Calcium-dependent potassium currents. In most cells, such as the large cell bodies of many molluscan neurons that have been used widely for voltage clamp studies of membrane currents, the total outward current carried by potassium exhibits a steady-state *I–V* relationship that is very different from that seen in the squid axon (*steady state* refers here to the sustained non-inactivating current, measured many tens or hundreds of milliseconds after the onset of a depolarizing pulse). The *I–V* curve has a characteristic N shape in the range of depolarized voltages (Fig. 7–6a), because it is the sum of several distinct current components (Fig. 7–6b,c). When the cell is injected with an agent that binds tightly to calcium, such as EGTA, or calcium entry is prevented during the depolarizations by phar-

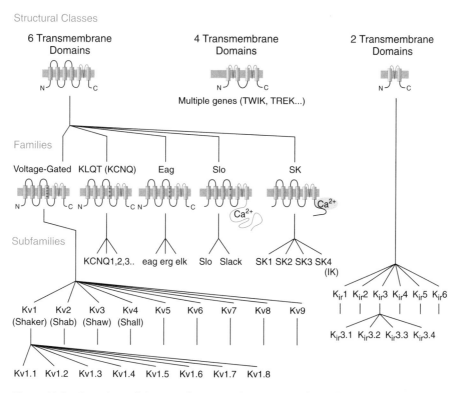

Figure 7–5. Overview of the vast diversity of potassium channels. There are three basic structural types of potassium channel subunits. The genes for potassium channels can be divided into different families and subfamilies. Only a few members of the subfamilies are shown for illustration (modified from Wei et al., 1996).

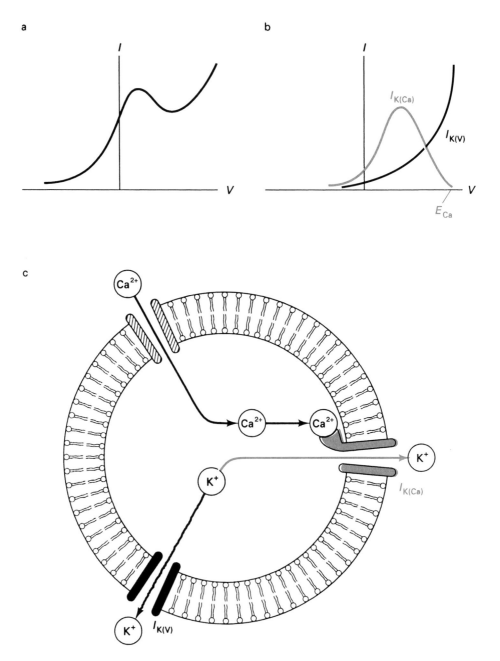

Figure 7–6. Different components of outward current. a: In most neuronal cell bodies, when the inward current is blocked, the current–voltage ($I–V$) relationship for the peak outward current has a characteristic N shape (see Meech and Standen, 1975). b: Two components of outward current. E_{Ca}, calcium equilibrium potential. c: The activation of two classes of potassium channels ($I_{K(V)}$, $I_{K(Ca)}$) is illustrated.

macological block of calcium channels, the resulting I–V curve (black in Fig. 7–6b) looks identical to that of the delayed rectifier potassium current in squid axon (compare with Fig. 6–6c). When its kinetics, voltage dependence, and pharmacology are examined, this current can be seen to exhibit the properties of a classic delayed rectifier, whose role in action potential repolarization we have already discussed in Chapter 6.

The other outward current component that contributes to the shape of the steady-state I–V curve at positive voltages is the one blocked by preventing calcium entry or binding intracellular calcium—a *calcium-dependent potassium current*. Its I–V curve (blue in Fig. 7–6b) is obtained by subtracting the delayed rectifier component from the total outward current. This current is activated not only by the depolarization per se but also by the calcium that enters during the depolarizing voltage pulse (Fig. 7–6c). A comparison of the I–V curve in Figure 7–6b with that in Figure 7–1c shows that the voltage dependence of the calcium-activated potassium current mirrors that of the calcium current; this of course arises from the requirement for calcium entry, through voltage-dependent calcium channels, to contribute to the activation of this potassium current. As the voltage approaches E_{Ca}, the driving force for calcium entry decreases, and hence there is less activation of the calcium-dependent potassium current (other calcium-dependent intracellular processes often exhibit a similar voltage dependence). This requirement for intracellular calcium also explains why the current is eliminated by blocking calcium entry during the depolarization. However, this current and other calcium-dependent intracellular events may still be evoked by intracellular injection of calcium or by physiological treatments that cause the release of calcium from intracellular stores (see Chapter 12).

Kinetic and pharmacological studies of voltage clamp currents had suggested that there might be some heterogeneity of the calcium-dependent potassium current, but the extent of this heterogeneity became apparent only from single channel experiments and more recently from molecular cloning. Many cell types contain a large-conductance, calcium-dependent potassium channel (a *maxi* or *BK* channel), but there are intermediate (*IK*) and small (*SK*) conductance ones as well (Fig. 7–5). Although the BK class exhibits voltage-dependent gating and indeed can be thought of as voltage-dependent channels whose voltage-dependence is influenced by calcium, voltage is not involved in the gating of the SK class. There is even heterogeneity within the BK class. For example, in rat brain plasma membrane preparations, there are at least two separate maxi channels that can be distinguished on the basis of their gating kinetics (Fig. 7–7) and pharmacology. It appears that more than one type of calcium-dependent potassium channel can be present in a single cell, but the functional significance of this heterogeneity remains to be determined. Since calcium-dependent potassium currents contribute (with the delayed rectifier) to action potential repolarization as well as to interspike currents that help to control the frequency of repetitive firing, it is possible that the different kinetic properties and voltage sensitivities of different calcium-dependent potassium channels enable them to undertake distinct functional roles. As we shall discuss in Chapter 14, a particularly well-understood example is the contribution of kinetically distinct calcium-dependent potassium channels to frequency tuning in cochlear hair cells of the inner ear.

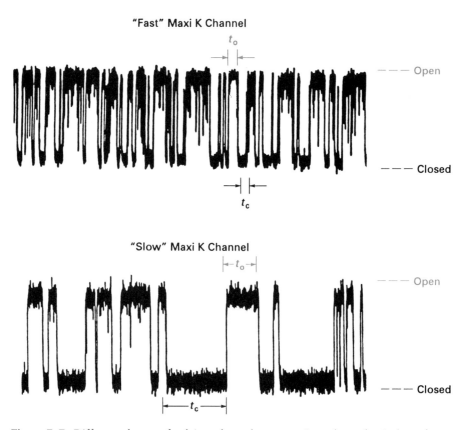

Figure 7–7. Different classes of calcium-dependent potassium channels. At least four distinct calcium-dependent potassium channels can be seen in plasma membrane fractions from mammalian brain. Two of them are shown here. They have very similar single channel conductances (240 pS), but differ in their gating kinetics (note the differences in t_o and t_c). These records were obtained following reconstitution of calcium-dependent potassium channels into artificial phospholipid bilayer membranes (see Reinhart et al., 1989).

The Slowpoke *locus encodes* BK *calcium-dependent potassium channels.* Once *Shaker* had been characterized, sequence homology cloning using *Shaker* sequences uncovered the large and still-growing family of voltage-dependent potassium channels in a wide variety of organisms, from bacteria to humans. However, this approach did not elucidate the molecular structures of the calcium-dependent potassium channels described above. Here again, *Drosophila* came to the rescue. A *Drosophila* mutant, called *Slowpoke*, lacks calcium-dependent potassium current in neurons and muscle cells. Positional cloning of the *Slowpoke* locus showed that it encodes a BK calcium-dependent potassium channel that shares many structural features with its *Shaker* family cousins, but is also different. The sequence of the Slowpoke cDNA predicts that the protein will have six membrane-spanning segments (Fig. 7–8), like Shaker, resembling one of the four homologous domains of the sodium and calcium channels (Fig. 5–3). There may also be a seventh membrane-spanning segment, S0, that places the amino terminus of the channel on the extracellular side of the membrane (Fig. 7–8). Furthermore, instead of terminating soon after the end of transmembrane segment S6, Slowpoke has an additional long stretch of amino acids that constitutes about two-thirds of the channel protein (Fig. 7–8). The functional significance of this portion of the channel protein is still under investigation, but it does appear to contain sequences that confer calcium sensitivity on channel activity. This carboxyl-terminal domain is also one region of the channel protein that interacts with certain kinds of auxiliary subunits that influence channel properties (see below).

Like Shaker, the Slowpoke messenger RNA can undergo alternative

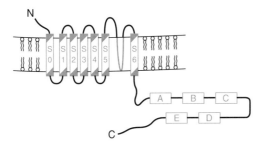

Figure 7–8. The Slowpoke calcium-dependent potassium channel cloned from *Drosophila*. In addition to the six membrane-spanning segments (S1–S6) also present in voltage-dependent potassium channels, Slowpoke may have a seventh membrane-spanning segment, S0, and also contains a long carboxyl-terminal tail. The boxes marked A to E are cassettes of amino acids that differ among different splice variants of the channel. (Modified from Adelman et al., 1992).

splicing to produce a number of different gene products. In fact, in the case of Slowpoke, the number is extraordinarily large—its sequence predicts a total of 144 possible splice variants arising from the single *Slowpoke* gene. Furthermore, as with Shaker, the functional calcium-dependent potassium channel is formed by a complex of four Slowpoke subunits. The total number of possible channels that can be derived from this single gene is 144^4 (almost 430,000,000)! Although it is not known how many of these channels actually exist in neurons, and only a very small number of the splice variants have been analyzed in any detail, the possibilities for functional heterogeneity are nevertheless nothing less than staggering. Modulation by different combinations of auxiliary subunits (see below) or by post-translational modification of the channel protein (Chapter 13) expands these possibilities even further. In addition, the IK and SK calcium-dependent potassium channels are encoded by genes distinct from *Slowpoke* (Fig. 7–5), and they also contribute substantially to the functional diversity of the calcium-dependent potassium currents in neurons.

Transient potassium current. In considering the repolarization of action potentials, we have been discussing potassium currents that inactivate very little if at all during a long depolarizing pulse. As we saw in the case of *Shaker*, however, there is also a transient potassium current in many neurons, often known as *A current*, that activates rapidly and then inactivates in a manner analogous to the sodium current. To measure this current, the membrane potential must first be set to a very negative holding potential for several hundred milliseconds to remove the voltage-dependent steady-state inactivation (this is reminiscent of the prepulse protocol for examining sodium current inactivation and removal of inactivation—see Fig. 6–10). When the membrane is depolarized from this very negative holding potential, an outward A current is seen (Fig. 7–9a) that mirrors the inward sodium current (Figs. 4–9 and 6–8), albeit with a more prolonged time course. The voltage dependence of A-current inactivation is such that, in neurons that have a relatively positive resting potential (more positive than about −45 mV), inactivation is more or less complete at the resting potential V_r (Fig. 7–9b; compare with Fig. 6–10c). Thus, in such cells, the steady-state inactivation must first be removed to examine this current.

The A current is active in the subthreshold region of membrane potential and helps to determine the frequency of repetitive firing in neurons. Although it is largely inactivated near the resting potential and completely inactivated during action potentials, some portion of the inactivation is removed by the afterhyperpolarization that normally follows an action potential. Hence the A current is active for a short while after an action potential and slows the return of the membrane potential toward the spike threshold. This in turn slows the firing frequency in a repetitively firing neuron.

Another role for A current is to allow a delay to occur between an excitatory stimulus and the onset of action potentials. This occurs in neurons with a relatively negative resting potential, in which there is little steady-state inactivation. When such a neuron is depolarized, the A current is activated and tends to oppose the change in membrane potential toward the threshold. As the A current inactivates during the depolarization, however, the neuron begins to depolarize more rapidly. Following a delay set by the kinetics of inactivation, the neuron finally reaches threshold. An example of this is found in the *Aplysia* ink gland motor neurons,

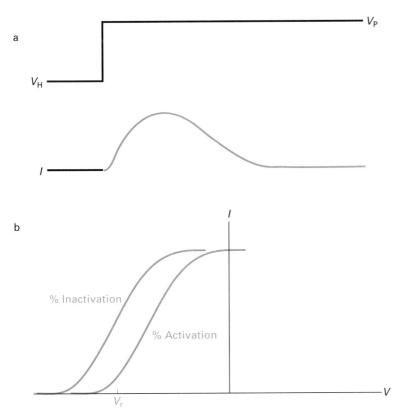

Figure 7–9. An inactivating potassium current. *a*: When the membrane is depolarized (V_P) from very negative holding potentials (V_H), a rapidly inactivating potassium current (I) can be observed. This potassium current has been termed the *A current*. *b*: Extent of activation and inactivation of the A current as a function of voltage (V). V_r, reversal potential.

which were depicted in Figure 3–13c. The prolonged noxious stimulus causes a depolarization that leads to progressive inactivation of A current. Only when the A current has undergone inactivation do the neurons fire the action potentials that trigger ink release.

Again, voltage clamp experiments have shown that there are multiple types of A currents in different cells. Shaker and its many cousins, the cloning and structure of which we described in Chapter 5, are rapidly inactivating A-current channels. These distinct A-current channels with different kinetic properties and voltage dependence, encoded by different genes or produced by alternative splicing from a single gene (as in the case of *Shaker*), contribute in different ways to the regulation of neuronal firing rates.

A potassium current activated by hyperpolarization. All the inward and outward currents we have discussed thus far are activated by depolarization, because either they are gated directly by voltage or depolarization-induced calcium entry is required for their activation, or both. This gives rise to rectification in the *I–V* relationship, an increase in the slope of the curve with depolarization. However, in many cells, there also exists a potassium current that is activated by hyperpolarization. This causes a *decrease* in the slope of the *I–V* curve with depolarization (Fig. 7–10), a phenomenon known as *anomalous* or *inward rectification.*

This all seems rather strange. Why would a cell bother with a channel that passes only inward but not outward potassium current? This question becomes particularly pressing when we remember that under normal

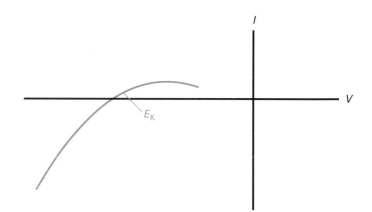

Figure 7–10. A potassium current that activates with hyperpolarization. Current–voltage (*I–V*) relationship for the inwardly rectifying potassium current, which displays a decrease in slope conductance with depolarization. E_K, potassium equilibrium potential.

conditions a neuron's V_m can never be more negative than E_K, since potassium is the charge carrier with the most negative reversal potential. Thus only under artificial hyperpolarizations imposed by the voltage clamp will the inward flow of potassium ever occur. One clue to the role of the anomalously rectifying potassium channels is the fact that they are not perfect rectifiers, and can pass some outward current in the voltage range up to about 30 mV depolarized from E_K (Fig. 7–10). Although the amount of current is not large, very few other membrane currents are active in this voltage range; accordingly, this current may play an important role in regulating the resting level of neuronal activity.

Cloning of the inward rectifier potassium channels. The inwardly rectifying potassium channels, like the calcium-dependent potassium channels, remained uncloned during the extensive homology screens that followed the initial characterization of Shaker. They finally fell to an approach called *expression cloning*, which we will describe in later chapters, and subsequent homology screens have uncovered a large family of inward rectifiers that clearly is distinct from the Shaker-like family of voltage-dependent potassium channels. The predicted structure of the inward rectifier potassium channels is interesting (Fig. 7–11). They contain only two putative membrane-spanning segments, flanking a pore domain that is very similar in sequence to that of the Shaker-like potassium channels; in this feature they resemble the bacterial KcsA channel, whose three-dimensional structure has been elucidated (Figs. 5–13 and 5–14). It is not entirely clear what mechanisms give rise to inward rectification, although voltage-dependent block of the channel pore by intracellular Mg^{2+} ion and/or other cytoplasmic factors appears to be involved. Inward rectifier potassium channels are subject to complex forms of modulation, which we shall discuss in Chapter 12.

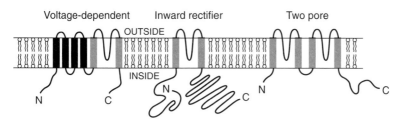

Figure 7–11. Predicted structures of other potassium channels. The inward rectifier and two pore potassium channels share some structural features (*blue*) with the six transmembrane voltage-dependent potassium channels. Compare with Figure 5–8.

Other potassium channels. We have by no means exhausted the complement of potassium channels with the description of the several classes of voltage-dependent channels above. An interesting and surprising discovery was that some potassium channels actually contain two P domains within the amino acid sequence of a single subunit (Fig. 7–11). These channels, which contribute to the resting membrane potential, form functional dimers and thus contain a total of four P domains like the other classes of potassium channels. There are other potassium-selective channels that are gated by ligands or intracellular metabolites; we have emphasized that some of these may exhibit voltage dependence as well. These other channels include the *M-current* and *S-current* potassium channels, whose activities can be modulated by the neurotransmitters muscarine (M current) and serotonin (S current), respectively. The M-current channel consists of KCNQ potassium channel subunits, mutations in which have been implicated in certain epilepsies as illustrated in Figure 7–12. We will describe in subsequent chapters the ways in which these currents contribute to important physiological phenomena. Among the fundamental questions that remain to be answered is why neuronal membranes require so many distinct conductance pathways for a single ion, potassium, and how these distinct pathways evolved as organisms required an increasing diversity and flexibility in the types of firing patterns that their neurons generate.

Auxiliary Subunits of Potassium Channels

As we have mentioned previously, it was evident from early protein purification experiments that sodium and calcium channel pore-forming α subunits copurify with a variety of auxiliary subunits, which are not essential for but often modulate channel function. Potassium channel purification, by contrast, has traditionally been extremely difficult because of the dearth of tissue sources containing sufficient potassium channel pro-

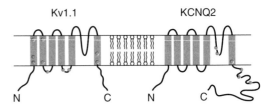

Figure 7–12. Mutations in potassium channels can cause epilepsy. The sites of naturally occurring mutations in the Kv1.1 and KCNQ2 channels that are responsible for certain cases of inherited epilepsy, are marked in blue.

tein—hence the need to clone Shaker by a positional cloning approach, which provides no information about associated subunits. It is now apparent, however, that association with auxiliary subunits is another characteristic that potassium channel α subunits share with the other voltage-dependent ion channels. Indeed, there is a long and growing list of potassium channel-associated proteins (Table 7–2) that influence channel properties in a variety of ways.

Auxiliary subunits modulate potassium channel function. The first potassium channel auxiliary subunit to be identified, Kvβ1, can confer rapid ball-and-chain type inactivation on a non-inactivating α subunit of a voltage-dependent potassium channel (Fig. 7–13) by providing the amino-terminal inactivation domain that this particular α subunit lacks. Roderick MacKinnon and colleagues have solved the three-dimensional structure of a Kvβ subunit, in association with a portion of the α subunit. The structure has several interesting features (Fig. 7–14 and Plate 5), including the surprising finding that the inactivation domain must find its way through a somewhat restricted lateral opening in the α subunit in order to gain access to and block the pore. As was already known from the Kvβ amino acid sequence and was confirmed by MacKinnon's structural studies, this β subunit is an oxidoreductase enzyme whose precise function is not understood. We shall see in Chapter 13 that other enzymes, most notably protein kinases and phosphatases that can participate in the modulation of channel function, also associate intimately with many ion channels.

The calcium-dependent potassium channels have their own complement of auxiliary subunits (Table 7–2) that differ in both structure and function from those associated with the voltage-dependent potassium channel family. As in the case of the calcium channels, the number of combinatorial possibilities and consequent functional heterogeneity afforded by

Table 7–2 Selected Examples of Auxiliary Subunits Associated with α Subunits of Potassium Channels

α Subunit	Auxiliary Subunit	Physiological Function
Kv family members	Kvβ1–Kvβn	Confer inactivation, influence membrane targeting
	Caspr2	Membrane targeting
Slowpoke family members	$K_{Ca}\beta$1–$K_{Ca}\beta$n	Modulate voltage and calcium dependence
	Slob, Slip	Modulate voltage and calcium dependence, influence membrane targeting

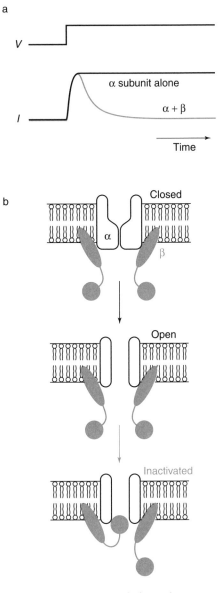

Figure 7–13. Potassium channel β subunits can contribute to rapid channel inactivation. *a*: A potassium channel α subunit that lacks a ball and chain (Fig. 5–11) does not inactivate when expressed alone (*black*), but does when it is co-expressed with β subunit (*blue*). I, current; V, voltage. *b*: The β subunit provides the ball and chain structure that confers inactivation (compare with Fig. 5–11). See Rettig et al., 1994.

multiple α-subunit genes, alternative splicing, and associated proteins is simply enormous.

Auxiliary subunits influence channel cell surface expression and membrane localization. Not all potassium channel auxiliary subunits modulate channel function directly. Instead, they may act as molecular chaperones to increase the insertion of active α subunits in the neuronal plasma membrane (a similar role has been demonstrated for some calcium channel β subunits), thereby increasing the whole-cell potassium current.

It has been known for many years that ion channels are not evenly distributed in the neuronal plasma membrane. For example, sodium channels are present at relatively low density in neuronal cell bodies, but at much higher density in the axon hillock, which as a result is often the site of action potential generation. How does this differential distribution of ion channels come about? It appears that many channels are targeted via their association with auxiliary subunits, which in turn may interact with local cytoskeletal elements. A particularly striking example of this is in myelinated axons. Recall from Chapter 3 that sodium channels are present at high density at the nodes of Ranvier and are sparse in the internodal region; potassium channels, in contrast, are concentrated adjacent to the nodes in the juxtaparanodal region. This channel distribution, which can be visualized with channel-specific antibodies coupled to fluorescent markers (see Fig. 3–10 and Plate 4), is what allows rapid saltatory con-

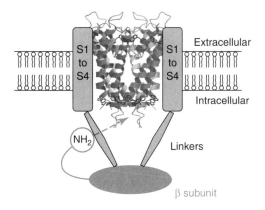

Figure 7–14. Structure of a potassium channel α–β complex. Rod MacKinnon and colleagues solved the crystal structure of a β subunit (*blue*) together with a portion of an α subunit (*gray*). Among the interesting features revealed by the structure is the path through a linker region that the β subunit ball must take to reach the pore of the channel. The pore region is based on the KcsA channel structure (Fig. 5–13), but the actual structure of S1–S4 is not yet known. (Based on Gulbis et al., 2000.) See also Plate 5.

duction of action potentials in myelinated axons. A protein called *Caspr2* colocalizes with the potassium channels, but not at all with the sodium channels. Biochemical experiments demonstrate that Caspr2 binds via an adaptor protein to the potassium channel α subunit, suggesting that it might act as an auxiliary subunit that targets the channel to the juxtaparanodal region of the membrane. The signals that tell Caspr2 itself to concentrate in this region and the mechanisms by which the sodium channels are targeted to the nodes remain to be determined.

Diseases Associated With Ion Channel Dysfunction

With the detailed molecular and functional characterization of ion channels has come the realization that ion channel dysfunction is often associated with serious disorders (*channelopathies*) in many cell types, including neurons. Such dysfunction may result from mutations in either the pore-forming α subunits or the modulatory auxiliary subunits of voltage-dependent ion channels. One form of human epilepsy, for example, is caused by a mutation in a sodium channel β subunit that normally speeds up channel inactivation (see Fig. 5–5). When this β subunit is defective, channel inactivation is slowed, sodium current is increased, and the neuronal membrane is thereby rendered hyperexcitable. Another way to generate hyperexcitability and epilepsy is by disrupting the function of potassium channels (recall that the phenotype of the *Shaker* mutant fly is hyperexcitability). Certain types of seizures in humans are associated with one of several mutations in different portions of the Kv1.1 or KCNQ2 potassium channel α subunits (Fig. 7–12). KCNQ2 associates with the closely related KCNQ3 α subunit to form heterotetrameric potassium channels responsible for the ubiquitous M current, which we have referred to briefly above and will discuss further in the context of channel modulation in Chapter 13. In view of the remarkable channel heterogeneity that we have stressed throughout this chapter, it is striking that a mutation in a single channel subtype can have such profound consequences for neuronal excitability. This strongly suggests that there is little functional redundancy among the multiple subtypes, and that each must play a unique and essential role in the physiology of the neuron.

Summary

Voltage clamp and patch clamp techniques have been used to reveal heterogeneity of ion currents carried through voltage-dependent sodium, calcium, and potassium channels. Advances in channel molecular biology have made it clear that the diversity of ion channels is even greater than was suspected from these electrophysiological measurements. This diversity is achieved by several different mechanisms, including the existence of multiple genes for the pore-forming α subunits of ion channels, alternative splicing of the messenger RNA transcribed from each individual gene, formation of heterotetramers containing different α subunits of potassium channels, and modulation of channel properties by auxiliary subunits that may themselves comprise a large and diverse family of proteins. The importance of this diversity for neuronal physiology is emphasized by the emerging evidence that many human diseases are associated with dysfunction of individual classes of ion channels in neurons.

III

INTERCELLULAR COMMUNICATION

The previous section of this book described the membrane specializations that permit the transfer of information from one part of a neuron to another. The next seven chapters address another fundamental aspect of nervous system function, *intercellular signaling*. This includes the mechanisms that neurons use to communicate with one another and with the outside world. Chapter 8 compares two fundamentally different modes of interneuronal communication. The first is the direct transfer of ions and small molecules from one neuron to another via *electrical synapses (gap junctions)*. The second involves the release or secretion from one cell of some chemical, a *neurohormone* or *neurotransmitter*, that diffuses to and affects the activity of a target cell. Often the membranes of the secreting and target cells are immediately adjacent to one another at the highly specialized structure known as the *chemical synapse*. As described in Chapter 9, mechanisms of release of neurotransmitters at chemical synapses are best understood from the study of two highly specialized synapses, the *nerve-muscle synapse* in vertebrates and the *giant synapse* in the stellate ganglion of the squid. The various classes of neurotransmitters and neurohormones that have been found in nervous systems and details of their synthesis and metabolism are presented in Chapter 10. The following two chapters describe the neurotransmitter and neurohormone *receptors*, which are specialized membrane proteins that recognize and bind signaling molecules and *transduce* the extracellular chemical signal into an electrical response in the target cell. Two distinct classes of transduction mechanism are considered. Chapter 11 discusses receptors in which the binding site is part of the same molecule or macromolecular complex as the ion channel whose activity is regulated by the neurotransmitter—the *directly coupled* receptor/ion channel systems. These are contrasted in Chapter 12 with the *indirectly coupled* systems, in which the occupation of the receptor by neurotransmitter sets in motion a chain of biochemical events. These events lead ultimately to a change in the activity of an ion channel that is not intimately associated with the receptor. Chapter 13 addresses the concept of *neuromodulation*, the long-term alteration of neuronal electrical properties as a result of neurotransmitter or neurohormone action, and the intracellular biochemical mechanisms that are responsible for these alterations. Finally, Chapter 14 describes neurons that act as *sensory receptors* by converting information from the outside world into electrical signals that can be passed on to other neurons in the brain. Sensory receptor neurons use the mechanisms discussed in Chapters 11 through 13 to convert sensory information into a change in the properties of membrane ion channels.

8

How Neurons Communicate: Gap Junctions and Neurosecretion

Within any organism, cells must be able to communicate. This is of course important in tissues other than the brain, but is essential for proper nervous system function. There are three general ways in which cells talk to each other:

1. Direct transfer of molecules and ions from the cytoplasm of one cell into that of another. As we mentioned in Chapter 1, this is mediated by *gap junctions*.
2. The release of a chemical that diffuses to, and acts on, another cell. This release process is termed *secretion*.
3. Direct physical contact. A cell can be influenced profoundly by events triggered when molecules in its plasma membrane interact with the membranes of adjacent cells.

This chapter will deal with the first two of these modes of communication, modes that neurons use on a day-to-day basis to generate specific behaviors. The third pattern of communication plays a very important role in the development of neurons and their connections, and we shall discuss it in more detail in Chapters 15 through 18.

Gap Junctions, Connexins, and Electrical Synapses

Intercellular communication through gap junctions is conceptually the very simplest form of cell-to-cell interaction. Small molecules and ions in one cell diffuse through pores in the plasma membrane directly into the cyto-

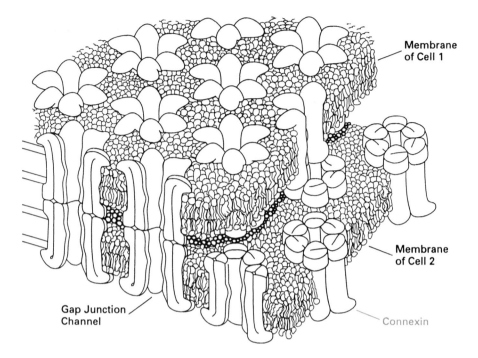

Membrane
of Cell 1

Membrane
of Cell 2

Gap Junction
Channel

Connexin

Figure 8–1. Gap junctions. Pores spanning two cell membranes are made of connexin proteins. This picture evolved from the X-ray diffraction work of Makowski et al. (1977).

plasm of a neighboring cell (Fig. 8–1). These pores can be visualized in the electron microscope and are found in clusters that sometimes have a crystalline appearance. Such an array was captured in the electron micrograph of Figure 8–2 by the technique of *freeze fracture*. In the preparation of tissues for freeze fracture, plasma membrane that has been frozen is allowed to break within the plane of the membrane itself. The exposed halves of the lipid bilayers are then coated with platinum and carbon to produce a form of bas-relief view of the inner plane of the membrane. These methods permit ready visualization of intramembranous particles, which represent integral membrane proteins such as receptors and ion channels. Figure 8-2 shows flattened sheets of membranes with arrays of

Figure 8–2. Freeze fracture replica of gap junction particles. *a*: Electron micrograph showing a bundle of processes of *Aplysia* neurons connected by gap junctions. *b*: Magnification of a single array of gap junction particles. Some of the arrays, marked with arrows in *a*, are shown in the drawing (*c*). (From Kaczmarek et al., 1979.)

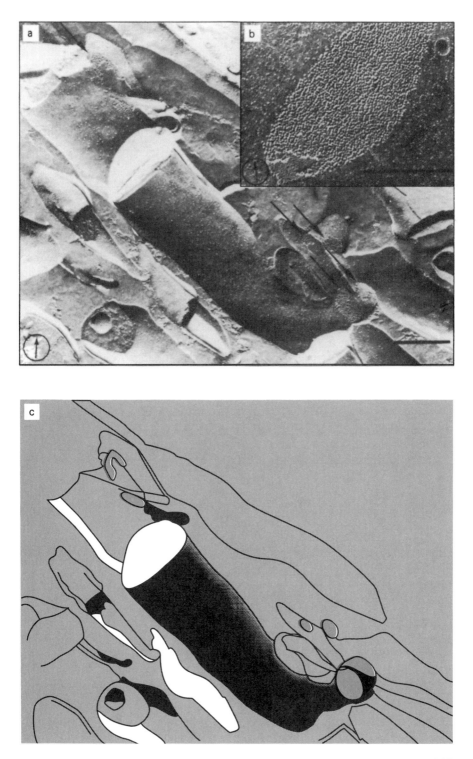

167

gap junction particles. These particles contain the proteins that form the cell-to-cell pore.

Gap junctions are abundant in tissues such as the liver and the lens, which have been used as sources for the purification of gap junction proteins. These proteins have been termed *connexins*. A pore is believed to be formed by a complex of six connexin proteins in the membrane. To link the pore to the cytoplasm of an adjacent cell, the connexins bind to another hexameric complex of connexins in that cell (Fig. 8–1). In liver, the major connexin protein has a molecular weight of 27,000. In other tissues, connexin proteins with different molecular weights may be found. This diversity may reflect the fact that the properties of gap junctions, and the way these properties are altered by neurotransmitters or hormones (see Chapter 19), vary in different cells.

Surprisingly, the electrical properties of gap junctions appear similar in many respects to those of the ion channels we have encountered in previous chapters. Despite the fact that gap junctions allow the passage of relatively large molecules, with molecular weights up to about 1000, recordings of the opening and closing of gap junctions resemble the gating of channels that allow specific ions to cross the plasma membrane. This can be measured by whole-cell patch clamp of a pair of cells that are coupled by only a small number of gap junctions (Fig. 8–3). When the membrane potential of one cell is maintained more negative than that of its partner, current flows across the pore only while the cell-to-cell channel is open. The conductance of the open channel, for example, in pairs of heart cells, is about 50 pS.

Despite the ubiquity of gap junctions, their biological role in most tissues is not well understood. Gap junctions are likely to function in the embryonic development of tissues, a time when many gap junctions are formed and then broken again. One of their roles may be to allow the transfer between cells of small molecules that are important for development and of second messenger molecules involved in intracellular signaling (see Chapter 12). This in turn allows a group of cells to act as one functional unit. In the nervous system and other excitable tissues, gap junctions take on a special significance. Connections between nerve cells via gap junctions are often called *electrical synapses*, in recognition of the fact that they are involved in rapid electrical signaling and information transfer. For example, they allow groups of neurons to synchronize their electrical activity. However, electrical synapses are also found between pairs of neurons that do not always fire in synchrony. In such cases, their role may be to allow synaptic inputs into one neuron to be registered in a neighboring neuron. Later in the book (see Chapter 19), we shall encounter specific examples of neurons that couple electrically through gap junctions.

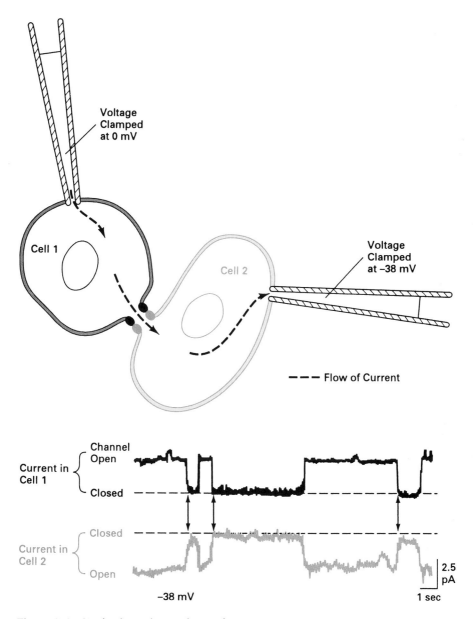

Figure 8–3. Single channel recordings of gap junctions. In an experiment carried out by Burt and Spray (1988), two cells are voltage clamped at different potentials. When the gap junction channel opens, the current that flows between the cells is recorded as outward current in cell 1 and inward current in cell 2.

169

Neurosecretion

Although gap junctions constitute a very basic and rapid form of communication, they are limited to bidirectional interactions between neighboring cells. When information has to be transferred from one cell to a distant cell, the usual mechanism is for the first cell to release a chemical into the extracellular space. This chemical then either diffuses, or is transported, to the target cell. A large number of different chemicals may act as extracellular signals. These include amino acids and other small organic compounds, lipids, small peptides, and large protein complexes. Chemicals that are released from a neuron and alter the excitability of another neuron or a muscle cell are termed *neurotransmitters*.

Figure 8–4 shows some of the mechanisms that allow molecules to leave a cell. Lipid molecules diffuse readily across a cell membrane. Once synthesized, they can leave the cell without requiring any specialized machinery (Fig. 8–4a). For certain other, more hydrophilic, molecules, carriers or pores exist in the plasma membrane to allow them to cross the membrane (Fig. 8–4b). The major pathway for the release of neurotransmitters, however, appears to be *vesicular secretion*. At the synaptic terminals of neurons, many secretory vesicles can normally be found (see Chapter 1). When a neuron is stimulated, these transmitter-containing vesicles fuse with the plasma membrane to release their contents into the synaptic cleft (Fig. 8–4c). This pathway probably evolved from the requirement of many cells to release large peptides and proteins that would not normally be able to cross the lipid membrane, and also from the need to insert proteins such as ion channels and other integral membrane proteins into the plasma membrane. Thus it is not surprising that many insights into the release of neurotransmitters have come from work with non-neuronal cells. In the remainder of this chapter we shall discuss the general mechanisms for secretion of proteins and other transmitters in neurons and exocrine cells.

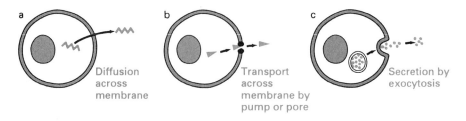

Figure 8–4. Three pathways (*a–c*) by which cells release substances into the external medium.

In the next chapter we shall consider in more detail the physiology of transmitter release at two well-studied chemical synapses.

Constitutive and Regulated Secretion of Protein

In all eukaryotic cells, proteins that are destined for release into the extracellular space are synthesized in the *rough endoplasmic reticulum* (Fig. 8–5). Newly synthesized proteins enter the *Golgi apparatus*, a tightly packed stack of intracellular membranes in which the proteins undergo a variety of post-translational modifications. The proteins are then transferred to vesicles that bud off the Golgi apparatus and move to the cell

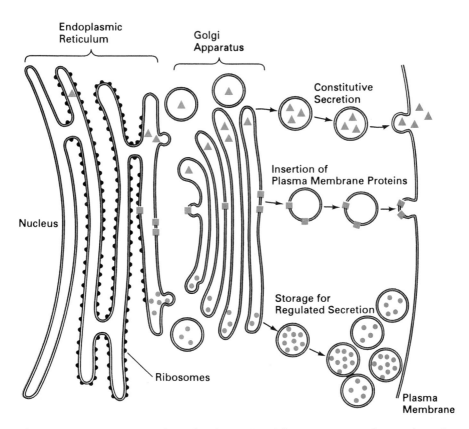

Figure 8–5. Constitutive and regulated secretion. The upper two pathways show the movement of proteins from ribosomes to the plasma membrane for constitutive release into the external medium or insertion into the plasma membrane. The lower pathway shows the buildup of protein-containing vesicles for regulated secretion.

surface. Here the vesicles release their contents into the extracellular space by fusion with the plasma membrane, a process known as *exocytosis*. In some cases, the arrival of the vesicles at the cell surface is followed immediately by exocytosis. This form of secretion has been termed *constitutive secretion*. The insertion of integral membrane proteins, including ion channels and receptor molecules, into appropriate regions of the plasma membrane also occurs by constitutive secretion (Fig. 8–5). Recall from Chapters 1 and 2 that the organelles involved in these processes are not restricted to neurons, and that the neuronal cell body has many features in common with other cells.

Neurotransmitters and hormones, in contrast, are not released immediately following their synthesis. They are packaged into vesicles, and the vesicles are transported along microtubules to the release sites, such as those at axon terminals. They are then stored at these sites until an appropriate stimulus is received by the cell. In neurons, this stimulus is usually a depolarization that causes calcium to enter the cell through voltage-dependent calcium channels. A large amount of neurotransmitter can then be released by the cell when the vesicles fuse with the plasma membrane. Such secretion, which is regulated acutely by external stimulation, has been termed *regulated secretion* (Fig. 8–5).

Even within these general classes of constitutive and regulated secretion there must be a large number of variants. For example, different proteins are inserted at different locations in the plasma membrane of a cell by constitutive pathways. In addition, neurons contain at least two kinds of secretory vesicles that participate in regulated secretion. *Large dense-core vesicles* contain primarily peptide neurotransmitters; *small synaptic vesicles* contain nonpeptide transmitters and the enzymes required for their synthesis. This diversity of intracellular traffic implies that newly synthesized proteins must somehow be assigned to the correct vesicle pathway. At least part of the information for the correct assignment may be found in the sequence of the protein itself. We shall now list some of the signals that may exist in a newly synthesized protein that determine whether part or all of the protein will be secreted, and by which secretory pathway. The focus in this section will be on peptide neurotransmitters.

Signals on Secreted Proteins

The signal sequence. The first part of a protein to be synthesized is the amino terminus. Proteins that are to enter one of the secretory pathways contain a stretch of hydrophobic amino acids at the amino terminus known as the *signal sequence* (Fig. 8–6). Although the exact signal sequence differs in different proteins, this hydrophobic stretch of amino acids is recognized by cytoplasmic factors (the *signal recognition particle*) and by components of the membrane of the rough endoplasmic reticulum. These factors then assist the protein to cross this membrane. Without crossing into the lumen of the endoplasmic reticulum, the protein could not eventually be packaged into membrane vesicles. Proteins that lack a signal sequence do not cross the membrane and thus become cytoplasmic proteins. The signal sequence is usually cleaved from the remainder of the protein by proteolytic enzymes shortly after it has crossed the membrane.

a   Vasopressin Precursor

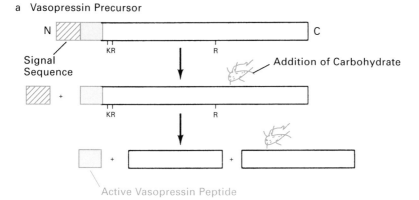

b   ELH Precursor

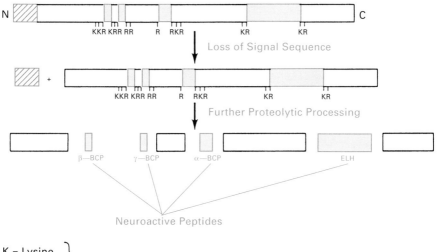

K = Lysine
R = Arginine } at cleavage sites

Figure 8–6. Processing of neuropeptide precursors. *a*: Formation of the hypothalamic peptide vasopressin. *b*: Formation of the *Aplysia* peptides α-, β-, and γ-BCP and ELH.

Sorting signals. Sorting of newly synthesized proteins must take place, so that different proteins are assigned to the appropriate vesicles and thus to the appropriate secretory pathway. In large part, this sorting appears to occur within the Golgi apparatus. The nature of the sorting signal is not understood. As we saw in Chapter 7, some proteins such as certain ion channels that are destined for specific plasma membrane compartments may be targeted there by specific auxiliary subunits (see Table 7–2). In other cases, however, the sorting signal may be intrinsic to the protein sequence itself. For example, DNA that encodes the protein precursor for insulin (proinsulin) can be introduced into a pituitary cell line that does not normally make insulin. When this is done, not only is the DNA faithfully transcribed and translated into proinsulin, but this protein is also packaged into vesicles of the regulated secretion pathway, and insulin can be secreted from the cell in response to an appropriate stimulus.

The sorting of peptide transmitters and hormones into vesicles frequently is associated with a condensation of the protein into a dense aggregate. Such aggregates presumably serve to increase the concentration of peptide in a vesicle. Because they appear electron opaque when viewed in an electron microscope, peptide-containing vesicles are frequently described as *dense-core vesicles* or granules (Fig. 8–7).

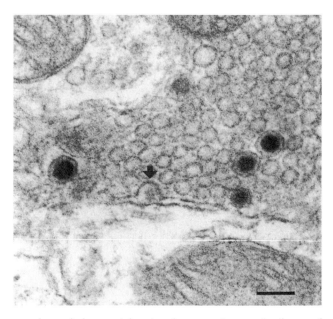

Figure 8–7. Dense-core granules and clear vesicles. An electron micrograph of part of the terminal of a rat neuron. Several larger dense-core granules coexist with smaller, clear synaptic vesicles. The arrow marks a vesicle that is undergoing exocytosis. The scale bar represents 100 μm (courtesy of Dr. Asa Thureson Klein).

Proteolytic processing. Most neuroactive peptides are not synthesized in the form in which they are eventually secreted. Instead, they are synthesized as part of a larger, inactive precursor protein, or *prohormone* (Fig. 8–6). A good example of this is the precursor of insulin, proinsulin, which we introduced above. Two others are the precursors for *vasopressin*, which is synthesized in certain neurons in the hypothalamus, and for *egg-laying hormone* (ELH), which is synthesized in *Aplysia* bag cell neurons. Proteolytic cleavage of the precursors to smaller fragments, including the active peptides, occurs in the secretory vesicles and also in the Golgi. In some cases, several different neuroactive peptides may be generated from a single precursor, for example, the production of the transmitters, α, β, and γ bag cell peptides (BCPs), together with ELH, from the ELH precursor (Fig. 8–6b). A sequence of two basic amino acids, either lysine or arginine, is frequently the site for proteolytic cleavage within the precursor (Fig. 8–6). Cleavage sites also exist, however, that are not marked by two basic amino acids.

Post-translational modifications. A newly synthesized protein and the peptide fragments generated from such a protein can be modified further by the action of enzymes in the Golgi or the secretory vesicles themselves. Table 8–1 lists the more common covalent modifications, some of which may be essential for the biological activity of a peptide. For example, one common modification is the amidation of the carboxyl terminal. This is carried out by the enzyme *peptidyl glycine (alpha)-amidating monooxygenase*, which is located within secretory granules. The enzyme acts on peptides that have a glycine residue at their carboxyl terminal by removing the glycine and amidating the penultimate amino acid residue. Figure 8-8 illustrates the amidation of the invertebrate neuropeptide FMR-Famide and of vasopressin. It has been found that the biological activity

Table 8–1 Some Covalent Modifications of Peptide Transmitters and Hormones

Modification	Possible Function	Example
Conversion of N-terminal glutamate to pyroglutamate	Increase stability to proteases	Neurotensin
Amidation of C-terminal amino acid	Increase stability to proteases	Substance P
Glycosylation (usually addition of sugar residues to asparagine)	Targeting to appropriate location?	Thyrotropin—also commonly found in integral membrane proteins
Sulfation	Unknown	Cholecystokinin

of neuropeptides such as vasopressin is very greatly reduced if the peptide is not amidated. This and other modifications may also influence the stability of the peptide once it has been released. Some post-translational modifications of newly synthesized proteins may participate in the sorting of the protein into the appropriate vesicles. A precedent for this is found in proteins of the lysosomes. Newly synthesized lysosomal proteins contain asparagine residues to which mannose phosphate groups are added.

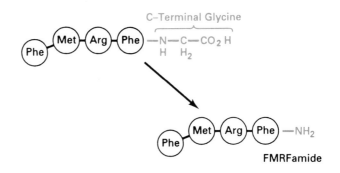

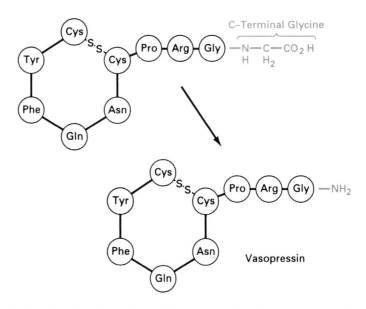

Figure 8–8. C-terminal amidation. Formation of the neuropeptides FMRFamide and vasopressin by removal of a C-terminal glycine.

These mannose phosphate groups are then recognized by receptors in the Golgi, causing these sugar-linked proteins to be targeted selectively to lysosomes.

"Classical" Neurotransmitters Use a Specialized Secretory Pathway

In contrast to peptide transmitters, small neurotransmitter molecules—including acetylcholine; the amino acid transmitters such as γ-aminobutyric acid (GABA), glycine, and glutamate; and the amines such as dopamine, norepinephrine, histamine, and serotonin—are not synthesized only at the soma (see Chapter 10). Instead it is the enzymes, which catalyze their synthesis, that are synthesized at the soma, then transported to the release sites at axon terminals. Depletion of neurotransmitter by electrical activity can therefore be followed by rapid resynthesis within the terminal. These small neurotransmitters are frequently termed *classical* neurotransmitters, because their function in neurons was recognized well before that of the neuropeptides.

Vesicles that contain these classical neurotransmitters are small and very homogeneous in size (typically 50 nm in diameter). These small synaptic vesicles are associated with the very rapid release of transmitter that occurs at specialized synaptic junctions (see Chapter 9). Because they do not generally contain a dense aggregate of neuropeptides, they are not electron dense and therefore appear as clear vesicles in electron micrographs (Fig. 8–7). Unlike the peptide-containing granules, which are formed at the soma and then transported to the synaptic endings, small synaptic vesicles are assembled within the nerve ending. The individual proteins in the membranes of small synaptic vesicles are first synthesized at the soma and then transported along axons to the terminals by the constitutive secretion pathway (see Fig. 8–5). On their arrival at nerve endings they are inserted into the plasma membrane and are then retrieved by endocytosis to form functional small synaptic vesicles (Fig. 8–9).

Both large dense-core vesicles and small synaptic vesicles release their neurotransmitter contents by exocytosis, resulting in the incorporation of vesicle membrane proteins into the plasma membrane. There is a fundamental difference, however, between these two types of vesicles. A dense-core vesicle is a "one-shot" apparatus; it can release its peptide neurotransmitter only once, after which the membrane proteins of the vesicle must be degraded or returned to the soma where new dense-core vesicles filled with peptide neurotransmitters are formed. In contrast, small synaptic vesicles can be recycled many times at the terminal, by repeated exocytosis followed by retrieval of vesicle proteins and refilling with neuro-transmitter.

Exocytosis of Neurotransmitter-Containing Vesicles

There is abundant evidence that regulated secretion in many non-neural cells occurs through exocytosis. For example, in a chromaffin cell of the adrenal medulla, stimulation by a transmitter causes the secretory gran-ules to fuse with the plasma membrane, releasing their contents to the ex-tracellular space. The vesicle membrane that has been added to the plasma membrane is then rapidly resorbed by endocytosis. In many such cells, the process of exocytosis can be observed by light microscopy of living cells.

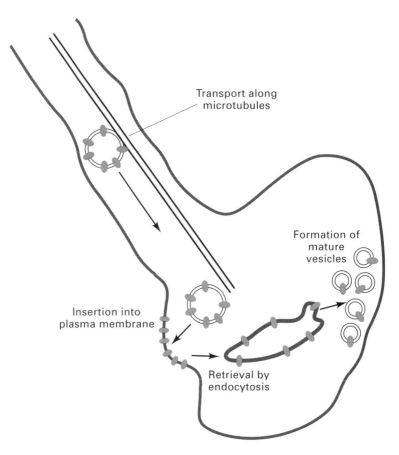

Transport along microtubules

Formation of mature vesicles

Insertion into plasma membrane

Retrieval by endocytosis

Figure 8–9. Formation of small synaptic vesicles. Vesicle proteins are transported down the axon to the terminals where they are inserted into the plasma membrane before being retrieved by endocytosis and then packaged into mature synaptic vesicles.

Release of neurotransmitter from small synaptic vesicles at synaptic junctions also occurs through exocytosis of transmitter-containing vesicles, but visualization of this process has been harder to achieve, largely because of the technical difficulties of working with small synaptic terminals. A fluorescent dye termed *FM1-43*, however, has proven to be a particularly useful tool for this (Fig. 8–10). This dye is not fluorescent in solution but becomes so when it binds to cellular membranes, which it is able to do very rapidly and reversibly. Thus, when a synaptic terminal is exposed to FM1-43, the external membrane becomes fluorescent. If the neuron is stimulated at this time, the membrane of small synaptic vesicles is temporarily added to the plasma membrane, where it encounters the FM1-43. When these vesicular membranes are taken up again by endocytosis, the synaptic vesicles within the terminal become fluorescent. If the external FM1-43 is then removed, the plasma membrane loses its fluorescence, but the internal synaptic vesicles remain labeled. Subsequent

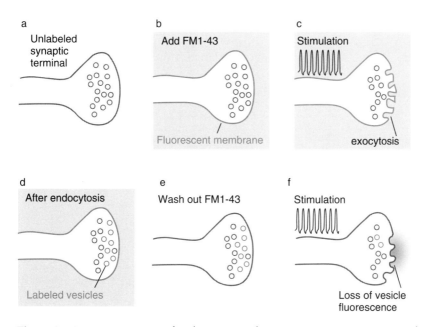

Figure 8–10. Measurements of endocytosis and exocytosis in synaptic terminals using FM1-43. The plasma membrane of a synaptic terminal (*a*) becomes fluorescent upon exposure to the dye (*b*). Stimulation (*c*) produces exocytosis and exposes the membrane of synaptic vesicles to the external FM1-43. Endocytosis of the synaptic vesicle membranes (*d*) causes them to become fluorescent, and they remain so after washout of the external dye (*e*). The exocytosis of these labeled vesicles can then be detected by subsequent stimulation in a dye-free solution (*f*).

stimulation of the terminal in an FM1-43-free solution allows one to measure the exocytosis of individual synaptic vesicles as a loss of the fluorescence of internal vesicles (Fig. 8–10). Further evidence for exocytosis at synaptic junctions is also presented in the next chapter.

Stages of transmitter release. As described above, exocytosis is the process of fusing one membrane, the vesicle membrane, to a second membrane, the plasma membrane. Such fusion of membranes is a very general biological process; it is required for the movement of vesicles from the endoplasmic reticulum to the Golgi apparatus, for example (see Fig. 8–5). Exocytosis is a special case of such fusion in which the acceptor membrane is the plasma membrane. In the case of neurotransmitter release, three distinct stages have been distinguished (Fig. 8–11).

Docking. Before the contents of a synaptic vesicle can be released, the membrane of the vesicle must first become tightly associated with the plasma membrane, a process termed *docking*. Before they are docked, vesicles are sometimes said to be in a *reserve pool*.

Priming. Simple association with the plasma membrane is not enough to ensure fusion. A priming reaction converts the vesicle to a form that can fuse when an action potential invades the terminal. The collection of primed vesicles at a presynaptic ending is frequently referred to as the *readily releasable* pool of vesicles.

Fusion. The active fusion of the vesicle membrane with that of the plasma membrane occurs when the calcium concentration is locally elevated to a high level by the opening of plasma membrane calcium channels during an action potential.

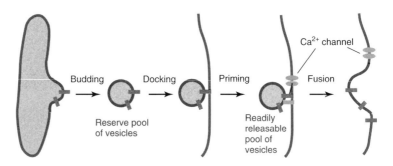

Figure 8–11. Steps in the movement of synaptic vesicles from internal membranes to fusion with the plasma membrane.

The fusion of synaptic vesicles is followed by retrieval of the vesicular membrane by endocytosis and its recycling to form a new vesicle that has been refilled with transmitter. We shall consider this recycling process later in this chapter.

Exocytosis and the SNARE Complex

Many discoveries are now being made through the study of the proteins that are in, or attached to, the membrane of synaptic vesicles. Relatively pure synaptic vesicles from the nervous system may be prepared by subcellular fractionation. In this technique nervous tissue is homogenized in a medium that allows subcellular organelles, such as mitochondria and synaptic vesicles, to remain intact. Because different organelles have different sizes, they can then be separated by centrifugation through layers of sucrose of different densities. In this way it is possible to obtain relatively pure preparations of vesicles from neuronal as well as other secretory tissues.

The availability of pure vesicles has enabled some of the key molecules in the process of exocytosis to be identified and the relationships between these molecules to be unraveled. Table 8–2 lists several of the proteins that are associated with secretory vesicles. Some of these will be discussed below, others will be covered in later chapters, while still others are listed for completeness. It should be pointed out that the small synaptic vesicles, which appear clear in electron micrographs (Fig. 8–7) and contain small neurotransmitter molecules such as acetylcholine, glutamic acid, GABA, or glycine, have a somewhat different protein composition than that of the slightly larger dense-core vesicles that are predominantly peptide containing. In particular, one set of proteins appears to be specific to the small vesicles.

Most of the biochemical interactions that comprise docking, priming, and fusion are not fully understood. Nevertheless, three molecules that are central to the exocytosis of synaptic vesicles are *synaptobrevin, syntaxin,* and *SNAP-25.* Of these, only synaptobrevin is a synaptic vesicle protein. It has a very asymmetric distribution across the membrane of the vesicle. Only a few amino acids, at the carboxyl-terminal end of the protein, are found inside the vesicle, and most of the mass of the protein is in the cytoplasm. Syntaxin has a very similar structure, but it is located in the plasma membrane of the synapse, with its bulk also in the cytoplasm. In contrast, SNAP-25 (named for **Sy**Naptosomal **A**ssociated **P**rotein of size 25 kDa) is not a true integral membrane protein but is firmly achored to the plasma membrane by palmityl chains. These palmityl groups are lipid chains that are attached at one end to the protein at a cluster of cysteine residues and insert firmly into the lipid environment of the plasma membrane. These three proteins together form a complex that links the synaptic vesicle to the plasma membrane and whose structure has been determined by X-ray crystallography (Plate 6). This structure is sometimes called the *fusion* or *SNARE complex*.

Table 8–2 Some Widely Studied Synaptic Proteins

Protein	Suggested Role in Secretion
Vesicle proteins	
Synaptobrevin	SNARE protein
Synaptotagmin	Calcium sensor
Synaptophysin	Genesis of vesicles—binding cholesterol, binding synaptobrevin
SV2	A protein with 12 membrane-spanning regions—homologous to transporters
Proton pump	See text
Neurotransmitter transporters	Uptake of transmitter into vesicle
Chloride channels	Not certain
Snapin	Regulates SNARE formation?
Proteins that associate with vesicles	
rab 3A, 3B, 3B, 3D	GTP-binding proteins—docking?
rabphilin	Binding to rab 3A
Synapsin I, II	Mobilization of reserve vesicles—see Chapter 9
α-, β-, and γ-SNAP	Dissolution of SNARE complex
NSF	Dissolution of SNARE complex
Cysteine-string protein	Ensures proper folding of other synaptic vesicle proteins?
Ca2$^+$/Cam kinase II	See Chapter 9
Plasma membrane proteins	
Syntaxin 1A, 1B	SNARE protein
SNAP-25	SNARE protein
Rim	Binding to rab 3A
Syntaphilin	Binds to SNAP-25—regulates SNARE formation?
Interacting cytoplasmic proteins	
Munc-18	Binds syntaxin when not in SNARE complex
Munc-13	Binds syntaxin and other synaptic proteins—activated by diacylglycerol (see Chapter 12); required for priming
Complexin	Binds SNARE complex
Tomosyn	Binds syntaxin

Prior to docking, the SNARE complex is not assembled. Instead, each of the components of the complex is bound to other proteins (Fig. 8–12a). For example, the synaptic vesicle SNARE protein synaptobrevin may be bound to other synaptic vesicle proteins such as *synaptophysin*, which is one of the most abundant proteins in the membrane of synaptic vesicles. Each synaptophysin protein spans the vesicle membrane four times and forms a homo-oligomer complex with other synaptophysin molecules. Synaptophysin binds the lipid cholesterol and may function to organize the membranes of synaptic vesicles into stable spherical organelles. Similarly, the plasma membrane SNARE proteins can have alternative partners when their vesicular mates are not around. Within nerve endings, munc-18 is a soluble protein that, like synaptophysin, is not part of the fusion complex but is able to bind syntaxin, and this binding reaction appears to prevent syntaxin from entering into a complex with its SNARE partners. Thus munc-18 may serve to regulate the formation of fusion complexes.

After docking brings the synaptic and vesicular membranes into close proximity, the SNARE components leave their alternative partners and form the fusion complex. This complex consists of four long bundles of helical regions of the three proteins (Plate 6). Even though this complex forms a close association between the vesicle and plasma membrane, its formation does not constitute either docking or priming. Instead, it appears to function in the fusion event itself, promoting the fusion of the

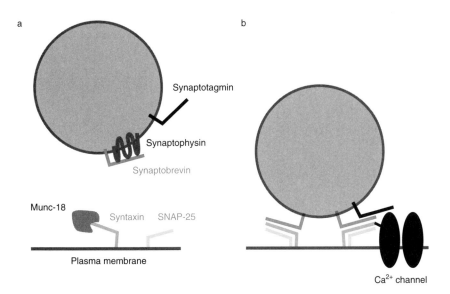

Figure 8–12. Some of the interactions of synaptic vesicle and plasma membrane proteins before (*a*) and after (*b*) formation of the SNARE complex.

two types of membrane. Indeed, the syntaxin molecule within the complex binds calcium channels directly (Fig. 8–12b) and is therefore at the site of greatest calcium elevation during an action potential. The SNARE complex itself, however, is not sensitive to calcium. The prime suspect for the calcium-sensor of neurotransmitter release is a synaptic vesicle protein termed *synaptotagmin* (Fig 8–12a). Two regions in the cytoplasmic part of the molecule, called *C2 domains*, closely resemble regions in other proteins that are known to bind both calcium and phospholipids. In fact, synaptotagmin binds to lipid membranes only when calcium levels are raised to the level that occurs in the synaptic terminal during vesicular release. Thus, synaptotagmin, which normally exists as a multimer of two or more synaptotagmin molecules bound together, has the properties expected for a protein that controls calcium-dependent fusion, most likely by regulating the SNARE complex.

Toxins have identified the SNARE proteins involved in exocytosis. As we have seen and shall see repeatedly in this book, important insights into the mechanisms of neuronal function have been gained through the use of toxins that poison the nervous system. In the case of neurotransmitter release, evidence that synaptobrevin and SNAP-25 are essential for exocytosis was obtained in studies using three deadly bacterial neurotoxins: tetanus toxin and botulinum toxins A and B. Poisoning by these agents, known as *clostridial neurotoxins*, after the bacteria that make them, causes paralysis by blocking neurotransmitter release. Tetanus toxin produces spastic paralysis, a characteristic rigidity of the body, by preventing transmitter release in the central nervous system, whereas botulinum B toxin causes flaccid paralysis by preventing acetylcholine release at the neuromuscular junction. The clostridial neurotoxins are produced by the bacteria as single proteins that are then cleaved into two different subunits, known as the *light chain* and the *heavy chain*. These subunits have different functions and are held together by disulphide bonds (Fig. 8–13a). The heavy chain binds to the external membrane of the neuron and facilitates the entry of the light chain into the cytoplasm of synaptic terminals. Thus the different heavy chains in tetanus toxin and the botulinum toxins determine which particular neurons they will affect.

It is the light chains of the toxins, which bind zinc ions, that actually do the damage. Once these light chains are released from the heavy chains and enter the cytoplasm, they act as proteases that rapidly destroy selected proteins within the synaptic endings. For example, botulinum toxin B and tetanus toxin destroy only synaptobrevin, whereas botulinum toxin A selectively cleaves SNAP-25 (Fig. 8–13b). Another toxin, botulinum toxin C1, destroys syntaxin. Because each of these toxins is very specific in its action, and all of them impair neurotransmitter release, they have provided direct evidence that synaptobrevin, syntaxin, and SNAP-25 are critical components of the exocytotic machinery.

Certain other toxins also regulate transmitter release. For example, α-laterotoxin, a component of the venom of the black widow spider, produces massive exocytosis of small synaptic vesicles. α-laterotoxin binds a protein termed *neurexin* in the plasma membrane of the presynaptic terminal. Neurexins are receptors that normally bind postsynaptic proteins termed *neuroligins*, forming a bridge across the synaptic gap, and may participate in the development of synapses (see Chapter 18). It appears, however, that the toxin uses neurexin only as a convenient binding site, and its mechanism of action on the exocytotic machinery is not yet known.

The SNARE complex is disassembled by NSF. The interaction between synaptobrevin, syntaxin, and SNAP-25 is a very tight one. For transmitter release to proceed normally, the SNARE complex must also become disassembled. This may occur at some point after exocytosis when the synaptic vesicle membrane is recovered and recycled. Some studies have suggested, however, that such ungluing occurs in the preparation of vesicles for release, perhaps during the priming step.

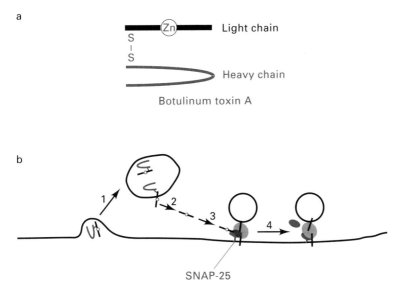

Figure 8–13. Blockage of neurotransmission by clostridial neurotoxins. *a*: Structure of botulinum toxin A. *b*: Uptake of botulinum toxin A into the nerve terminal, followed by release of the light chain and proteolysis of SNAP-25.

Another set of proteins is responsible for this ungluing process (Fig. 8–14). These include a homotrimeric protein, made up of three 76 kDa subunits, termed *NSF* (named for one of its chemical properties, N-ethylmaleiimide Sensitive Factor), and Soluble NSF Accessory Proteins (SNAP). By a true perversity of scientific nomenclature, these SNAPs are entirely unrelated to SNAP-25. Three different SNAPs, α-, β-, and γ-SNAP, are known to exist and a functional ungluing complex requires the presence of γ-SNAP together with either α- or β-SNAP. Indeed, the SNARE proteins were first named for their association with these proteins (**SNAP-REceptors**). Electron microscopic and structural studies have shown that the SNAPs wrap around the elongated SNARE complex and that several NSF molecules assemble at one end of this complex. The conformation of the NSF complex is altered by ATP, and this change in shape may serve to unravel the SNARE complex (Fig. 8–14).

GTP-binding proteins regulate transmitter release. A set of proteins that bind GTP are known to regulate the budding and fusion process that controls the traffic of all membranous vesicles through cells (Fig. 8–15). These GTP-binding proteins are termed *rab* proteins (see Table 8–2), and different members of this family associate with different membranes such as those of the Golgi apparatus or the endoplasmic reticulum. The synaptic vesicle member of this protein family, which is termed *rab3*, binds to proteins in

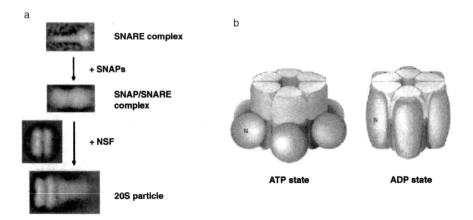

a

SNARE complex

+ SNAPs

SNAP/SNARE complex

+ NSF

20S particle

b

ATP state   ADP state

Figure 8–14. Ungluing the SNARE complex by NSF and the SNAPs. *a*: Electron microscopic images of the SNARE complex and its interactions with SNAPs and NSF to form a large complex termed the *20S particle* (Hohl et al., 1998). *b*: Diagram of the change in the structure of the NSF complex produced by ATP (Hanson et al., 1997). This change may cause the unraveling of the interactions between the plasma membrane and vesicular SNARE proteins.

the fusion complex and is thought to catalyze the formation of this complex at the appropriate sites at the plasma membrane.

The rab3 protein leads a dual life (Fig. 8–15). Much of the time it is anchored to the membrane of synaptic vesicles through a lipid chain, termed a *geranylgeranyl* group, which is attached to the rab3 protein at specific cysteine residues in a manner similar to the attachment of palmityl groups to the SNAP-25 molecule. This attachment to the membrane only occurs when the protein is bound to GTP. When vesicle fusion occurs, the bound GTP is hydrolyzed to GDP and rab3 dissociates from the vesicle membrane to begin its second life as a soluble protein in the cytoplasm of the nerve ending. To become solubilized, the GDP-bound form of rab3 binds a soluble protein termed *GDI* (for **GDP-Dissociation Inhibitor**). The GDP on the rab3 protein is subsequently exchanged for GTP in the cytoplasm, allowing rab3 with its lipid modification again to bind vesicles that have not yet docked at the plasma membrane. Thus each cycle of budding and fusion at the synaptic terminals is associated with one cycle of GTP hydrolysis (Fig. 8–15).

Rab3 is known to bind *rabphilin*, a protein that resembles synaptotagmin in that it contains two C2 domains. Unlike synaptotagmin, however, rabphilin is not a membrane-spanning protein but becomes anchored to the vesicle membrane solely through binding rab3. During the fusion cycle, rab3 probably also interacts with *Rim*, a protein associated with the plasma membrane. Although its exact function in neurotransmitter secretion is not known, it appears to be an important component of the release process and may be required for docking of synaptic vesicles at the plasma

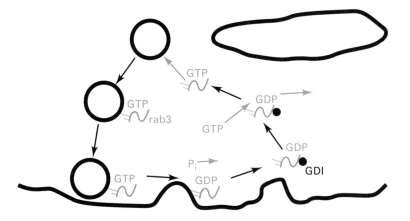

Figure 8–15. Cycle of GTP-dependent association and dissociation of rab3 from synaptic membranes.

membrane. The consequences of manipulating rab3 at the synapse will be considered again in the next chapter.

Recycling of Small Synaptic Vesicles

Once a vesicle has released its contents by fusing with the plasma membrane, the membrane of the vesicle, together with the synaptic vesicle proteins that have entered the plasma membrane, must be retrieved. This process occurs for both the small synaptic vesicles containing classical neurotransmitters and for the larger neuropeptide-containing dense-core granules. In the case of small synaptic vesicles, the retrieved membrane can be recycled to form new small vesicles filled with neurotransmitter. In contrast, the membrane proteins of the neuropeptide-containing granules must be destroyed or returned to the soma.

The recovery of small synaptic vesicles from the plasma membrane involves several new rounds of budding and fusion and introduces a new set of protein components (Fig. 8–16). A major pathway for recovery involves coating the membrane to be removed in a layer of protein termed *clathrin*. The structure of this coat resembles a cage made of chicken wire. Each link in the cage is a "three-legged" protein complex consisting of

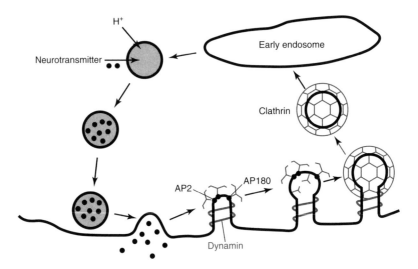

Figure 8–16. Recycling of synaptic vesicle membranes. After exocytosis, membranes are retrieved by the motor protein dynamin and are coated with clathrin. The membranes are then transported to the early endosome and reformed into new vesicles, which are refilled with neurotransmitter.

three heavy chains and three light chains of the clathrin molecule. The first step in this process is the binding of an adaptor protein, AP2, to the membrane that is to undergo endocytosis. AP2 binds directly to synaptotagmin, and this binding may target endocytosis selectively to membrane that contains recently fused vesicular components. A second adaptor protein, AP180, which, like AP2, binds clathrin also contributes to endocytosis in neurons.

Another protein that is required for the budding of the vesicle membrane from the plasma membrane is *dynamin*. Like kinesin and related proteins that we considered in Chapter 2, dynamin is a motor protein and is capable of generating movement in the presence of GTP. This force-generating protein, however, does not belong to the same protein family as the kinesins. As membrane that contains the synaptic vesicle proteins begins to bud off from the plasma membrane, dynamin forms a collar of protein around the neck of the newly budding vesicle (Fig. 8–16). This collar presumably allows the bud to pinch off from the remainder of the membrane. In cells that have defective dynamin proteins, vesicle proteins fail to be retrieved from the plasma membrane. An example of this occurs in the *Drosophila* strain *shibire*. These flies are defective in that their dynamin proteins fail to function at elevated temperatures, so that raising the temperature produces rapid and reversible paralysis because synaptic vesicles cannot be recycled.

The formation of the clathrin coat and the removal of the underlying membrane involves close interactions of the exocytosis proteins with the lipids of the membrane. Two other proteins, *synaptojanin* and *endophilin*, are enzymes that act on phospholipids in the budding vesicles and are important regulators of these interactions. Finally, *amphiphysin*, a protein that binds to dynamin, may aid in the organization of lipids into the tube-like structures that form during budding.

After the coated vesicle buds off the plasma membrane it moves to another membranous structure known as the *early endosome* (Fig. 18–16). This is the structure from which new synaptic vesicles are formed. After fusion of the coated vesicles with the early endosome, the retrieved synaptic vesicle proteins are ready to be reorganized into new small synaptic vesicles. To form mature synaptic vesicles, the vesicles that bud from the early endosomes must be replenished with neurotransmitter. Before this happens the interior of the vesicle is first acidified by the activity of a proton pump. Such a proton pump uses ATP in the cytoplasm to pump protons across the membrane into the lumen of the vesicle. The acidic environment produced by this pump is essential, in that it drives the uptake and storage of neurotransmitter by specific transport proteins present in the membrane of the vesicles.

Detection of Exocytosis and Endocytosis by
Capacitance Measurements

There are still many unanswered questions about the dynamics of exocytosis and endocytosis, even in those non-neuronal cells in which the process can be visualized readily in the microscope. For example, must the membrane of a vesicle undergo complete fusion into the plasma membrane to release transmitter? Alternatively, can a vesicle fuse with the plasma membrane transiently, release its neurotransmitter through a pore that spans the two membranes, then reseal without losing its integrity? The latter form of hypothetical release mechanism has been termed a *kiss-and-run mechanism* (Fig. 8–17a). A variant of the patch clamp technique, devised by Erwin Neher and colleagues, is providing answers to these sorts of questions. The technique is based on the fact that a cell's capacitance, which can be measured using the whole-cell configuration of the patch clamp, is directly proportional to the surface area of the cell membrane. To provide a continuous measure of cell capacitance, a high-frequency (~800 Hz) sinusoidal voltage command is applied to the cell. The current that flows across the membrane is measured with an amplifier known as a *lock-in amplifier*. This determines the magnitude of the currents that are in phase with the voltage oscillation and those that are 90° out of phase. The latter can be related directly to the capacitance of the cell. When a vesicle fuses with the plasma membrane, there is a small increase in the size of the surface membrane (Fig. 8–17b). This is registered as an increase in cell membrane capacitance, allowing the whole-cell patch clamp apparatus to detect directly the exocytosis of single secretory vesicles.

Figure 8–17c shows measurements of capacitance in a mast cell from the peritoneum of a mouse. When stimulated, mast cells release massive amounts of histamine from their secretory granules and their activity is responsible for many of the symptoms of an allergic attack. In whole-cell recordings, introduction of a nonhydrolyzable analog of GTP into the patch pipette is sufficient to trigger this release, suggesting that a GTP-binding protein (see Chapter 12) may contribute to the onset of secretion. A stepwise increase in capacitance is recorded as each vesicle fuses with the plasma membrane (Fig. 8–17c, left). Stepwise decreases in membrane capacitance can also be observed (Fig. 8–17c, right); these represent membrane retrieval by endocytosis.

For this technique to work the secretory vesicles must be large, as is the case in chromaffin cells and mast cells, so the amount of added membrane will be detectable as an increase in capacitance. Although it has not yet been possible to apply the technique to the exocytosis of synaptic vesicles in intact nerve terminals, the approach has provided several insights into the process of exocytosis in non-neuronal cells. An early step in exocytosis in mast cells is the formation of a pore between the inside of the vesicle and the external medium. The initial conductance of the pore is about 230 pS. With time, the conductance increases as the pore dilates and the vesicle fuses with the plasma membrane. The initial stages of pore

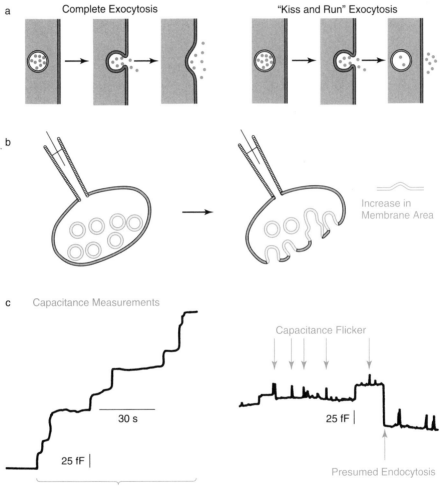

Figure 8–17. Exocytosis and capacitance measurements. *a*: Diagram contrasting total exocytosis with a "kiss-and-run" mode of exocytosis. *b*: Exocytosis leads to an increase in the area of plasma membrane. *c*: Capacitance measurements in a mast cell demonstrating stepwise increases (*left*) in capacitance at the onset of exocytosis, capacitance flicker, and stepwise decreases (*right*) in capacitance. Experiments of this sort have been carried out by Erwin Neher, Wolf Almers, and their colleagues.

formation, however, appear to be reversible. This is observed as the occurrence of *flicker*, in which the capacitance fluctuates between two levels (Fig. 8–17c). This indicates that vesicles can fuse with the plasma membrane and dilate partially, but then return to a "closed" state without undergoing full exocytosis. It is not yet known if the contents of secretory vesicles are released during such partial fusions. Nevertheless, such findings lend some support to the hypothesis that release can occur during a kiss-and-run mode of exocytosis.

Testing the Roles of Synaptic Proteins

In this chapter we have introduced some of the molecules that are important players in the game of exocytosis at synaptic endings. The exact roles of most of these proteins are not fully understood. As can be seen in Table 8–2, there are multiple forms of many of the proteins. For example, there are three forms of the synaptobrevin protein. Although the three proteins are very similar to one another, each is encoded by a separate gene, and different cells may possess different amounts of each form. Moreover, each synaptobrevin has preferred partners among the six different syntaxin molecules. These findings suggest that certain characteristics of transmission, such as kinetics and regulation, may differ at synapses that contain different variants of these proteins.

Most of the information on synaptic proteins presented in this chapter has been gained through biochemical studies of the interactions among these proteins. We have seen that naturally occuring toxins have played a critical role in identifying which proteins are essential to the exocytotic process. There are other experimental approaches to test the function of specific synaptic proteins. These include techniques such as the injection of proteins into synaptic endings or the production of mutant animals that lack a specific protein. To understand these approaches, however, we must first understand in more detail the physiology of synaptic transmission. This will be covered in the next chapter, which will also introduce some additional molecules that regulate transmitter release.

We should emphasize here that much of what we have learned about the biochemical interactions involved in exocytosis has come from the study of the small synaptic vesicle proteins. This is because these are much more abundant in the brain than are the neuropeptide-containing dense-core granules. The mechanism of exocytosis of dense-core vesicles almost certainly involves a slightly different set of proteins. For example, the priming of dense-core granules involves the action of an enzyme that transfers phosphate groups from ATP to membrane lipids. Whether the basic mechanisms of secretion differ for the peptide neurotransmitters has yet to be resolved.

Nonvesicular Release of Neurotransmitters

Exocytosis is the major form of transmitter release at most synaptic junctions. Nonetheless, there are several examples of the release of transmitter by neurons that are likely to result from mechanisms other than calcium-dependent exocytosis. One such example is found in the retina. Some of the synapses made by the *photoreceptors*, as well as synapses made by a retinal cell termed the *horizontal cell*, lack synaptic vesicles. Moreover, in contrast to most synapses, these synapses do not require extracellular calcium to release their neurotransmitter. Using one type of horizontal cell from the retina of the catfish, it has been shown that graded release of the neurotransmitter GABA occurs in response to depolarization of the presynaptic membrane, with no change in intracellular calcium concentration. It has been proposed that a carrier protein exists in the plasma membrane and that, in response to depolarization, this protein transports GABA from the cytoplasm to the extracellular space. Other examples of apparent nonvesicular release of transmitter also exist.

Summary

Two ways neurons communicate with one another are by direct electrical coupling and by the secretion of neurotransmitters. Electrical coupling arises from the existence of proteins, known as connexins, that form pores linking the cytoplasm of adjacent cells. Ions (as well as small molecules) can carry signals from one cell to another through these pores. Neurosecretion is a more complex process in which different categories of molecules are sorted into vesicles in the cytoplasm. A variety of chemical processes within these vesicles ensures that they contain biologically active transmitters or hormones. Stimulation of cells, which usually leads to an elevation of intracellular calcium, allows the vesicles to fuse with the plasma membrane and to release their contents in the extracellular space. Elucidation of the molecular mechanism by which this occurs is an ongoing challenge for cell biologists.

9

Synaptic Release of Neurotransmitters

*I*n the previous chapter we saw that secretion of proteins occurs through the exocytosis of membranous vesicles. This is a process that has been elaborated throughout evolution in endocrine, exocrine, and neuronal cells. It allows cells to send specific chemical signals that diffuse to, and act on, recipient cells. In many cases, the properties of neurons are very much like those of endocrine cells, whose business is chemical communication. Some neurons release peptides directly into the blood, just as an endocrine cell does. Other neurons release their transmitters locally into the extracellular space, where the transmitter diffuses slowly over some distance and influences many other neurons. Many neurons, however, differ from these other cell types in that they have been under evolutionary pressure to develop very rapid chemical communication with specific target neurons and muscle cells. To this end they have developed long axons that bring the source of the messenger substance right up to the membrane of their target cell. In addition, neurons often use small chemical transmitters that can be synthesized directly at the terminal rather than being transported from the soma, as is the case with peptide transmitters. The characteristics of the release of such transmitters at synaptic terminals differ from those of many other secretory cells. In this chapter we give an account of transmitter release at two thoroughly studied synaptic junctions, the *vertebrate neuromuscular junction* and the *giant synapse of the squid.*

Transmitter Release Is Quantized

We have seen that in many cells secretion occurs through the exocytosis of packets of peptide or hormone that are stored inside vesicles. As expected for a process that involves the exocytosis of synaptic vesicles, the release of neurotransmitter at most chemical synapses also occurs in small packets, or *quanta*. This was first demonstrated by Bernard Katz and colleagues through electrophysiological studies at the neuromuscular junction. They placed electrodes in the postsynaptic muscle cell and measured the extent of depolarization of the muscle in response to synaptic stimulation. This depolarization provides a direct measure of the amount of synaptic transmitter released under various experimental conditions.

The vertebrate neuromuscular junction. Figure 9–1 is a drawing of the frog neuromuscular synapse, which uses acetylcholine as its transmitter. Large numbers of synaptic vesicles are associated with specialized areas of the presynaptic membrane that have been termed *active zones*. These are located close to structures called *dense bars*, which are at the cytoplasmic side of the presynaptic membrane, but whose nature is not well understood. The dense bars may serve to align the synaptic vesicles at the sites of neurotransmitter release. Behind the active zones is a high density of *mitochondria* that provide the energy for secretion, reuptake of vesicles, and, as we shall see later, also regulate calcium levels in the terminal. On the muscle cell, clusters of *receptor molecules*, to which the released acetylcholine binds, are located in the areas of membrane closest to the active zones of the presynaptic terminals.

EPPs *and* MEPPs. When the presynaptic nerve is stimulated, an action potential travels along the axon to the presynaptic terminal. The depolarization of the terminal causes the release of acetylcholine. This in turn acts on the receptors in the postsynaptic membrane to depolarize the muscle by mechanisms that will be discussed in Chapter 11. This depolarization is termed an *end-plate potential* (EPP) (Fig. 9–2). Under normal conditions the end-plate potential is many tens of millivolts in size, sufficient to trigger an action potential and the subsequent contraction of the muscle. However, even in the absence of nerve stimulation, small depolarizations can be recorded with an electrode in the muscle (Fig. 9–2). These spontaneously occurring depolarizations are only about 0.5 mV in amplitude, but in most other respects they are very similar to the larger end-plate potential evoked by nerve stimulation. In particular, the time course of the small depolarizations matches that of the end-plate potential. In addition, the spontaneously occurring potentials, like the end-plate potential, can be blocked by antagonists of the acetylcholine receptor such as curare (see Chapter 11). The potentials can also be prolonged by agents that prevent the hydrolysis of acetylcholine by the enzyme acetylcholinesterase in the synaptic cleft. Finally, the frequency of occurrence of these small depolarizations increases on depolarization of the presynaptic terminal. These and other findings indicate that these small potentials are due to the spontaneous release, at random intervals, of a small amount of acetylcholine from the presynaptic terminal. The small potentials were therefore named *miniature end-plate potentials* (MEPPs).

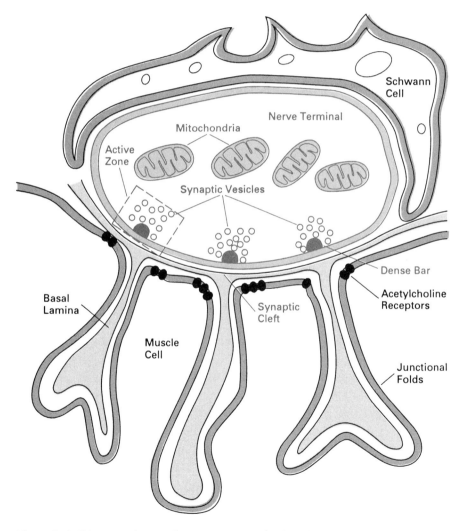

Figure 9–1. Diagram of a vertebrate neuromuscular junction.

EPPs *are made up of multiple* MEPPs. Katz then showed that the stimulus-evoked synaptic potential, that is, the end-plate potential, was caused by the simultaneous occurrence of a large number of individual potentials each of which appeared identical to a MEPP. To analyze the synaptic potentials in detail, the neuromuscular junction was bathed in a medium that contained lower than normal levels of calcium ions and a higher concentration of magnesium ions. As we shall see, such a medium reduces the amount of transmitter that is released on stimulation. In these particular experiments, release was reduced to such an extent that the average amplitude of the postsynaptic potential following nerve stimulation was a few millivolts, only a few times larger than a spontaneously occurring MEPP. Under these conditions the evoked end-plate potential did not have a fixed amplitude with each stimulus to the nerve. Instead, some stimuli failed to generate an end-plate potential, some generated end-plate potentials that were equal in amplitude and duration to a single MEPP, while others generated end-plate potentials that were equal in amplitude to two or more individual MEPPs (Fig. 9–3a). When a count is made of the number of

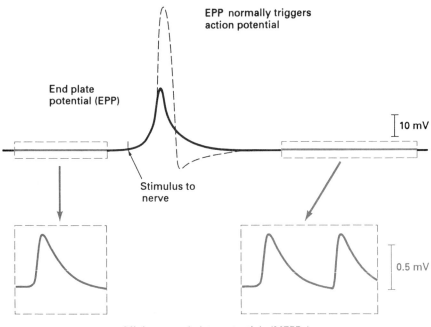

Figure 9–2. End plate potentials (EPPs) and miniature EPPs (MEPPs). Membrane potential recordings in a muscle cell. An EPP evoked by a nerve stimulus normally triggers a postsynaptic action potential. When its amplitude is decreased or the action potential is blocked, however, its time course matches that of MEPPs.

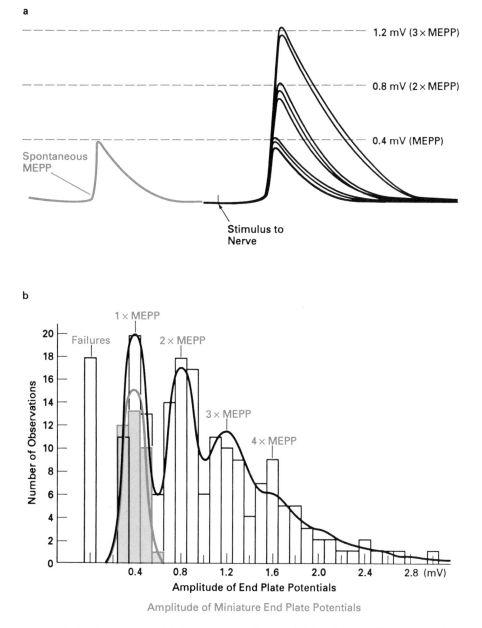

Figure 9–3. End plate potentials (EPPs) are made of multiple miniature EPPs (MEPPs). *a*: Under conditions of low transmitter release, nerve-evoked EPPs have amplitudes that correspond to a unit number of MEPPs. *b*: Histogram showing the relation between the size of EPPs and MEPPs in an experiment by Boyd and Martin (1956) on the cat neuromuscular junction.

times that end-plate potentials of different amplitudes occur in such an experiment, a histogram such as that in Figure 9–3b is generated. Although there is some variability in the size of individual MEPPs, the peaks in the histogram of evoked responses clearly correspond to the amplitudes of integral numbers of MEPPs.

A simple calculation shows that a single MEPP arises from the simultaneous action of a large number of acetylcholine molecules in the synaptic cleft. We now know that the conductance of the channel that is opened by acetylcholine is about 40 pS, and that the current flowing through the open channel is in the range of 5 pA near the muscle resting potential. The resistance of the muscle membrane is such that the opening of a single acetylcholine-gated channel in the postsynaptic membrane can produce a depolarization of less than 1 μV. Because much of the acetylcholine released into the synaptic cleft is hydrolyzed before it is able to interact with the receptor, and two molecules of acetylcholine are required to open a single acetylcholine-gated channel (see Chapter 11), it can be estimated that approximately 5000 acetylcholine molecules are released synchronously into the synaptic cleft to generate a single MEPP.

We shall see later that many factors can alter the strength of synaptic transmission. The fact that transmitter release occurs in quanta can sometimes make it possible to determine whether an alteration in the strength of synaptic transmission results from a change in the amount of transmitter that is released (rather than from a change in the sensitivity of the postsynaptic cell to the transmitter). In particular, if a change in number of quanta released on stimulation is detected, this immediately implies that some alteration has occurred in the presynaptic terminal. This quantal analysis is therefore a highly useful technique for investigating the properties of those relatively few synapses where such measurements can be made.

Morphological Evidence for Exocytosis During Synaptic Transmission

In the 1950s, Katz and colleagues suggested that the packets or quanta of acetylcholine released from the presynaptic terminals at the neuromuscular junction correspond to the content of acetylcholine within single synaptic vesicles. They suggested further that, even at rest, vesicles occasionally fuse with the presynaptic membrane, resulting in exocytosis of the contents of a single vesicle and the generation of a MEPP in the postsynaptic muscle cell. Depolarization by a presynaptic action potential greatly increases the probability of exocytosis of vesicles, leading to the simultane-

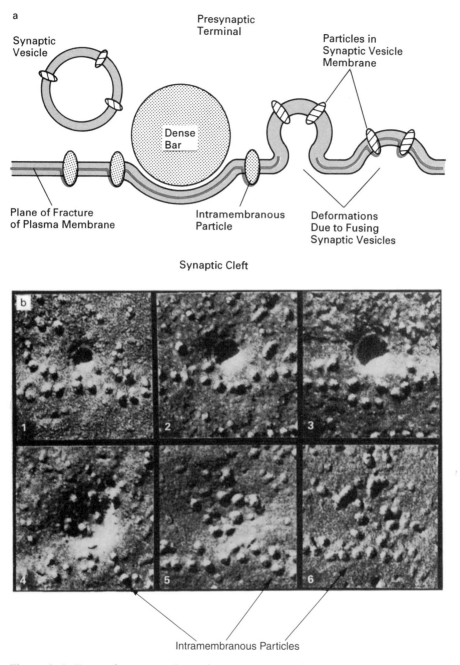

a

Synaptic Vesicle

Presynaptic Terminal

Particles in Synaptic Vesicle Membrane

Dense Bar

Plane of Fracture of Plasma Membrane

Intramembranous Particle

Deformations Due to Fusing Synaptic Vesicles

Synaptic Cleft

b

1 2 3

4 5 6

Intramembranous Particles

Figure 9–4. Freeze fracture evidence for exocytosis at the neuromuscular junction. *a*: Deformations of the plane of the plasma membrane are made by intramembranous particles, underlying structures, and fusing vesicles. *b*: Images of freeze fracture replicas of the presynaptic membrane, made by Tom Reese and colleagues, showing progressive stages (1–6) in the exocytosis of a single vesicle (courtesy of Tom Reese).

201

ous release of the contents of many vesicles. A normal end-plate potential would result from the exocytosis of several hundred synaptic vesicles. Direct visualization of exocytosis at the neuromuscular junction was achieved only 20 years later, by using electron microscopy combined with the freeze fracture technique (Fig. 9–4).

In the last chapter, we saw the use of freeze fracture to detect arrays of gap junction particles. When applied to presynaptic membranes at the neuromuscular junction of a frog, this technique reveals deformations of the plasma membrane, due to the presence of the dense bars under the presynaptic membrane. Aligned in two rows on either side of the dense bar are strings of intramembranous particles that correspond to the calcium channel proteins (Fig. 9–4). The electron micrographs of Figure 9–4 were made using freeze fracture coupled with a technique that allows the terminals to be frozen very rapidly, and at precise times, following the stimulation of the motor nerve. In a terminal at rest, or in one that has been stimulated but that has not yet begun to release transmitter, the dense bar and the two rows of particles can be detected. At the very time that acetycholine release occurs, however, further deformations of the membrane can be seen. These newly formed "pits" are thought to represent fusion of synaptic vesicles with the plasma membrane. The presence of these pits strongly suggests that release of transmitter occurs through exocytosis.

For technical reasons it has not been possible to stimulate nerves when a small number of quanta are released, and then to compare directly the number of quanta with the number of pits formed by exocytosis of synaptic vesicles. However, the neuromuscular junction has been stimulated in the presence of the potassium channel blocking agent 4-aminopyridine, which prolongs the action potential and greatly increases the amount of transmitter released. In this condition the amount of acetylcholine released does match the number of pits observed in freeze-fracture replicas.

Synaptic Transmitter Release Is Dependent on Calcium

It has been known since the work of Sidney Ringer in the nineteenth century that calcium ions in the extracellular medium are required for the normal function of the neuromuscular junction and other synapses. At most chemical synapses, eliminating calcium from the external medium prevents the release of transmitter evoked by nerve stimulation. In contrast, an increase in the external concentration of calcium frequently enhances the amount of neurotransmitter that is released.

The squid giant synapse. A major drawback to the investigation of neuro-transmitter release is the small size of most vertebrate presynaptic terminals, including those of the neuromuscular junction. This precludes normal electrophysiological recordings from the terminals. A synapse at which this is not a problem is the giant synapse in the stellate ganglion of the squid (Fig. 9–5). This synapse is used in escape behavior; when stimulated, this synaptic pathway triggers the ejection of water through the mantle of the squid, propelling the animal rapidly away from a source of danger. Several cell bodies of the average molluscan neuron and many of the average mammalian neuron can be enclosed comfortably in the presynaptic terminal of the giant synapse (the terminal is about 50 μm in diameter and 700 μm in length). Accordingly, two or more independent microelectrodes can be placed in the presynaptic terminal as well as in the postsynaptic cell (Fig. 9–5a). As in the case of the neuromuscular junction, the amplitude of the postsynaptic voltage change is taken as a measure of the amount of transmitter released.

Work with the squid giant synapse confirmed and extended the findings of Katz on the neuromuscular junction and definitively established a role for calcium and for voltage-dependent calcium channels in the release of transmitter following a presynaptic action potential. For example, it is possible to evoke transmitter release at this synapse by direct injection of calcium ions into the presynaptic terminal. As in the somata of many neurons, voltage-dependent calcium currents can be recorded in the presynaptic terminal of this synapse (together with the much larger, voltage-dependent sodium and potassium currents that shape the action potential). Stimulation of an action potential in the terminal usually liberates sufficient transmitter to depolarize the postsynaptic axon to threshold and to trigger a postsynaptic action potential (Fig. 9–5b). If, however, the voltage of the postsynaptic cell is clamped near its resting potential, then the stimulation of the synapse generates an inward current in the postsynaptic cell (Fig. 9–5c). This inward current represents the current flowing through the transmitter-activated ion channels in the postsynaptic membrane.

It is possible to block the sodium and potassium channels in the presynaptic membrane, leaving calcium flux as the only voltage-dependent ion current. This is accomplished by applying the sodium channel blocker tetrodotoxin (TTX) to the external medium, and by injecting the potassium channel blocking agent tetraethylammonium (TEA) into the terminal (see Chapters 4 and 5). In this condition, postsynaptic responses can still be recorded when the presynaptic terminal is depolarized (Fig. 9–5d). Of course, in the presence of TTX and TEA, normal action potentials no

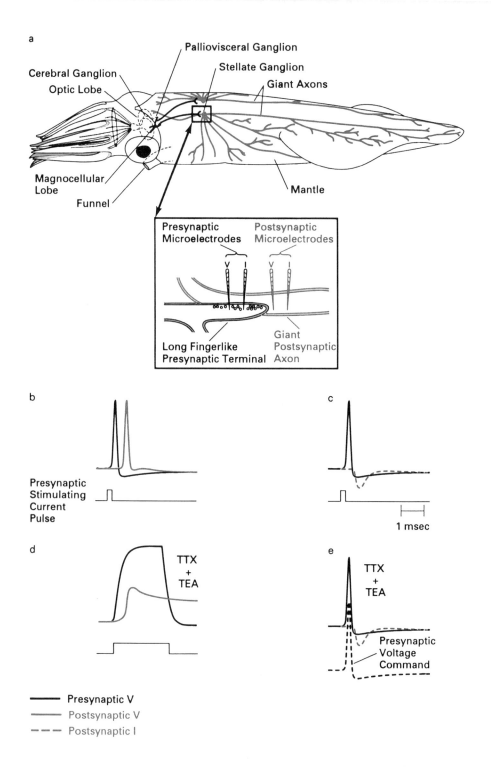

a

Cerebral Ganglion
Optic Lobe

Palliovisceral Ganglion
Stellate Ganglion
Giant Axons

Magnocellular
Lobe
Funnel

Mantle

Presynaptic
Microelectrodes

Postsynaptic
Microelectrodes

Long Fingerlike
Presynaptic Terminal

Giant
Postsynaptic
Axon

b

Presynaptic
Stimulating
Current
Pulse

c

1 msec

d

TTX
+
TEA

e

TTX
+
TEA

Presynaptic
Voltage
Command

⎯⎯ Presynaptic V
⎯⎯ Postsynaptic V
--- Postsynaptic I

204

longer occur in the presynaptic terminal. However, when the voltage in the terminal is driven by the voltage clamp to follow the normal shape of an action potential, the postsynaptic current exactly matches the normal postsynaptic response (Fig. 9–5e). This indicates that the normal presynaptic sodium and potassium fluxes are not required for release of neurotransmitter, but that calcium entry alone is sufficient.

Calcium channels are clustered near release sites. In the last chapter we saw that the SNARE complex is able to bind calcium channels. Accordingly, the spatial distribution of calcium channels in the squid terminal closely matches the sites of transmitter release. This was first suggested by the fact that the calcium current recorded in the presynaptic terminal is very much greater than that in regions of the axon leading to the terminal. Direct measurement of calcium levels in the terminal, however, required the use of substances that could be introduced into the terminal to measure changes in calcium concentration. The first of these to be used was a protein known as *aequorin*, which emits light when it binds calcium. This protein was used to provide direct evidence that the calcium concentration in the terminal is raised during transmission. Subsequently, other calcium-indicator dyes have been used for this purpose, including the dye Arsenazo III, and the now widely used calcium indicator fura-2. In its structure fura-2 resembles the common chelator of calcium ions, EGTA (Fig. 9–6a). It is, however, a fluorescent compound, whose excitation spectrum changes when it binds calcium (Fig. 9–6b).

Using a fluorescence microscope coupled to a computer, digital images can be made of changes in calcium concentration occurring during transmitter release. Figure 9–6c and Plate 7 illustrate the application of fura-2 imaging to the squid giant synapse. During a brief burst of action potentials, calcium levels within the terminal rise. This elevation occurs first at the active zones that are closely apposed to the postsynaptic fiber. During the burst, a steep gradient of calcium concentration develops across the terminal. After stimulation ceases, the gradient dissipates. Such images il-

---

Figure 9–5. The squid giant synapse. *a*: Position of the giant synapse within the stellate ganglion. *b–e*: Presynaptic and postsynaptic responses recorded in experiments by Bernard Katz and Ricardo Miledi, and by Rodolfo Llinas and co-workers. *b*: The normal response. *c*: The postsynaptic axon is voltage clamped and the postsynaptic current is recorded. *d, e*: Presynaptic sodium and potassium currents have been blocked by tetradotoxin (TTX) and tetraethylammonium (TEA). *d*: The prolonged postsynaptic potential evoked by a long presynaptic depolarization. *e*: The presynaptic voltage is driven to follow that of a normal action potential, resulting in a normal postsynaptic current.

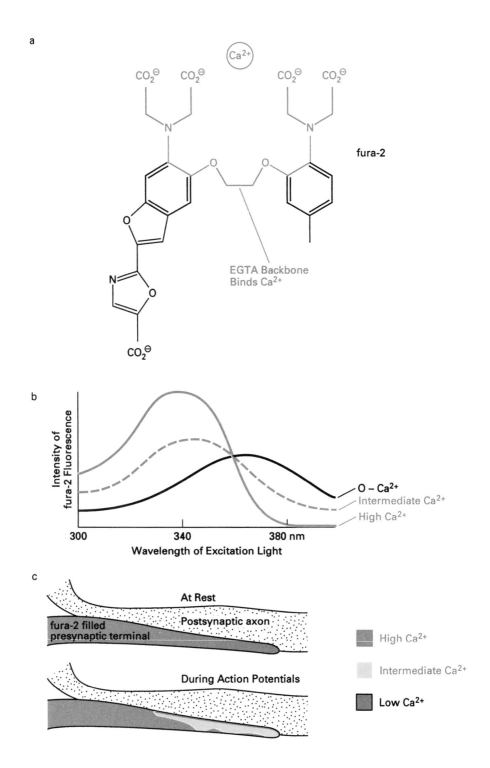

a

CO$_2^\ominus$ CO$_2^\ominus$ CO$_2^\ominus$ CO$_2^\ominus$

Ca^{2+}

N   N

fura-2

O   O

EGTA Backbone
Binds Ca^{2+}

N
O

CO$_2^\ominus$

b

Intensity of
fura-2 Fluorescence

300   340   380 nm

Wavelength of Excitation Light

O – Ca^{2+}
Intermediate Ca^{2+}
High Ca^{2+}

c

At Rest

fura-2 filled
presynaptic terminal

Postsynaptic axon

During Action Potentials

High Ca^{2+}

Intermediate Ca^{2+}

Low Ca^{2+}

lustrate further that calcium channels are clustered near the release sites, a finding that has also been confirmed at the neuromuscular junction by direct labeling of calcium channel proteins.

Three Important Features of Calcium-Dependent Transmitter Release

Electrical measurements, coupled with measurements of intracellular calcium, have provided three further important conclusions about the mechanism of transmitter release: (1) transmitter release depends on a high power of the calcium concentration; (2) transmitter release is more sensitive to calcium ions than to other divalent cations; and (3) release occurs very rapidly following calcium entry. We shall now discuss briefly the evidence for each of these conclusions.

Transmitter release requires binding of several calcium ions. As described above, transmitter release depends on the presence of extracellular calcium. At low concentrations of extracellular calcium, release of transmitter at the frog neuromuscular junction depends on the fourth power of the external calcium concentration. Experiments at the squid giant synapse, in which calcium currents and increases in calcium concentration can be measured directly, indicate that calcium entry into the terminal does not depend on the fourth power of the external calcium concentration, but rather that the release process itself depends on a high power of intracellular calcium (Fig. 9–7a). The simplest interpretation of such findings is that some reaction in the terminal, perhaps the interaction of synaptotagmin with the SNARE complex, requires the binding of several calcium ions before release of transmitter occurs.

The release mechanism prefers calcium over other divalent cations. When the extracellular calcium at a synapse is replaced by other divalent cations, transmitter release is usually reduced or abolished. Ions such as nickel, cadmium, manganese, cobalt, and the trivalent ion lanthanum act as calcium channel blockers and would not be expected to evoke release. However,

---

Figure 9–6. Measurement of intracellular calcium. *a*: Structure of the calcium indicator dye fura-2, which was synthesized by Roger Tsien. *b*: The intensity of fura-2 fluorescence varies with calcium concentration (Grynkiewicz et al., 1985). *c*: Diagram of how calcium levels in the squid presynaptic terminal, measured using fura-2 fluorescence, change during stimulation (Smith and Augustine, 1988; see also Plate 7).

the ions barium and strontium readily enter the cell through voltage-dependent calcium channels. Even for these ions, release of transmitter at the squid synapse is very much lower than for an equivalent amount of calcium influx. Such experiments suggest that the ion-sensitive step in the release process prefers calcium strongly over the other ions in the order Ca>Sr>Ba.

Transmitter release occurs very rapidly following calcium entry. When the presynaptic terminal of the squid is depolarized to allow calcium channels to open, release generally increases after a delay of a few milliseconds. This, however, is not a good measure of the rate at which the release process

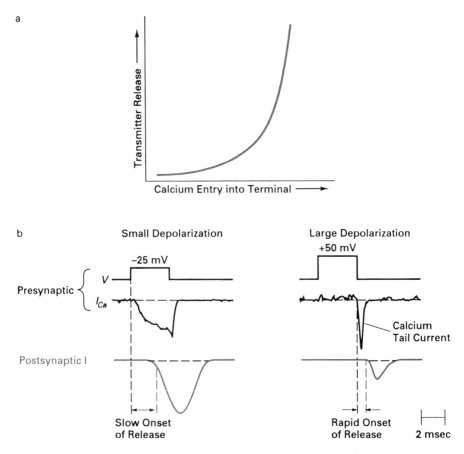

Figure 9–7. Calcium dependence of release. *a:* Steep dependence of release on amount of calcium entry into the squid terminal. *b:* The postsynaptic response occurs very rapidly after a calcium tail current (after Augustine et al., 1985). I_{Ca}, calcium current; V, voltage.

itself is activated by calcium, because the presynaptic calcium current activates over a period of milliseconds. A more direct measurement of the response time of release can be obtained during measurements of calcium tail currents.

If in a voltage-clamp experiment the presynaptic terminal is stepped from its resting potential to a very positive potential close to the equilibrium potential for calcium ions, then calcium channels open in response to the depolarization. Nevertheless, at this potential calcium ions do not enter the terminal, because there is little or no driving force for calcium entry (Fig. 9–7b). Thus no transmitter release occurs with such large depolarizations. The voltage-clamp circuitry can then be used to step the membrane potential very rapidly back to the resting potential. Immediately after this step, the calcium channels remain open for a finite time at the resting potential, before they eventually close. Because the driving force for calcium entry is large at the resting potential, calcium ions enter through the still open calcium channels, resulting in a rapid but transient calcium tail current, measured after the end of the depolarizing pulse. This tail current is accompanied by transmitter release, measured as a postsynaptic depolarization. The delay between the onset of the sharp tail of calcium current in the presynaptic terminal and the onset of the postsynaptic response has been found to be as little as 200 μsec (Fig. 9–7b). This means that the release process at this synapse is so rapid that the actions of calcium are unlikely to involve complex, multistep biochemical reactions.

Domains of calcium entry. Because calcium channels are discrete membrane proteins, calcium concentrations do not rise uniformly throughout the terminal following a depolarization. Instead, calcium levels are initially much higher directly under the membrane where the calcium channels are located (see Fig. 9–6c). It is important to consider this spatial inhomogeneity when thinking about the relation between the amount of calcium that enters a cell and the effect of that calcium on processes such as transmitter release.

Quantitative models have been useful in predicting the way calcium is distributed in the presynaptic terminal after entry through calcium channels. Figure 9–8a shows the pattern of intracellular calcium expected near the mouth of a calcium channel that has been open for a millisecond or so. The computed profile of calcium concentration takes the form of a volcano centered on the mouth of the channel. Near the channel itself, calcium concentrations may reach as high as 100 μM (the resting level of calcium is usually about 0.1 μM). As calcium diffuses from the channel, its concentration drops. Proteins located close to the mouth of the channel, such as synaptotagmin and the other vesicular proteins, may therefore be exposed to higher concentrations of calcium ions than those seen further from the channel.

This idea of calcium domains allows certain predictions about transmitter release. For example, it suggests that the same amount of calcium entering a cell at two different voltages can, in theory, produce different effects on transmitter release or on other calcium-sensitive reactions. We know that as a cell is progressively depolarized, calcium current first in-

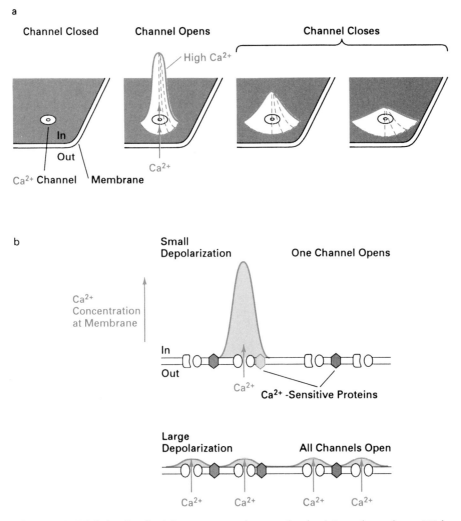

Figure 9-8. High levels of calcium occur at the mouth of calcium channels. *a*: "Volcanos" of calcium forming inside a cell near the mouth of an open channel. *b*: Comparison of the spatial profiles of intracellular calcium expected with small and large depolarizations.

creases as calcium channels open and then decreases as the voltage approaches the equilibrium potential for calcium ions. Figure 9–8b shows the profile of calcium concentrations expected at two different voltages that produce the same net calcium influx into the terminal. In the first case, a small depolarization of the membrane allows only a few calcium channels to open. Because the driving force on calcium ions is high, however, relatively high concentrations of calcium are achieved near the mouths of these few open channels. In the second case, a large depolarization causes the opening of nearly all of the channels. At this very positive potential, however, calcium driving force and hence flux through each open channel is greatly reduced. In the first case, large but spatially inhomogeneous transients of calcium are attained. These will act on calcium-sensitive proteins such as synaptotagmin or other vesicle proteins near the open channels. In the second case, although a more uniform change in calcium levels is attained, levels at any one site may not reach the critical level needed for triggering key calcium-activated processes. Although we have considered the consequences of this localization for synaptic release, exactly the same considerations apply to other neuronal processes that are sensitive to calcium entry, such as the activation of calcium-activated potassium channels (Chapter 7) or enzymes that trigger changes in gene transcription (see Chapter 18). The relative localization of calcium channels and calcium-sensitive proteins is a very important factor in the efficient organization of each of these processes.

Homosynaptic Plasticity: Facilitation, Potentiation, and Depression of Transmitter Release

As a series of action potentials invades a nerve terminal, the amount of neurotransmitter released with each action potential does not always remain constant. Depending on the synapse that is studied and the frequency at which it is stimulated, a train of action potentials in the presynaptic terminal may produce either a progressive increase or a progressive decrease in the amount of release. This property, which allows the amount of transmitter release to change as a result of previous activity in the terminal, has been termed *homosynaptic plasticity*. Three major forms of homosynaptic plasticity are *facilitation*, *potentiation*, and *depression*. These may be contrasted with a change in release induced by the action of other cells. The latter phenomenon has been termed *heterosynaptic plasticity*, and examples will be provided in Chapter 20. Facilitation, potentiation, and depression may all occur at a single type of synapse, resulting in a complex time course of changes in neurotransmitter release following the onset of a train of action potentials. Figure 9–9 shows the relative time course of these different homosynaptic processes. We will now describe each of them in turn.

Facilitation describes a progressive increase in the amount of transmitter released by successive action potentials *during* a brief stimulus train lasting up to a few seconds (Fig. 9–9). A leading hypothesis for the cause of facilitation is that the calcium concentration at the release sites does not have time to return to basal levels between the action potentials. Thus, at the occurrence of each action potential after the first, a small amount

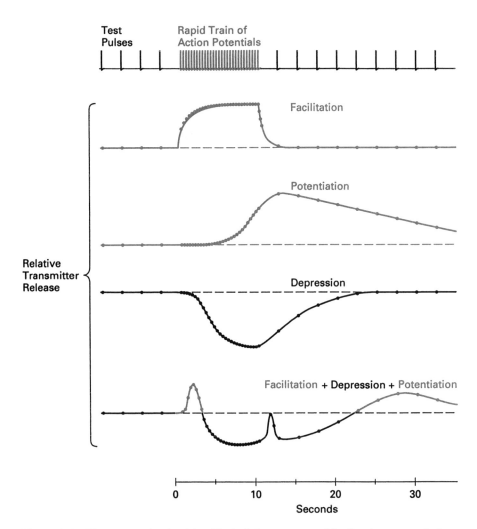

Figure 9–9. Homosynaptic plasticity. Typical time courses of facilitation, potentiation, and depression.

of residual calcium remains near the release site. The level of residual calcium is, by itself, insufficient to cause a significant amount of transmitter release during the interval between action potentials. Because release is very nonlinearly dependent on calcium concentration (Fig. 9–7a), the residual calcium adds to the calcium that enters during the next action potential to produce a progressive increase in release. Recovery from facilitation is rapid, occurring within a few hundred milliseconds after the end of stimulation.

Potentiation describes an increase in transmitter release by an action potential *following* repetitive stimulation of a synapse (Fig. 9–9). Unlike facilitation, potentiation is long-lasting and is slow in onset, usually requiring seconds to develop. For example, following a rapid train of action potentials, termed a *tetanus*, the amount of release in response to a single action potential may be enhanced over that prior to the tetanus for up to several minutes. This phenomenon can be observed at a wide variety of synapses including the neuromuscular junction, and has been termed *posttetanic potentiation* (PTP). At least at some synapses, potentiation, like facilitation, is due to an elevation of resting calcium levels over those in the terminal prior to stimulation. The long-lasting nature of this residual calcium results from the activity of mitochondria. In most synapses, there is a high density of these organelles behind the active zones (see Fig. 9–1). In addition to providing energy for transmission in the form of ATP, mitochondria are able to take up large amounts of calcium. During the tetanus, calcium that enters through calcium channels spreads throughout the terminal and is rapidly accumulated into the matrix of the mitochondria (Fig. 9–10). After the end of the tetanus, this accumulated calcium is slowly released back into the synaptic cytoplasm, providing residual calcium that

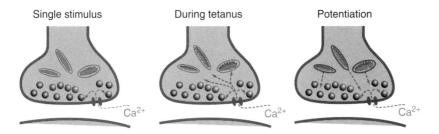

Figure 9–10. Calcium accumulation by synaptic mitochondria during a tetanus. Initially, a single action potential elevates calcium locally near the mouth of the channel (*left*). During the tetanus, calcium rises in the cytoplasm and is taken up by the mitochondria (*center*). After the tetanus, calcium released from the mitochondria adds to that entering through calcium channels (*right*) (Tang and Zucker, 1997).

can potentiate transmitter release by action potentials for several minutes. At many central synapses, potentiation may endure for periods ranging from tens of minutes to hours or days, depending on the duration and intensity of the stimulus train. This has been termed *long-term potentiation* (LTP). The mechanisms of LTP appear to be distinct from those of PTP, and differ from synapse to synapse. The phenomenon of LTP has been studied as a model for the establishment of memories by the nervous system, and we will discuss LTP further in this context in Chapter 20.

Synaptic *depression* describes a progressive decrease in the amount of transmitter released during a train of action potentials (Fig. 9–9). This phenomenon is often encountered when a synapse is stimulated at a high rate and, in many cases, results from the depletion of the readily releasable pool of neurotransmitter at active zones (see Fig. 8–11). The proportion of synaptic vesicles that are released by a single action potential (also termed the *release probability*) differs widely for synapses in different parts of the nervous system. In general, the amount of depression at a synapse depends on this initial release probability. Synapses with a high probability of release tend to suffer depression with repetitive stimulation, whereas low-release probability synapses enjoy facilitation and post-tetanic potentiation.

Testing the Roles of Synaptic Proteins in Neurotransmission

We have now described some of the dynamic features of transmitter release at synaptic terminals. In the previous chapter, we covered the biochemistry of some of the proteins of synaptic vesicles and their partners on the plasma membrane. An ongoing task for neurobiologists is to discover how each of these proteins contributes to neurotransmission and, perhaps even more importantly, determine how the modulation of these proteins may alter characteristics of release such as potentiation and depression.

One approach that is being widely adopted to test the importance of a particular protein in the process of synaptic release is the genetic manipulation of animals such as mice or fruit flies to produce a *knockout* of a selected protein. By a technique known as *homologous recombination* it is possible to replace the normal gene for a selected mouse protein by a nonfunctional mutant gene. Such mutant animals can then be bred to produce strains of mice that lack the functional protein. As might be surmised, if an important protein is selected, the mutant animals may fail to develop normally, and experimental tricks often have to be employed to keep embryos alive long enough to isolate cells to study. Nevertheless, results have been generated from this approach and some of them have been surprising. For example, the elimination of synaptotagmin I, one of the two major forms of this presumed calcium sensor, does not eliminate synaptically evoked transmitter release but significantly alters the timing of the release following invasion of an action potential. This suggests that calcium-sensitive proteins other than synaptotagmin I may also contribute to the calcium sensitivity of release. Similarly, the knockout of rab3A, the major form of rab3 protein in the brain, does not prevent synaptic release but seems merely to accelerate the rate of synaptic depression during repeated stimulation of a synapse (Fig. 9–11). Such findings will eventually have to be incorporated into our understanding of how processes such as docking, priming, fusion, and reuptake contribute to the rate and amount of transmitter release from a synapse during physiological patterns of activity.

One of the difficulties in the interpretation of genetic knockout experiments is that compensatory changes may occur in the levels of other synaptic proteins. An alternative to the genetic strategy is the injection of reagents that block the function of specific synaptic proteins into the giant presynaptic terminal of the squid. For example, injection of a GTP analog, GTPγS, irreversibly blocks transmitter release. This analog would be expected to bind irreversibly to rab3 proteins and other GTP-binding proteins, and therefore inhibit the cycling of synaptic vesicles depicted in Figures 8–15 and 8–16. Similarly, the injection of small fragments of the synaptotagmin molecule, which may interfere with the normal binding of synaptotagmin to other proteins, also prevents transmitter release. We shall now provide an example of the combined use of knockout and injection

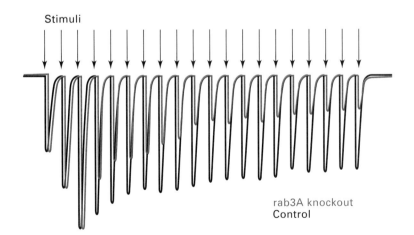

Figure 9–11. Effects of genetic knockout of the rab3A protein on synaptic currents. In response to a train of stimuli, synaptic depression occurs more rapidly at synapses from the mutant animals (Geppert et al., 1994).

experiments in testing the role of another synaptic vesicle protein, synapsin I (see Table 8–2).

Synapsins, Calcium/Calmodulin-Dependent Protein Kinases, and Neurotransmitter Release

There are three known synapsin proteins: synapsins I, II, and III. Synapsin III is present in cells before synapses are formed and its function is not known. Synapsins I and II are proteins that associate with the cytoplasmic surface of synaptic vesicles. In electron microscopy experiments they have been found to be associated primarily with the clusters of vesicles that are located away from active zones, those that are sometimes referred to as the *reserve pool* (see Fig. 8–11). In addition to binding to the surface of synaptic vesicles, synapsins are able to bind the cytoskeletal protein actin. The properties of synapsins can be substantially modified by the action of several enzymes termed *protein kinases*. Before we discuss the effect of these modifications we must cover some basic biochemistry of protein kinases.

Protein kinases. Members of this large family of enzymes transfer the terminal phosphate group from ATP to a variety of proteins. The addition of phosphate to a protein alters the electrical charge on the protein (phosphate groups are negatively charged) and may also change the three-dimensional shape, or *conformation*, of the protein. This in turn may induce a change in the biological activity of the phosphorylated protein (for a more detailed discussion, see Chapter 12). The activity of protein kinases can be detected in a homogenate of the nervous system by incubating the homogenate with ATP that has been radiolabeled in the terminal (γ) phosphate. The transfer of the radioactive phosphate group to specific proteins can then be measured readily. If calcium ions are also added to the homogenate, the incorporation of phosphate into certain proteins is very much enhanced. Further enhancement is also usually observed with the addition of *calmodulin*, a small (16.7 kDa) calcium-binding protein that is found in all eukaryotic cells. The calcium-dependent phosphorylation of proteins is carried out by several different protein kinases, one of which is termed the *calcium/calmodulin-dependent protein kinase type II* (abbreviated Ca^{2+}/Cam kinase II). This enzyme is one of the myriad of cellular activities that are regulated by calcium and calmodulin.

Ca^{2+}/Cam kinase II phosphorylates synapsin I. Ca^{2+}/Cam kinase II is found in most cells. It is particularly abundant in the nervous system, however, where it accounts for 0.5%–1.0% of total protein, an extraordinarily high

concentration for an enzyme. It is a large, multisubunit complex consisting of two different subunits, α and β, with molecular weights of 50,000 and 60,000, respectively. The active enzyme appears to contain 12 subunits (Fig. 9–12), and the relative ratio of α to β subunits in the active enzyme varies in different types of cells. For example, in some cells, the enzyme is composed entirely of α subunits, whereas in other cells the larger β subunit predominates.

Following an elevation of the calcium concentration inside a cell, the calcium ions bind to calmodulin in the cytoplasm. The calcium/calmodulin complex, in turn, binds to the individual subunits of the Ca^{2+}/Cam kinase II. When the enzyme is bound in this way, it becomes active and is

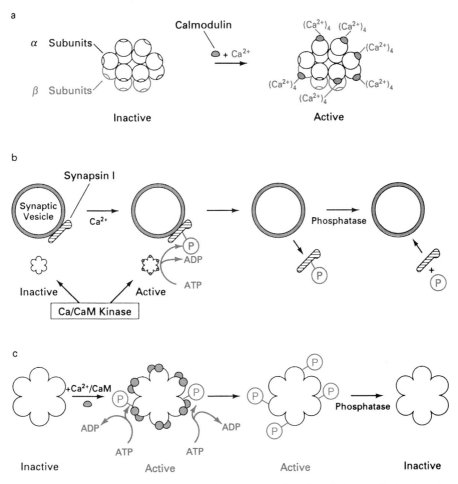

Figure 9–12. Calcium/calmodulin-dependent protein phosphorylation. a: Activation of Ca^{2+}/Cam kinase II. b: Phosphorylation of synapsin I. c: Autophosphorylation of Ca^{2+}/Cam kinase II.

able to transfer phosphate groups from ATP to a wide variety of proteins. One interesting feature of Ca^{2+}/Cam kinase II is that it is also able to phosphorylate itself. This is termed *autophosphorylation*. When this happens, the enzyme remains active but becomes independent of calcium and calmodulin until the phosphate groups on the enzyme are removed by other enzymes, termed *phosphoprotein phosphatases*. The autophosphorylation may therefore allow Ca^{2+}/ Cam kinase II to remain active for a considerable time even after the calcium concentration in the cell has returned to its basal level (Fig. 9–12c).

Because Ca^{2+}/Cam kinase II is so abundant, it is likely to regulate many different functions of cells. It is, for example, the major protein to be found in the region of a neuron immediately under the neurotransmitter receptors at the postsynaptic junction, where its role is not yet known. Nevertheless, a major part of the Ca^{2+}/Cam kinase II within the nerve terminal is found on the surface of synaptic vesicles, where it is known to bind synapsin I. Indeed, synapsin I is one of the best substrate proteins for this enzyme. As mentioned above, synapsin normally binds the surface of synaptic vesicles as well as to actin. When it undergoes phosphorylation by Ca^{2+}/Cam kinase II, however, this association is greatly weakened and the phosphorylated synapsin I may be released from the surface of the vesicles (Fig. 9–12b).

Role of synapsin I and Ca^{2+}/Cam kinase II in transmitter release. Evidence that Ca^{2+}/Cam kinase II plays a role in regulating neurotransmitter release has been provided by injecting this enzyme into the giant presynaptic terminal of the squid (Fig. 9–13). This causes an increase in neurotransmitter release. However, there is no change in the amplitude of the presynaptic calcium current, suggesting that the injection of the enzyme increases the efficiency of transmitter release. We have already seen that the rapid release of neurotransmitter at synaptic junctions occurs too rapidly to be mediated by a complex enzyme reaction. Ca^{2+}/Cam kinase II is therefore unlikely to be involved in triggering release directly, but instead may determine the amount of transmitter that is available for release by an action potential.

It is possible that this action of Ca^{2+}/Cam kinase II at the squid synapse occurs through the phosphorylation of synapsin I or a related molecule. A variety of experimental approaches, including genetic knockouts in mice, protein injections into squid and lamprey synapses, and electron microscopy, suggest that unphosphorylated synapsin I acts as a glue that holds together the reserve pool of synaptic vesicles behind the active zone. Phosphorylation of synapsin I may free some of these vesicles, allowing them to approach the plasma membrane and dock at release sites. For exam-

ple, injection of unphosphorylated synapsin I into the presynaptic terminal decreases release, whereas injection of synapsin I that has previously
been phosphorylated by Ca^{2+}/Cam kinase II has no apparent effect on release. This would be expected if excess unphosphorylated protein kept the
reserve pool glued together and unavailable for release. Genetic knockout
of the synapsin gene in mice or injection of anti-synapsin antibodies into
synaptic endings disrupts the tight clusters of reserve vesicles (Fig 9-14).
These manipulations do not, however, prevent normal synaptic transmission, but rather decrease release at high rates of synaptic stimulation, when
the reserve pool is most likely to be needed.

Studies such as these suggest that phosphorylation of synapsin I by
Ca^{2+}/Cam kinase II plays a role in ensuring continued neurotransmitter
release during high rates of synaptic activity. There are still many questions remaining about the role of phosphorylation in the control of
synapsins as well as other synaptic proteins. For example, the synapsin II

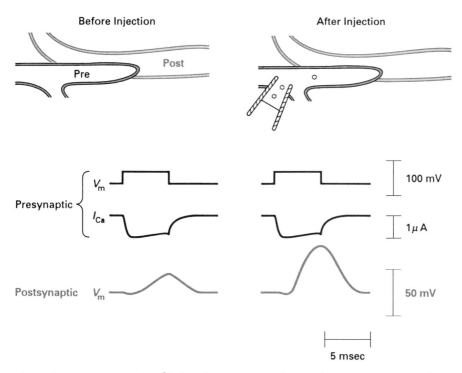

Figure 9–13. Injection of Ca^{2+}/Cam kinase II into the squid presynaptic terminal. In
a collaborative experiment between the laboratories of Paul Greengard and Rodolfo
Llinas, injection of this enzyme caused increased transmitter release, measured as an
increase in the postsynaptic depolarization (Llinas et al., 1985). I_{Ca}, calcium current;
V_m, voltage.

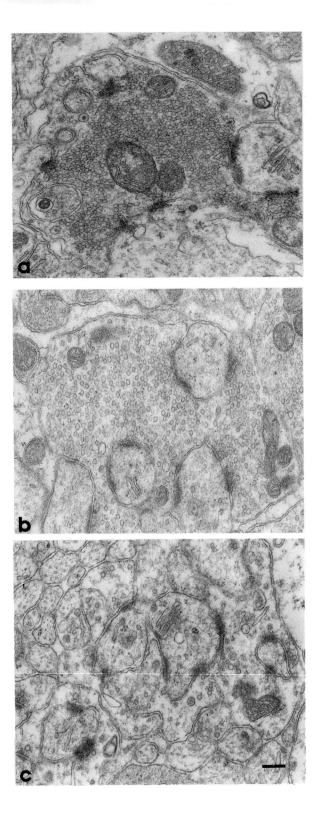

220

protein resembles synapsin I in its structure but is not phosphorylated by Ca^{2+}/Cam kinase II. However, both of these proteins are phosphorylated by other protein kinases, many of which we shall encounter in subsequent chapters. Each of the different kinases may alter the characteristics of neurotransmission in specific ways.

Summary

Two specialized synapses, one in the squid stellate ganglion and the other at the frog neuromuscular junction, have been instrumental in advancing our understanding of the release of neurotransmitters from presynaptic terminals. Studies of rapid synaptic transmission have shown that neurotransmitters are released in packets or quanta, which may correspond to the exocytosis of individual synaptic vesicles. Following an action potential, release is very closely linked in space and time to the entry of calcium though voltage-dependent channels. The amount of transmitter that is released by a single action potential is not fixed, but can increase or decrease after repetitive stimulation of a synapse. We are still far from a complete understanding of the mechanisms that induce neurotransmitter release and of the factors that modulate release. Furthermore, the characteristics of the release of transmitter from small synaptic vesicles at active zones may differ substantially from those of neuropeptides in large dense-core vesicles. Biochemical experiments that characterize the components of synaptic vesicles and release sites, coupled with physiological experiments that test the effects of these components at specific synapses, are providing further insights into the release process.

Figure 9–14. Genetic elimination of synapsins. *a*: Synaptic terminals on neurons in the hippocampus of normal mice are densely packed with small clear synaptic vesicles. Experiments by Magarinos, Pieribone, and Greengard have shown that terminals in mice lacking synapsin I have fewer synaptic vesicles and that these pack together less densely (*b*), while elimination of synapsin II causes a dramatic loss of vesicles in synaptic terminals (*c*).

10

Neurotransmitters and
Neurohormones

Ｗe have seen in the previous two chapters that a neuron is in
large part an elaborate and intricately regulated machine for the
secretion of a variety of chemicals. Why do cells go to all this
trouble? Although direct electrical connections between nerve cells also
play an essential role (see Chapter 8), it is chemical signaling that mediates much of the intercellular communication among nerve cells within the
central nervous system. In addition, the transfer of information into the
nervous system from sensory organs and the output from the nervous system in the form of muscular contraction are mediated by extracellular
chemical messengers. In this chapter we will discuss in a systematic way
the different classes of neurotransmitters and neurohormones, some of
which we have already met in other contexts. Subsequent chapters will
deal with receptors on the target cell that recognize and bind these substances and with the transduction mechanisms that are involved in converting the extracellular chemical signal into an appropriate response (usually electrical) in the target cell.

What Is a Neurotransmitter and What Is a Neurohormone?

Which neuroactive substances are transmitters and which are hormones?
Classically, synaptic *neurotransmitters* have been thought of as substances
that are released locally into an anatomically well-defined synaptic cleft,
and influence the activity of only one or a few adjacent cells (Fig. 10–1).
The prototype neurotransmitter is acetylcholine, which was first demon-

strated to be the chemical mediating nerve-to-muscle synaptic transmission in cardiac and skeletal muscle (see Chapter 1) and was subsequently found to be an important neuron-to-neuron transmitter as well. In contrast, *hormones* have been defined as substances that are released from the tissue in which they are synthesized, and travel via the blood to other (often remote) organs whose activities they influence (Fig. 10–1). Another criterion that has often been used to distinguish between transmitters and hormones is a temporal one: transmitters have been thought to produce

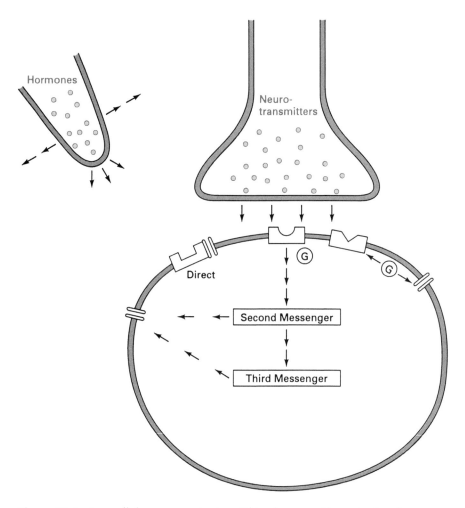

Figure 10–1. Intercellular communication. This chapter will emphasize the neurotransmitters and hormones (*blue*) that mediate much cell-to-cell communication in the nervous system. G, guanyl nucleotide binding protein.

rapid-onset and rapidly reversible responses in the target cell, whereas the actions of hormones can be slower and much longer lasting.

Because hormone synthesis and secretion had been studied most thoroughly in organs such as the adrenal gland and the gonads, it came as something of a surprise when it was demonstrated many years ago that the nervous system also synthesizes and releases hormones—neurohormones—that act on remote organs. The classical neurohormones are the closely related nine amino acid peptides *oxytocin* and *vasopressin*, which are (1) synthesized in the so-called *magnocellular neurons* in the hypothalamus, (2) transported down the axons of these neurons to the posterior pituitary where they are released, and (3) dispersed via the bloodstream to regulate smooth muscle contraction and water balance, respectively.

More recently it has become evident that oxytocin, vasopressin, and other neuroactive peptides can have local transmitter-like actions as well. In addition to being secreted into the blood, they may be released at synapses instead of—or even together with—more classical transmitter substances. Furthermore, we know now that the actions of some classical neurotransmitters may be slow in onset and long in duration, and indeed they may be released into the bloodstream to act as true hormones, whereas many peptide "hormones" may produce rapid transmitter-like effects on target cells. In other words, the classical distinctions between neurotransmitters and neurohormones are becoming obsolete. One person's transmitter is another person's hormone, and it may be more useful to classify neuroactive substances on the basis of other criteria—for example, the nature and mechanism of the response they evoke in the target cell (see Chapters 11 and 12).

Acetylcholine

The first chemical to be implicated as a neurotransmitter was *acetylcholine*, the structure of which is shown in Figure 10–2. It had been known since the early part of this century that acetylcholine could influence the physiological properties of nerve and muscle cells. In the 1920s it was demonstrated that acetylcholine is the transmitter at *neuromuscular synapses*, which are synapses between neurons and cardiac, smooth, and skeletal muscle, as well as at a variety of neuron–neuron synapses in the central and peripheral nervous systems. It is instructive to recall at this time the first experiment to demonstrate unequivocally the chemical mediation of synaptic transmission by acetylcholine, the classic double heart experiment published by Otto Loewi in 1921 (see Fig. 1–7), because it is so beautiful an example of a *bioassay*, the use of a physiological response to assay for a biologically active compound. The bioassay remains an essential tool by which neuropharmacologists identify and quantitate neuroactive substances for which no sufficiently sensitive or specific chemical assay is available.

Synthesis and release. Unlike the other neurotransmitters and neurohormones that we shall discuss below, acetylcholine is not simply one member of a class of closely related compounds. Rather, it has some unique properties that place it in a class by itself. It is synthesized in nerve terminals from acetyl-CoA and choline, in a reaction catalyzed by the enzyme *choline acetyltransferase* (Fig. 10–3). Although acetyl-CoA and choline are common metabolites present in all cells, choline acetyltransferase (and hence acetylcholine) is not. In fact, the presence of choline acetyltransferase in a neuron is sufficient to define it as a cholinergic neuron. The acetylcholine is packaged in synaptic vesicles (see Chapter 8) and is released following the arrival of an action potential at the nerve terminal via vesicle exocytosis. However, not all the acetylcholine in nerve terminals is in vesicles. Some is in the cytoplasm, and evidence exists for the direct release of acetylcholine from these cytoplasmic stores at some synapses.

Degradation and resynthesis. Following its release into the synaptic cleft, acetylcholine can bind to at least two distinct classes of receptor molecule and produce different responses in different target cells (see Chapter 11). However, the neurotransmitter does not remain at a high concentration in the synaptic cleft for very long. The fate of the released acetylcholine is to be destroyed by a powerful hydrolytic enzyme, *acetylcholinesterase*, which produces acetate and choline (Fig. 10–3). This enzyme is clustered at high concentrations in the synaptic cleft. In addition, its catalytic rate (of the order of 10^4 to 10^5 substrate molecules hydrolyzed per second) ranks it among the most rapid enzymes known, ensuring that the concentration of acetylcholine in the cleft drops very quickly following its re-

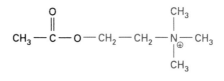

Acetylcholine

Figure 10–2. Chemical structure of acetylcholine.

lease. Much of the choline is then taken up again into the nerve terminal and utilized for the replenishment of the terminal's acetylcholine. Cholinergic nerve terminals contain a high-affinity sodium-dependent choline uptake system (Fig. 10–3) that provides a large proportion of the choline in the terminal and the activity of which is probably rate limiting for acetylcholine synthesis. As we shall see below, sodium-dependent uptake systems (or *transporters*) specific for particular neurotransmitters or for their precursors or metabolites are ubiquitous in nerve terminals and play an essential role in regulating the amount of neurotransmitter available for release.

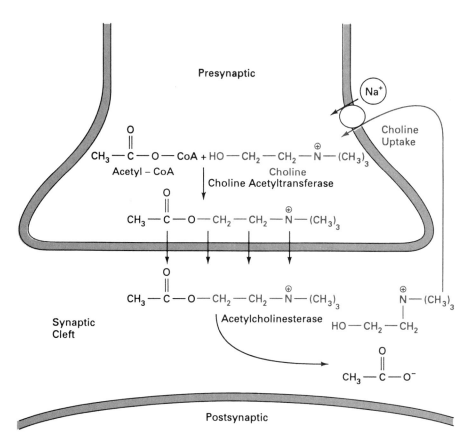

Figure 10–3. Synthesis, release, and degradation of acetylcholine. The transmitter is synthesized from choline and acetyl-CoA by the enzyme choline acetyltransferase. Following its release it is broken down rapidly by the enzyme acetylcholinesterase to choline and acetate. The choline can be taken back up into the terminal via a sodium-coupled choline transport system.

The Amine Neurotransmitters

Epinephrine and norepinephrine. During the period when Loewi and others established that acetylcholine is the chemical transmitter in peripheral *parasympathetic* nerves such as the vagus nerve, other neuropharmacologists were investigating the nature of synaptic transmission in the *sympathetic* nervous system, another component of the peripheral *autonomic* nervous system. There is a classic set of criteria that must be fulfilled to conclude that a particular compound is indeed a physiological transmitter substance. It was demonstrated early that the compound *norepinephrine* (Fig. 10–4) fulfills all the criteria for the sympathetic neurotransmitter, in that

1. it is synthesized and stored in high concentration in sympathetic nerve terminals;
2. it is released on stimulation of sympathetic nerves; and
3. it mimics the action of the endogenous transmitter when it is applied exogenously to target organs.

In addition, pharmacological agents that block the response to sympathetic nerve stimulation also antagonize the actions of exogenously applied norepinephrine. Norepinephrine can bind to several different classes of *adrenergic receptor* on the postsynaptic cell; these receptors can be distinguished on the basis of their pharmacological properties and the mechanisms they use to transduce the signal from the neurotransmitter into a response in the target cell (see Chapter 12).

For technical reasons it was much more difficult to establish a neurotransmitter role for norepinephrine in the central nervous system, but now this role is also widely accepted. Most of the brain synapses that use norepinephrine arise from neurons whose cell bodies lie in the *locus ceruleus*, a cluster of only several thousand neurons located in the midbrain.

Adrenergic synapses use either norepinephrine (noradrenaline) or its N-methylated derivative *epinephrine* (adrenaline) as their neurotransmitter (Fig. 10–4). The fuzziness in the distinction between neurotransmitters and hormones arises even in this most classic case of adrenergic transmission. Although most adrenergic synapses use norepinephrine as their

---

Figure 10–4. Biosynthesis of the catecholamines. The starting point for the synthesis of the catecholamines is the amino acid tyrosine. Hydroxylation of tyrosine to dihydroxyphenylalanine by the enzyme tyrosine hydroxylase is the rate-limiting step in the biosynthetic pathway.

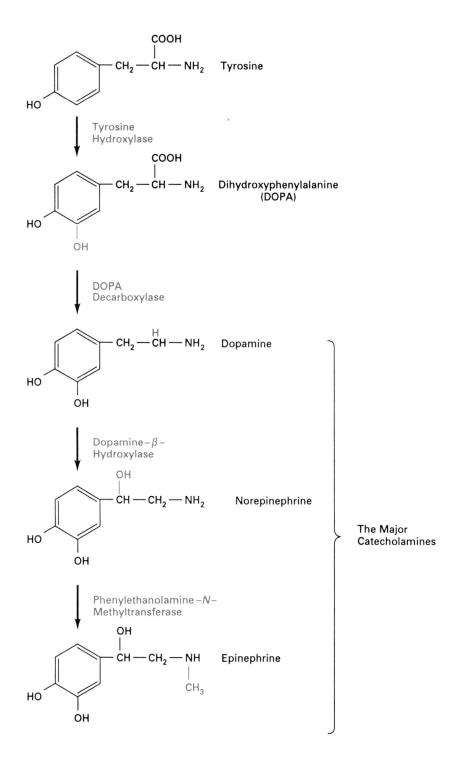

COOH
|
CH₂—CH—NH₂ Tyrosine

HO

↓ Tyrosine
Hydroxylase

COOH
|
CH₂—CH—NH₂ Dihydroxyphenylalanine
(DOPA)

HO

OH

↓ DOPA
Decarboxylase

H
|
CH₂—CH—NH₂ Dopamine

HO

OH

↓ Dopamine–β–
Hydroxylase

OH
|
CH—CH₂—NH₂ Norepinephrine

HO

OH

↓ Phenylethanolamine –N–
Methyltransferase

OH
|
CH—CH₂—NH Epinephrine
|
CH₃

HO

OH

The Major
Catecholamines

neurotransmitter, epinephrine is synthesized and stored at high concentrations in the *chromaffin cells* of the adrenal medulla and is released into the bloodstream to act as a hormone on many of the same target organs that receive sympathetic innervation. During embryonic development the adrenal medulla arises from the same precursor cells as the sympathetic neurons. They share many properties with sympathetic neurons and thus are widely used as a readily accessible model system for investigating adrenergic transmission (see Chapter 16).

Dopamine. Both norepinephrine and epinephrine belong to the general family of compounds known as *catecholamines*, organic molecules that contain an amine group as well as a catechol nucleus (a benzene ring with two adjacent hydroxyl substitutions—see Fig. 10–4). Another important member of this family is *dopamine*, which is an intermediate in the biosynthesis of norepinephrine and epinephrine, and is a major central nervous system neurotransmitter in its own right. In contrast to the relatively few adrenergic neurons in mammalian brain, there are several distinct nuclei—large collections of neurons—that contain dopamine, and dopaminergic axons are distributed in complex patterns to many parts of the brain. Dopamine systems play an essential role in certain motor functions as well as in behavior, mood, and perception. As we shall discuss briefly below, a number of debilitating diseases, including Parkinson's disease, schizophrenia, and bipolar illness, can be attributed at least in part to a dysfunction in dopaminergic pathways.

Synthesis, storage, and release of the catecholamines. The biosynthetic pathway for the catecholamines is diagrammed in Figure 10–4. The first step is the hydroxylation of the common amino acid tyrosine to dihydroxyphenylalanine (DOPA) via the enzyme *tyrosine hydroxylase*, which is found only in adrenal chromaffin cells and sympathetic neurons, and thus its presence is diagnostic of an adrenergic cell (analogous to choline acetyltransferase for cholinergic cell types). Tyrosine hydroxylase is the rate-limiting enzyme for catecholamine biosynthesis and is subject to complex regulatory control; for example, its activity can be modulated by products in the biosynthetic pathway, and its synthesis is controlled by factors (such as nerve growth factor, see Chapter 16) that affect the growth and differentiation of sympathetic neurons.

The subsequent step in the pathway involves the removal of the carboxyl group from DOPA via the enzyme *DOPA decarboxylase* to produce dopamine, the first of the major catecholamine neurotransmitters. Dopamine can then be hydroxylated on the β carbon by dopamine β-hydroxylase (dopamine β-oxidase) to produce norepinephrine, which can in turn be methylated to epinephrine by a phenylethanolamine-N-methyltrans-ferase (Fig. 10–4).

The catecholamines, like acetylcholine, are packaged into vesicles. The properties of catecholamine-containing vesicles have been studied most thoroughly in adrenal chromaffin cells (where they are called *chromaffin granules*) and sympathetic noradrenergic neurons, and it is assumed that the properties of the storage vesicles in central catecholaminergic neurons are similar. In addition to the neurotransmitter, catecholamine storage vesicles contain high concentrations of ATP (perhaps as high as 100 mM, about one-quarter the intravesicular concentration of the neurotransmitter) as well as a protein called *chromogranin*, whose function is only poorly understood but which may be involved in packaging and storage. Dopamine β-hydroxylase is also present in the granules, suggesting that at least one of the steps in the biosynthesis of norepinephrine occurs within the vesicles themselves.

The release of catecholamines from chromaffin cells occurs by exocytosis following the entry of calcium into the cell, presumably via voltage-dependent calcium channels as is the case for cholinergic neurons. Because of the large size of chromaffin granules (in the range of 0.1 μM, exocytosis can be observed directly in the microscope and can be studied with techniques such as capacitance measurements, as described in Chapter 8. Exocytosis has not yet been established, however, for other catecholamine-releasing neurons. In fact, it seems somewhat puzzling that a neuron would dump the energetically expensive contents of its adrenergic granules into the extracellular space. There is evidence that the ATP may play some role in communicating with adjacent cells, but this is probably not the case for the chromogranin and dopamine β-hydroxylase, which would have to be replaced via new protein synthesis and axonal transport, processes that are slow and might place an apparently unnecessary demand on the cell's energy resources. It is possible that the proteins remain associated with the vesicle membrane in some way that allows their reuptake, perhaps via active transport or endocytosis. Alternatively, the suggestion has arisen, as in the case of acetylcholine, that non-exocytotic release of the transmitter occurs.

Uptake and metabolism of the catecholamines. The actions of catecholamines on their target cells are terminated much more slowly than those of acetylcholine. There is no rapidly acting extracellular enzyme analogous to acetylcholinesterase. Instead, catecholamines are removed from the synaptic cleft by reuptake into the presynaptic cell. The uptake is the sodium-dependent transport process we have come across in our discussion of choline uptake and will meet again often before this chapter ends. The high-affinity active transport mechanism moves catecholamines against a concentration gradient and causes them to accumulate inside the pre-synaptic cell at a much higher concentration than that in the extracellular space.

The two major enzymes involved in the catabolism of catecholamines are *monoamine oxidase* (MAO) and *catechol O-methyltransferase* (COMT). The former catalyzes the metabolism of catecholamines to their corresponding aldehydes (Fig. 10–5), which can then be broken down further to products that leave the brain and are excreted. MAO is localized in the mitochondrial membrane of catecholaminergic terminals and helps to regulate the levels of catecholamines in these terminals. It is also present in other cell types in which its function is not understood. COMT catalyzes the methylation of one of the hydroxyl groups of the catechol nucleus (Fig. 10–5), again producing a product that is metabolized further and then excreted. Although COMT functions to metabolize catecholamines throughout the body, its precise localization and function in catecholaminergic transmission have yet to be determined. Inhibitors of MAO and COMT are important psychoactive drugs.

Catecholamine pharmacology and nervous system dysfunction. There is evidence that dysfunction in brain catecholamine pathways contributes to bipolar disorder and schizophrenia. The evidence is indirect, however, and is based largely on the fact that drugs that ameliorate the symptoms of these diseases interact with catecholamine systems. The classic finding is that a variety of MAO inhibitors such as pargyline, which cause a rise in brain catecholamine levels, are clinically effective antidepressants. A separate class of clinically effective compounds, the *tricyclic antidepressants*, such as imipramine, appear to prolong catecholamine action (predominantly at noradrenergic synapses) by inhibiting the high-affinity reuptake system. Findings such as these have given rise to the *catecholamine theory of affective disorder*, which in essence states that decreased activity at certain central noradrenergic synapses causes behavioral depression. In addition, according to this theory, mania results from excess activity at these synapses. The latter hypothesis is supported by the fact that the stimulant drug amphetamine increases activity in noradrenergic pathways, most likely by inhibiting the reuptake of the neurotransmitter. All of these data point to the sodium-dependent, high-affinity neurotransmitter uptake systems as essential for the proper functioning of central nervous system synapses (see below). More recently, serotonin has also been implicated in bipolar disorder.

The *catecholamine theory of psychotic illness* focuses on dysfunction at dopaminergic synapses. A variety of antipsychotic drugs, the classic example being chlorpromazine, are effective blockers of postsynaptic dopamine receptors. It is particularly compelling that several chemically diverse

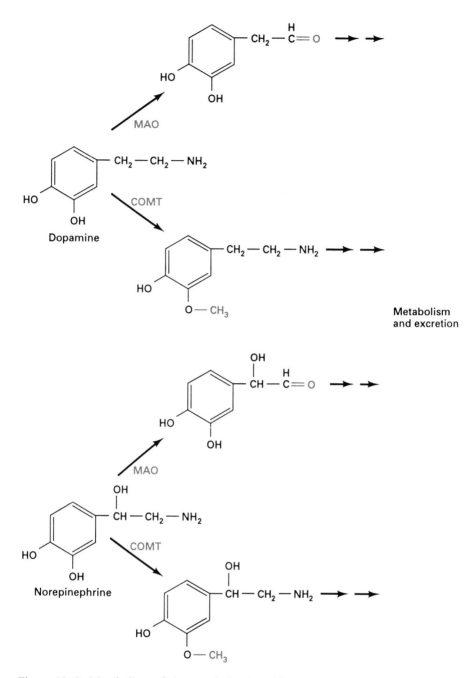

Figure 10–5. Metabolism of the catecholamines. Two enzymes, monoamine oxidase (MAO) and catechol-O-methyltransferase (COMT), catalyze the first steps in the degradation of the catecholamines.

233

groups of compounds (such as the butyrophenones, thioxanthenes, and phenothiazenes) all block dopamine receptors and ameliorate the symptoms of schizophrenia, giving rise to the hypothesis that excessive activity in dopaminergic pathways is responsible for schizophrenia. Again the evidence is indirect, but this has not deterred pharmaceutical companies from devoting enormous resources to the search for novel dopamine receptor blockers that might serve as antipsychotic drugs.

The role of dopaminergic pathways in certain motor functions is more firmly established in that there are anatomical findings to correlate with the pharmacology. The *basal ganglia*, several *nuclei*, or collections, of nerve cells deep in the brain, play an essential role in the control of body movements. The basal ganglia themselves receive inputs from the *substantia nigra*, a major dopamine-containing center in the brain, and influence the activity of the motor cortex via the thalamus (Fig. 10–6a).

Dopamine released by this pathway is essential for normal motor activity. The dopamine neurons that project from the substantia nigra to the *caudate nucleus*, one of the basal ganglia, can undergo pathological degeneration of unknown cause. As a result, the influence of the substantia nigra is removed (Fig. 10–6b), and this leads to characteristic motor dysfunction, including low-frequency tremor of the extremities at rest and impairment of postural reflexes. This degenerative disorder is called *Parkinson's disease*, after the English physician James Parkinson who first described the symptoms more than a century ago. With the realization that Parkinson's disease involves a degeneration of dopaminergic neurons, Arvid Carlsson and colleagues reasoned that it might be possible to alleviate the symptoms by introducing dopamine into the brain. Because dopamine cannot readily enter the brain from the blood, the treatment of choice is to administer DOPA, which does enter the brain and is converted to dopamine via the action of DOPA decarboxylase (Fig. 10–4). When Parkinson's patients are administered DOPA, together with an MAO inhibitor (Fig. 10–6c), there is a dramatic, albeit temporary, alleviation of symptoms. This is a striking example of a disease of the nervous system that is attributable to the loss of a particular neurotransmitter and that responds to a rational treatment. Carlsson was awarded the Nobel Prize for his role in identifying dopamine as a neurotransmitter and introducing DOPA therapy for Parkinson's patients. Unfortunately, DOPA treatment does not reverse the course of the disease, which involves a progressive degeneration and deterioration over a period of several years, but simply relieves the symptoms for some brief interval. As we shall see in subsequent chapters, the degeneration seen in Parkinson's disease shares certain features with other neurodegenerative disorders, including Alzheimer's disease, and there has been exciting recent progress in defining some of the molecular events that lead to neurodegeneration in these disorders.

Serotonin. Serotonin, or *5-hydroxytryptamine* (5-HT), is another neuroactive compound that is neither exclusively a hormone nor exclusively a classical neurotransmitter. Large quantities of serotonin are found in the circulation, for example, in platelets, as well as in the central nervous systems of vertebrates and invertebrates. Like the catecholamines, serotonin is synthesized from one of the common amino acids, in this case, tryptophan, which is taken up into neurons via a specific sodium-dependent uptake system and is hydroxylated in a reaction catalyzed by *tryptophan hydroxylase* (Fig. 10–7). As in the case of catecholamine biosynthesis, this initial reaction is the rate-limiting step in the formation of serotonin. The resulting 5-hydroxytryptophan is then immediately decarboxylated to produce serotonin. Serotonin is packaged into secretory granules and is pre-

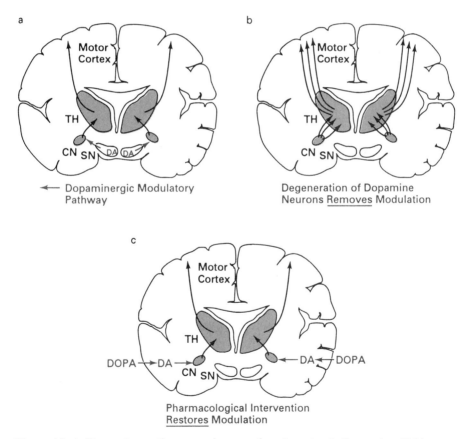

Figure 10–6. Dopamine pathways and motor functions (*a–c*). Dopamine (DA) neurons in the substantia nigra (SN) provide an important influence on motor functions. The DA neurons project to the caudate nucleus (CN), which in turn communicates with neurons in the thalamus (TH) that influence output from the motor cortex.

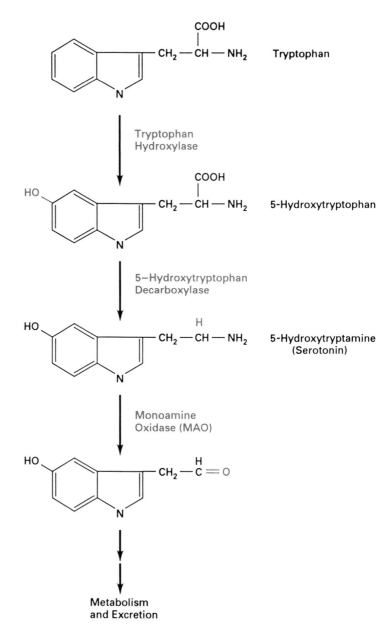

Figure 10–7. Synthesis and metabolism of serotonin (5-hydroxytryptamine, or 5-HT).

sumed to be released by a calcium-dependent exocytotic mechanism, then taken back up into the presynaptic terminal where it can be degraded by MAO (Fig. 10–7).

Serotonin is localized in discrete groups of neurons, largely in the brain stem, that send projections all over the brain. However, the precise role of serotonergic pathways remains obscure. Serotonin has been implicated in the regulation of sleep and "vigilance", and it is widely believed that hallucinogenic drugs such as lysergic acid diethylamide (LSD) may produce their effects by interacting with serotonin pathways. The experimental evidence is complex and does not fall into a readily interpreted pattern, but it appears that LSD may antagonize some and mimic other actions of serotonin. The drug Prozac and its relatives such as Zoloft, all of which are selective blockers of serotonin reuptake, are highly effective and widely used antidepressants, and have also been used successfully to treat a variety of less severe syndromes usually characterized as neuroses. The effectiveness of serotonin reuptake inhibitors such as Prozac indicates that dysfunction in serotoninergic pathways must contribute to affective disorders, but again, both the anatomical and molecular details are only poorly understood. In some invertebrates, for example, lobsters and the marine snail *Aplysia*, serotonin acts as a neurotransmitter/neurohormone to influence certain behaviors via mechanisms that are becoming reasonably well understood at the cellular and even molecular level (see Chapters 19 and 20).

More amines. We have not yet exhausted the category of amine neurotransmitters. For example, evidence is rapidly accumulating that histamine can affect neuronal activity in the mammalian (as well as in the invertebrate) central nervous system. Another important compound in many species is octopamine, which is closely related to dopamine and norepinephrine. The nucleotide ATP may be released at certain synapses together with catecholamines and influence neuronal properties, and the nucleoside adenosine can also regulate neuronal activity. Although we will not discuss these other candidates further, we remind the reader that the list of amine neurotransmitters is almost certain to be extended in the future.

Amino Acid Neurotransmitters

It should come as no surprise that it was at first difficult to demonstrate a neurotransmitter role for amino acids. Although such a role had been suspected for many years, how does one test the relevant criteria, for example, the presence of the compound in synaptic terminals, for compounds that occur in high concentration not only in neurons but in all cell types?

Of the three major amino acid neurotransmitters in the mammalian nervous system, γ-aminobutyric acid (GABA), glycine, and glutamic acid (Fig. 10–8), this problem has been particularly acute for the latter two, which are ubiquitous constituents of proteins; GABA, in contrast, is present almost exclusively in brain and was recognized early on as a probable neurotransmitter. In any event, accumulating evidence has put the doubts to rest, and it is now widely accepted that the large majority of central nervous system synapses use amino acids as their neurotransmitters.

Glutamate and other excitatory amino acid transmitters. Glutamic and aspartic acid and various synthetic analogs of these amino acids produce excitatory (depolarizing) responses on neurons in virtually every part of the mammalian brain. Glutamate has long been established as an excitatory neurotransmitter at insect and crustacean neuromuscular junctions, and it has now become widely accepted that its pharmacological actions in mammalian brain reflect the fact that it is the major excitatory brain neurotransmitter. Much of the evidence has been based on the demonstration of several different classes of receptor for glutamate in brain (see Chapter 11), and there is a great deal of current excitement about the possibility that one of these receptor classes may play an essential role in long-term plastic changes at synapses, both during development and in the adult (see Chapters 18 and 20). It is not clear whether aspartate can be classified as

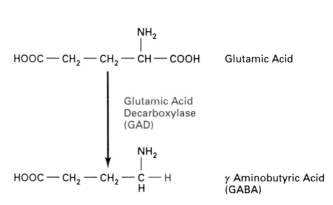

Figure 10–8. The major amino acid neurotransmitters.

a physiological neurotransmitter in its own right or whether it simply interacts with one or more of the glutamate receptor classes.

The details of glutamate synthesis and catabolism may be found in any standard textbook of biochemistry, so we will not dwell on them here. The way in which the synaptic actions of glutamate are terminated is not completely understood, but, as is the case for all the neurotransmitter candidates we have discussed, there is a sodium-dependent high-affinity glutamate transport system in neurons (as well as one in glia) that is likely to be involved (see below).

GABA *and glycine: the inhibitory amino acid neurotransmitters.* The involvement of GABA in neurotransmission has been much easier to determine. Again it was first established as an inhibitory neurotransmitter at an invertebrate synapse, in crustacean muscle. Attention was focused on its role in mammalian brain when it was found that its concentration there is much higher than in any other tissue. GABA is synthesized from glutamic acid via a reaction catalyzed by the enzyme *glutamic acid decarboxylase* (GAD) (Fig. 10–8), the presence of which is considered to be positive identification of a GABAergic neuron.

The location of proteins within the brain (or other tissues) can be found using a technique called *immunohistochemistry*, an important technique that we have seen before (see Plate 2) and shall encounter again, particularly in the chapters dealing with neuronal development and plasticity (Part IV). An antibody that binds specifically to a protein is incubated with fixed or frozen sections of brain tissue. The sections are then incubated again with a fluorescent or colored reagent that binds to and reveals the location of the antibody, and the pattern of distribution of the protein to which the antibody binds can be observed in the microscope. Such immunohistochemical investigations, using specific anti-GAD antibodies, have revealed that GABAergic terminals are present throughout the brain. Thus GABA appears to be the major inhibitory neurotransmitter in the mammalian central nervous system.

Synaptic terminals contain a sodium-dependent high-affinity GABA uptake system, and the major route of catabolism is via a mitochondrial GABA-α-oxoglutarate transaminase that regenerates glutamic acid. GABA is a particularly interesting neurotransmitter because its actions are subject to modulation by a variety of pharmacological agents that have profound effects on brain function; in the next chapter we shall discuss the ways some of these agents interact with GABA receptors to modulate GABAergic transmission.

The role of glycine in neurotransmission has not been easy to determine because, like glutamate, there is too much of it. It appears, however, to be the most important inhibitory neurotransmitter in the spinal cord and lower brain stem (and probably in the retina as well). As in the case of glutamate, much recent progress has come from the identification and isolation of specific receptors that mediate the postsynaptic actions of glycine. Glycine can also interact with at least one class of brain glutamate receptor and modulate glutamatergic transmission. The actions of glycine in the spinal cord are terminated by a specific sodium-dependent transport system in presynaptic endings (see below).

Neurotransmitter Transporters

We have emphasized throughout this chapter that a characteristic common to all of the small neurotransmitters is the existence of neuronal and glial plasma membrane uptake systems, which are responsible for halting neurotransmitter action and replenishing their supply in presynaptic terminals. In the case of acetylcholine at the neuromuscular junction, its action is terminated by enzymatic hydrolysis as we have seen earlier in this chapter, but the choline that is produced is then taken up by a specific transport system as well (see Fig. 10–3). The individual uptake systems are mediated by distinct transporter proteins, each of which is specific in that it prefers to transport a particular neurotransmitter. However, the various transporters do have common features. In particular, all require sodium to be present in the external medium and use the energy provided by the sodium concentration gradient across the membrane to concentrate neurotransmitters within the nerve terminal. That is, the movement of the neurotransmitter molecule into the cell is coupled obligatorily to the movement of sodium ions across the membrane.

Families of neurotransmitter transporters. Through molecular cloning we have learned that, like the ion channels, neurotransmitter transporters can be grouped into several families that exhibit distinct features of structure and function. One family contains transporters present in the membranes of synaptic vesicles. They are responsible for concentrating neurotransmitters from the cytoplasm into the vesicle prior to exocytosis during synaptic transmission; we will not discuss them further here. A second family contains the plasma membrane transporters for GABA, glycine, and a number of amines including norepinephrine, dopamine, and serotonin. The members of this family exhibit substantial sequence homology with one another and from hydrophobicity plots are predicted to have 12 membranespanning segments (Fig. 10–9a). For all of them, chloride ion is also an obligatory cosubstrate. The *stoichiometry* of the transport, the ratios of the three cotransported species, is 2 Na$^+$:1 Cl$^-$:1X, where X is the neuro-transmitter (Fig. 10–9b). As a result, the transport is *electrogenic*—that is, it will tend to change the membrane voltage, and indeed it is possible to record transmembrane currents associated with the activity of some of these neurotransmitter transporters. The combination of the chloride and sodium gradients allows the neurotransmitter to be concentrated in the synaptic terminal to concentrations as much as 10,000-fold higher than those in the extracellular space.

Interestingly, the transporters for glutamate fall into a distinct family of their own. Their sequences exhibit little homology to those of the Na$^+$- and Cl$^-$-dependent carriers, and they are predicted to have fewer membrane-spanning segments. In addition, their stoichiometry is differ-ent. Transport of glutamate is still associated with the cotransport of so-dium, but chloride cotransport is not required. Instead, there is counter-transport of potassium out of the cell, probably together with hydroxyl ions (Fig. 10–9b), with a stoichiometry of 2 Na$^+$:1 K$^+$:1 OH$^-$:1 gluta-mate. Thus, in addition to being electrogenic, activity of the glutamate transporters may produce a decrease in intracellular pH.

Diversity of neurotransmitter transporters. Although the diversity of the neu-rotransmitter transporters does not (yet) rival that of the calcium or potas-sium channels, there do appear to be several distinct transporters for most of the small molecule neurotransmitters. For example, multiple different transporters for GABA, glycine, and glutamate have been cloned. As in

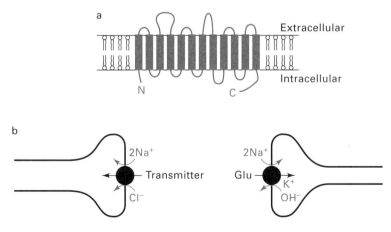

Figure 10–9. Neurotransmitter reuptake. *a*: Predicted structure of the sodium/chloride-dependent neurotransmitter transporters. *b*: Stoichiometries of the sodium/chloride-dependent (*left*) and the glutamate (*right*) transporters.

the case of ion channels, both multiple genes and alternative splicing of messenger RNA for a single gene contribute to the diversity. This molecular heterogeneity was not unexpected, because it has been known for a long time that there are differences in the affinity of the transporter for the neurotransmitter and in transporter pharmacology in different brain regions. In addition, there are differences in the cellular distribution of the different transporters for a given neurotransmitter. Experiments using immunohistochemistry as described above, as well as a companion technique known as *in situ hybridization*, through which a specific messenger RNA can be localized, have demonstrated that some transporters are expressed in neurons whereas others are restricted to glial cells. Recall from Chapter 2 that one of the important functions of glia is thought to be the regulation of synaptic transmission by the uptake and metabolism of neuronal neurotransmitters.

Structure and function in neurotransmitter transporters. As in the case of the ion channels, molecular approaches have been used to elucidate the relationship between sequence and function in the neurotransmitter transporters. Because the amine transporters are the physiological targets for a number of important drugs, including clinical antidepressant compounds and such stimulants as amphetamines and cocaine, there is much interest in using mutagenesis to identify the molecular determinants of drug action. An example of this approach is illustrated in Figure 10–10. Because

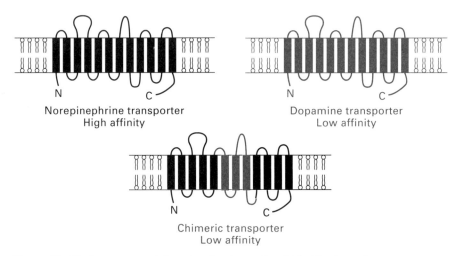

Norepinephrine transporter
High affinity

Dopamine transporter
Low affinity

Chimeric transporter
Low affinity

Figure 10–10. Structure and function in the sodium/chloride-dependent neurotransmitter transporters. The predicted structures of the dopamine and norepinephrine transporters are very similar, but they differ in their affinities for tricyclic antidepressants. A chimeric transporter reveals that the central domain is important for determining the affinity.

the transporters for dopamine and norepinephrine share substantial sequence identity but differ markedly in their affinities for the tricyclic antidepressants, chimeric transporters formed by combining pieces of each have been useful in identifying specific functional domains in the proteins (Fig. 10–10). For example, it has been found that the central section of the transporter, including the sixth, seventh, and eighth transmembrane segments, is the region of the protein that binds to these clinically important drugs. This finding that there are discrete structural modules in transporters that are largely responsible for specific functions is reminiscent of the situation for ion channels that we described in earlier chapters.

The Peptides

By the early 1970s a consistent pattern was emerging of neurotransmitter candidates in the central nervous system. Acetylcholine, serotonin, and the catecholamines were well established as major brain neurotransmitters, and although the transmitters at many central synapses remained unidentified, suspicions were beginning to arise that amino acids might fill this gap. The recognition that *neuroactive peptides* are more than simply hormones that are released to carry out actions on targets outside the brain, that they play a crucial role within the central nervous system, has made it clear just how naive this simple picture was.

Neuropeptides share some of the characteristics of the small molecule neurotransmitters. For example, like many classical transmitters, some neuropeptides are released to the circulation and act at a distance, while others are confined to a discrete synaptic cleft. As mentioned at the beginning of this chapter, it will not be profitable to focus on the largely semantic distinction between neurotransmitters and neurohormones. Nevertheless, the neuropeptides do differ in many respects from their smaller counterparts. Table 10–1 lists some of the properties of peptide neurotransmitters that tend to distinguish them from the classical neurotransmitters. Because

Table 10–1 Properties of Peptide Neurotransmitters

Synthesized as a larger precursor protein at the soma and transported to release sites; must be replenished by synthesis at soma

Slow postsynaptic effects

Actions terminated by extracellular proteases or by diffusion

Coreleased with classical neurotransmitters

Can trigger complex coordinated behaviors

Actions do not require point-to-point synaptic connections

these are not all true at every location at which peptidergic transmission occurs, they are more appropriately termed trends rather than properties.

The roster of putative peptide neurotransmitters continues to grow at an enormous pace (Table 10–2), and we cannot do justice to this rapidly developing field in a short space. We will limit ourselves here to describing just a few of the neuroactive peptides, with emphasis on the historic development of this field and some examples of the trends listed in Table 10–1.

Substance P. The story of the peptides actually began as far back as the 1930s, with the accidental discovery of substance P. While screening various tissues for acetylcholine, Ulf von Euler and John Gaddum found a compound in brain and intestine that caused a lowering of blood pressure and contraction of intestinal smooth muscle. Because its actions were not blocked by the cholinergic antagonist atropine, they concluded that this compound could not be acetylcholine, and named it substance P (for *powder*). Although von Euler suggested as early as 1936 that substance P might

Table 10–2 Samples of Some Thoroughly Studied Neuroactive Peptides

Peptide	Sequence[a]
Substance P	RPKPQQFFGLM-NH$_2$
Neurotensin	pELYENKPRRPYIL
Vasoactive intestinal peptide	HSDAVFTDNYTRLRKQMAVKKYLNSILN
Thyrotropin-releasing hormone (TRH)	pEHB-NH$_2$
Luteinizing hormone–releasing hormone (LHRH)	pEHWSYGLRPG-NH$_2$
Oxytocin	CYIQNCPLG-NH$_2$
Vasopressin	CYFQNCP$_K^R$G-NH$_2$
α-Endorphin	YGGFMTSEKSQTPLVT
Met-enkephalin	YGGFM
FMRFamide	FMRF-NH$_2$
Proctolin	RYLPT
Egg-laying hormone (ELH)	ISINQDLKAITDMLLTEQIRERQRYLADLRQRLLEKG-NH$_2$

[a]Single letter amino acid code: A, Ala; R, Arg; N, Asn; D, Asp; C, Cys; Q, Gln; E, Glu; G, Gly; H, His; I, Ile; L, Leu; K, Lys; M, Met; F, Phe; P, Pro; S, Ser; T, Thr; W, Trp; Y, Tyr; V, Val. A small p at the N-terminal indicates a pyroglutamate; some C-terminals are amidated (NH$_2$).

be a protein, it was to be more than 30 years before its structure was determined. Substance P is an 11 amino acid peptide that is present, as determined by direct bioassay and immunohistochemical studies, throughout the mammalian brain. It is thought to be a synaptic transmitter in sensory pathways concerned with pain and touch. It is, in fact, found in neurons that innervate tooth pulp, where the only known sensory modality is pain. Substance P was the first, and remains among the best understood, of the so-called brain-gut peptides, neuroactive substances found in both the central nervous system and the gastrointestinal tract. There are now numerous examples of this localization pattern, which reflects the fact that the gut is densely innervated.

Hypothalamic peptides. As mentioned previously, the hypothalamus is the site of synthesis of the two classical neurohormones, oxytocin and vasopressin. In addition to affecting peripheral tissues, oxytocin and vasopressin can alter the firing patterns of central neurons, and vasopressin in particular has been reported to have behavioral effects in rats and humans. The magnocellular neurons in which these peptides are synthesized project not only to the pituitary circulation but also to a variety of sites within the brain, and the immunohistochemical localizations of oxytocin and vasopressin are consistent with their involvement in synaptic transmission (Fig. 10–11).

Also synthesized in the hypothalamus are other biologically active peptides, the *releasing factors* or *releasing hormones.* The releasing hormones enter the portal circulation, which brings them to the anterior pituitary where they regulate the release of another group of pituitary peptide hormones. These in turn act on peripheral tissues. For example, the release of *thyroid-stimulating hormone* (thyrotropin or TSH), which enters the general circulation from the pituitary to act on the thyroid gland, is promoted by *thyrotropin-releasing hormone* (TRH) from the hypothalamus (Fig. 10–11). Much TRH is also found in other brain regions where it may act as a local hormone or neurotransmitter. This is true for other releasing factors as well.

Luteinizing hormone–releasing hormone (LHRH) is another of the releasing factors. It was in fact the first peptide to be shown convincingly to be the neurotransmitter at a particular synapse, an excitatory synapse in the frog sympathetic ganglion. This synapse illustrates many of the trends listed in Table 10–1. Stimulation of the presynaptic fibers produces a complex set of responses in the postsynaptic ganglion cells. In addition to a slow synaptic inhibition that we will not discuss here, three distinct temporal phases of synaptic excitation are evoked by the stimulation; the fast excitatory postsynaptic potential (EPSP), the slow EPSP, and the late slow EPSP (Fig. 10–12a). The fast and slow EPSPs are both due to the action of acetylcholine, acting at two distinct receptors (see Chapters 11 and 12). The late slow EPSP, which can last for 5 min or longer, is due to the action of an LHRH-like peptide. It is mimicked by application of LHRH (Fig. 10–12b) and can be blocked by drugs that are known to block other (non-neuronal) actions of LHRH. The LHRH-mediated postsynaptic potential is observed in two types of sympathetic ganglion neurons, the large B cells and the smaller C cells. Interestingly, the LHRH-containing presynaptic fibers do not synapse on the B cells directly. The postsynaptic re-

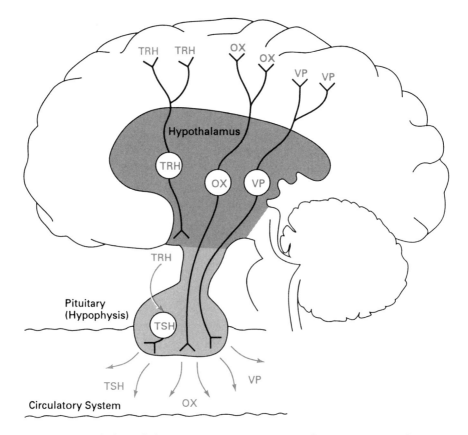

Figure 10–11. The hypothalamus is an important source of neuroactive peptides. Oxytocin (OX) and vasopressin (VP) neurons project to the posterior pituitary (also called the *neurohypophysis*) where the peptides are released to the general circulation. Releasing hormones, here exemplified by thyrotropin-releasing hormone (TRH), reach the anterior pituitary (*adenohypophysis*) via the portal circulation and stimulate release of hormones such as thyrotropin (TSH). The hypothalamic peptides can also act as brain neurotransmitters (see Silverman and Zimmerman, 1983).

sponse in the B cells occurs because the released LHRH can diffuse to them from the release sites micrometers away. This illustrates that point-to-point wiring of synapses is not required for this synaptic response.

The slow time course of the postsynaptic response can also be shown to be due to the lingering presence of LHRH at the postsynaptic cells. If a drug that blocks the actions of LHRH is applied during a postsynaptic potential, the response is terminated immediately, indicating that the continued action of LHRH is required to maintain the response. Finally, LHRH is one of the peptides that can produce prolonged and complex behavior in an animal. There is no "acetylcholine behavior" or "GABA behavior," but there is an "LHRH behavior." If LHRH is administered into the brains of female rats, it evokes a complex and stereotyped pattern of sexual behavior.

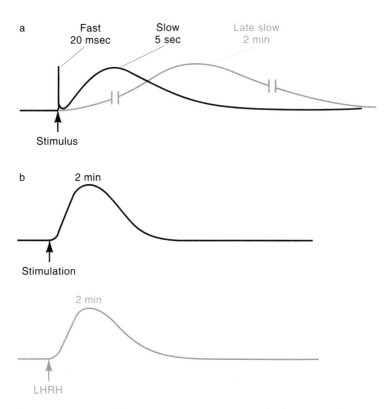

Figure 10–12. Long-lasting synaptic responses in the frog sympathetic ganglion. *a*: Preganglionic stimulation results in three excitatory (and one inhibitory) synaptic responses in ganglionic neurons. Their time courses differ by four orders of magnitude. *b*: Application of luteinizing hormone–releasing hormone (LHRH) mimics the late slow excitatory postsynaptic potential (EPSP).

Opioid peptides. The age of the peptides was ushered in with a vengeance in the mid-1970s with the description of the *enkephalins* and other opioid peptides. The story of the opioid peptides is particularly interesting because their discovery was not simply serendipitous but resulted from a rational search for endogenous compounds that might mimic the actions of morphine and other opiates.

Throughout recorded history it has been known that the juice of the poppy produces feelings of euphoria and is a highly effective painkiller. The active ingredient, morphine (named after Morpheus, the Greek god of dreams), was first isolated almost 200 years ago. By the early 1970s it was reasoned that the actions of morphine and other opiates must result from their binding to specific receptor sites in the brain, and it became possible to demonstrate the binding of radioactive opiates to brain membranes. The next assumption was that if the brain contains specific receptor sites, there must be endogenous ligands that bind to and activate these receptors.

Two compounds with such properties were indeed found. They were first isolated by their ability to produce *analgesia*, relief from pain, in bioassays for pain relievers. These compounds are pentapeptides of similar structure, which were named *Met-enkephalin* and *Leu-enkephalin* because they differ only in their carboxyl-terminal amino acids:

Tyr-Gly-Gly-Phe-*Met*   *Met*-enkephalin

Tyr-Gly-Gly-Phe-*Leu*   *Leu*-enkephalin

Synthetic enkephalins were also soon shown to be potent opiates in the standard bioassays for analgesics.

It was noted that the entire structure of Met-enkephalin is contained in amino acid residues 61–65 of a much larger pituitary hormone, the 91 amino acid β-lipotropin, which had been isolated and sequenced several years earlier but whose function was obscure. Within a year after the description of the enkephalins it had become evident that at least three additional longer peptides with opioid-like activity, the *endorphins*, are contained within the sequence of β-lipotropin. Immunohistochemical experiments have demonstrated that the enkephalins and endorphins are distributed widely in the brain, but do not appear to be colocalized within the same neurons.

The enkephalin/endorphin story emphasizes another important way the peptides differ from the more classical neurotransmitter candidates (see Table 10–1). The latter tend to be small molecules that can be synthesized and metabolized by enzymes present in nerve terminals, whereas the peptides must be synthesized by the protein biosynthetic machinery, presumably in the cell bodies, and undergo complex processing and packaging (see Chapter 8) before they can be released to exert their biological effects. Questions as to how peptide stores can be replenished rapidly to sustain release for long periods of time have not yet been resolved; this replenishment does not seem to be a problem for the classical neurotransmitters.

The finding that the endorphins and enkephalins are contained within a larger precursor was not entirely surprising, since it was known that many peptide hormones, for example, insulin and the original neurohormones oxytocin and vasopressin, are synthesized as larger prohormones and then processed proteolytically to produce the active hormone (see Chapter 8). In fact, β-lipotropin is contained within a much larger and more complex precursor. Molecular cloning approaches have enabled investigators to demonstrate that the actual precursor is a polypeptide that contains within its sequence the structure of the pituitary hormone corticotropin (ACTH) as well as of the opioid peptides and several other naturally occurring peptides of unknown function. This rather astonishing discovery has many ramifications. For example, in Chapter 19 we shall discuss the physiology of neurons that use several peptide neurotransmitters. Each of these is cleaved from a different part of a single precursor protein (see Fig. 8–6b).

Some invertebrate peptides. Invertebrates have been a rich source of neuroactive peptides, some of which are also present in vertebrate nervous systems (Table 10–2). Among the best studied of the invertebrate neuropeptides are the pentapeptide *proctolin*, first isolated from the cockroach hindgut, the snail tetrapeptide *FMRFamide*, and the 36 amino acid *Aplysia egg-laying hormone* (ELH). The genes encoding the precursors for some of these peptides show remarkable homologies to certain mammalian neuropeptides. Furthermore, the large size and ready identifiability of many invertebrate neurons are experimental advantages that have allowed the physiological roles of some of these peptides to be investigated in considerable detail. For example, the synthesis, processing, and release of ELH by the neurosecretory bag cell neurons of *Aplysia*, as well as its mechanism of action on target neurons, are becoming well understood. Similarly, the actions of proctolin in modulating behavioral patterns in the lobster have been thoroughly analyzed at the cellular level. Some of these systems will be discussed in more detail in subsequent chapters.

Colocalization of peptides and classical neurotransmitters. The pharmacologist Henry Dale suggested many years ago that a given neuron synthesizes only a single neurotransmitter and releases only that transmitter at all its terminals. However, there is now convincing histochemical evidence that some neurons contain one or more neuropeptides *and* a classical neurotransmitter, packaged in different vesicles but often present in the same synaptic terminal.

It is not known precisely what advantages this offers a neuron. It has become clear, however, that the different transmitters need not be released at the same time. In several cases it has been found that only the classical transmitter is released by low-frequency stimulation, and corelease of the peptide requires short bursts of high-frequency stimulation. It is not evident how the selective release of one transmitter, and not another, comes about, but it may have to do with the very different patterns of calcium distribution expected in a nerve terminal invaded by low- and high-frequency action potentials. At low firing frequency there will be brief and highly localized changes in calcium immediately under the membrane and adjacent to the voltage-dependent calcium channels, whereas calcium levels elsewhere, for example, away from the membrane, will be little affected. At higher rates of stimulation, however, calcium levels will increase progressively with each action potential during a burst, and a substantial elevation will also occur away from the immediate vicinity of the calcium channels. Thus if the peptide-containing vesicles undergo exocytosis only at high levels of calcium, or if they are preferentially located at a distance from the membrane, peptide release will occur only with higher frequencies of presynaptic stimulation (Fig. 10–13). We can see, then, that the coexistence of different neurotransmitters in distinct vesicle populations within a single neuron allows that neuron to produce different effects on a postsynaptic target, depending on the precise pattern of stimulation.

Questions about the functional significance of such colocalization of neurotransmitters can be broadened to ask why, in fact, there are so many neuroactive substances. In principle a nervous system could function with just two neurotransmitters, one to mediate excitation and the other for inhibition. Indeed, as we shall see in the next two chapters, since there are multiple receptors for most (if not all) neurotransmitters, even a *single* neurotransmitter might in principle be sufficient and the excitatory or inhibitory nature of the response could be determined by the type of receptor that happens to be present on the target cell. We do not have a definitive answer to this dilemma, but again a reasonable explanation is that multiple neuroactive substances provide both a wide range of times over which the response endures and a wide range in the character of the response. It is a mistake to think of neurons as simply on or off, active or inactive, excited or inhibited. Rather, as we have seen in Chapters 3–7, neurons contain a variety of different ion channels that allow their activity to be modulated in subtle ways, and it may be that a multiplicity of transmitters (and receptors) has evolved to participate in this fine tuning of neuronal function.

Summary

A multitude of chemicals called *neurotransmitters* mediate intercellular communication in the nervous system. Some of them have been well understood for well over half a century, yet new ones are still appearing. Although they exhibit great diversity in many of their properties, all are stored in vesicles in nerve terminals and are released to the extracellular space via a process requiring calcium ions. Their actions are terminated

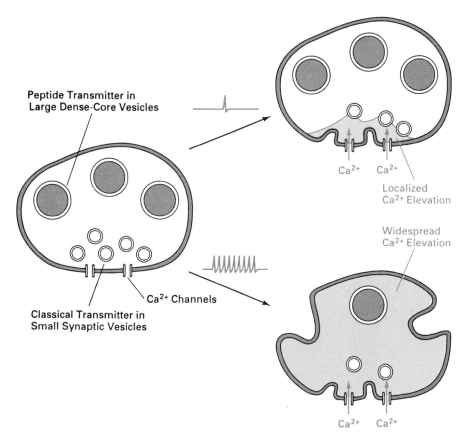

Figure 10–13. The release of classical and peptide neurotransmitters at synaptic endings. A hypothesis for the selective release of classical neurotransmitters at low frequencies of stimulation and for corelease of both types of transmitters during rapid bursts of action potentials.

by reuptake into the presynaptic terminal or nearby glial cells, by specific transporter proteins. The role of neurotransmitters is to alter the properties, chemical and/or electrical, of some target cell. With the arrival on the scene of the peptides, it has become evident that signaling in the nervous system occurs through the use of rich and varied forms of chemical currency, and that some neurons use more than one type of currency simultaneously.

Receptors and Transduction Mechanisms I: Receptors Coupled Directly to Ion Channels

*A*ll of the neuroactive substances we discussed in the previous chapter alter some property of a target neuron. This effect on the target cell is highly specific for the particular neurotransmitter or neurohormone. How does a neuron know just which of the many possible chemical signals it is being tickled by, and how does it decide on a response appropriate for that signal? Obviously the answers to these questions are crucial for understanding intercellular communication in the nervous system. In this and the following chapter we will discuss the neurotransmitter and hormone receptors that recognize the signaling molecules, and the transduction mechanisms that convert the extracellular signal into a response, usually (but not always) electrical, in the target neuron. The focus of this chapter is on neurotransmitter receptors that are coupled *directly* to the ion channels whose activity they regulate (Fig. 11–1). In the next chapter we will discuss *indirect* receptor–channel coupling mechanisms (compare Fig. 12–1). We emphasize here, as we have previously, that these mechanisms are not restricted to nerve cells. Other cell types have receptors for intercellular signaling molecules and convert the signal into some biological response. Neurons are unusual in that their biological response is normally a change in voltage that ultimately alters transmitter release, allowing the signal to be passed along from one neuron to another in a multineuronal pathway.

Specificity of Responses

The pharmacological concept of specific receptor structures has been with us for almost a century. Pharmacologists recognized many years ago that drugs that produce specific effects must interact with specific sites on or in the cell. It became possible to build up a pharmacological profile of a receptor by identifying drugs that produce a particular response (receptor *agonists*), and other drugs that inhibit the response to agonists (receptor *antagonists*). Furthermore, the concentrations at which these various agonists and antagonists are effective can be measured, to provide a quan-

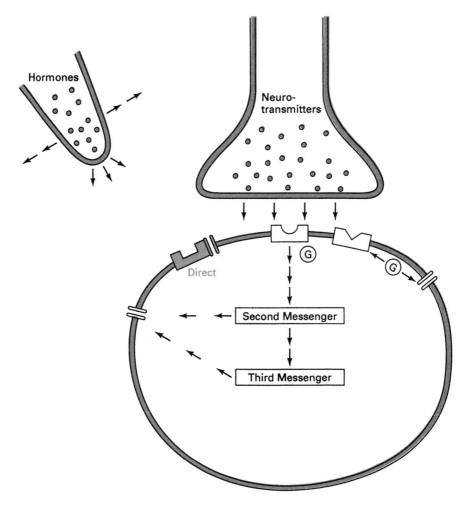

Figure 11–1. Intercellular communication. This chapter will discuss receptors for neurotransmitters that are coupled directly to the ion channels that they regulate (*blue*).

titative pharmacological profile. The earliest examples of such pharmaco-logical distinctions arose from studies with the first identified neurotrans-mitter, acetylcholine.

Although acetylcholine was found to be the transmitter substance at neuromuscular junctions, in sympathetic and parasympathetic ganglia of the peripheral autonomic nervous system, and in postganglionic parasym-pathetic neurons, the pharmacological profile was not identical for all re-sponses to acetylcholine. Instead it was found that nicotine and related compounds can act as agonists at neuromuscular junctions in skeletal mus-cle, but not in cardiac muscle, and only at some cholinergic synapses in the autonomic nervous system (Fig. 11–2). Furthermore, responses at these *nicotinic* synapses, but not at the others, could be blocked by compounds such as hexamethonium and the plant alkaloid curare (Table 11–1). It is

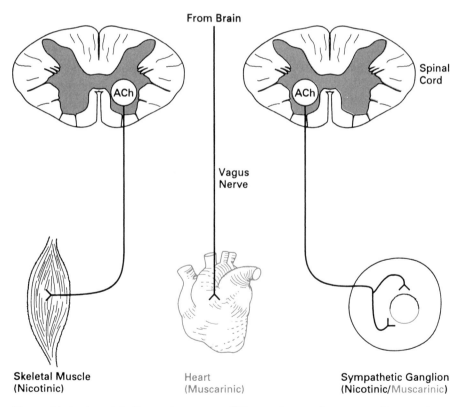

Figure 11–2. Acetylcholine activates two different classes of receptors. Some actions of acetylcholine (ACh) released from cranial or spinal neurons can be mimicked by nicotine, whereas others can be mimicked by muscarine. The receptors that mediate these different classes of response are termed *nicotinic* and *muscarinic*, respectively.

worth noting that this pharmacology has been understood for a very long time by South American tribes that use curare at the tips of their arrows to paralyze prey.

In contrast, the action of acetylcholine at other cholinergic synapses can be mimicked by muscarine but not by nicotine (Fig. 11–2) and blocked by atropine and quinuclidinylbenzylate but not curare (Table 11–1). It now appears that such *muscarinic* synapses account for a large proportion of the cholinergic synapses in the mammalian central nervous system. The two cholinergic synaptic responses in frog sympathetic ganglion that we discussed in the last chapter, the fast and slow excitatory postsynaptic potentials (EPSPs; see Fig. 10–12), result from the actions of acetylcholine at nicotinic and muscarinic receptors, respectively (see also Fig. 11–2).

Although this breakdown of acetylcholine responses into two distinct groups seems to make life much more complicated for the harassed neuroscientist trying to understand transmitter actions, it is only the tip of the iceberg. As shown in Table 11–2, virtually every neurotransmitter is now known to interact with more than a single class of receptor; acetylcholine, for example, not only has two major classes of receptor but within the muscarinic and nicotinic classes multiple different subtypes exist. About the time the pharmacology of acetylcholine responses was being clarified, norepinephrine was also shown to interact with more than a single class of receptor, and the number of adrenergic receptor subtypes has increased over the years as new, more specific pharmacological tools have become available. Similarly, the amines, the excitatory and inhibitory amino acids, and the peptides all can mediate multiple responses in target cells (Table 11–2). As we shall see below, the structural basis for these multiple responses is becoming understood as methods for measuring receptor properties have become available and as the techniques of molecular cloning have been brought to bear on the receptor molecules.

Table 11–1 Two Pharmacologically Distinct Receptors for Acetylcholine

| Receptor Type | Some Examples of | | Responding Cell Type |
	Agonists	Antagonists	
Nicotinic	Acetylcholine	Hexamethonium	Skeletal muscle
	Nicotine	Curare	Sympathetic neurons
			Parasympathetic neurons
			Some brain neurons
Muscarinic	Acetylcholine	Atropine	Smooth muscle
	Muscarine	Scopolamine	Sympathetic neurons
	Oxotremorine	Quinuclidinylbenzylate	Gland cells
			Heart cells
			Many brain neurons

Receptor-Binding Assays: From Concept to Physical Entity

We have mentioned that the pharmacological concept of specific receptor sites for transmitters has been around for some time. It is only in the last 30 years, however, that techniques have become available for the direct measurement of membrane receptors. The development of *ligand-binding assays* for this purpose has confirmed the diversity of receptors inferred from the pharmacology of neurotransmitter responses. Furthermore, binding assays have enormously expanded our understanding of receptor structure and function, and so it is important to understand this approach and the kinds of information it can provide.

The fundamentals of the ligand-binding assay are shown in Figure 11–3. The term *ligand* (from the Latin *ligare*, to tie or bind) is used to denote a molecule that will bind to the receptor under study. The ligand is labeled in some way, usually with radioactivity but occasionally with a fluorescent probe, and is incubated together with plasma membrane fragments from cells that contain the receptor (Fig. 11–3a). After an appropriate period of time to allow the ligand to bind to receptors on the plasma membrane fragments, the bound ligand is separated from the remaining free ligand (the ligand is added in large excess, so that even when all receptor sites are occupied there will still be some free ligand). The amount

Table 11–2 Examples of Neurotransmitters and Neuromodulators That Interact With More Than One Class of Receptor

Neurotransmitter/Neuromodulator	Receptor Class
Acetylcholine	Nicotinic
	Muscarinic
Adenosine	A_1, A_2, A_3
Norepinephrine	α-Adrenergic
	β-Adrenergic
Histamine	H_1, H_2, H_3
Dopamine	Multiple subtypes
Serotonin	Multiple subtypes
GABA	$GABA_A$
	$GABA_B$
	$GABA_C$
Glutamate	NMDA
	KA/AMPA
	Metabotropic
Opioid peptides	μ, δ, κ

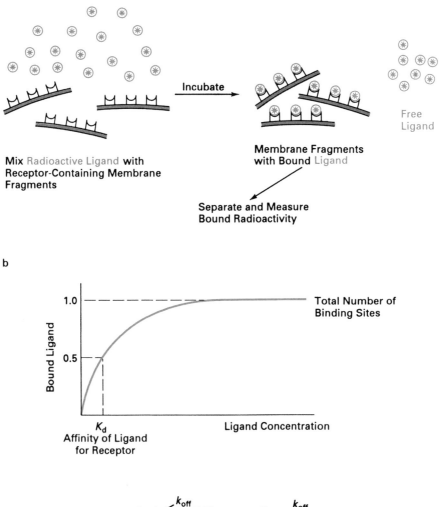

a

Incubate →

Free Ligand

Membrane Fragments with Bound Ligand

Mix Radioactive Ligand **with Receptor-Containing Membrane Fragments**

Separate and Measure Bound Radioactivity

b

Bound Ligand

1.0

0.5

K_d
Affinity of Ligand
for Receptor

Ligand Concentration

Total Number of Binding Sites

$$R + L \xrightleftharpoons[k_{on}]{k_{off}} RL \qquad K_d = \frac{k_{off}}{k_{on}}$$

Figure 11–3. Ligand-binding assays for receptors. *a*: Radioactive ligands (L, *blue*) that bind to the membrane receptor under investigation (R, *black*) can be used to characterize some properties of the receptor. *b*: Under appropriate conditions the ligand-binding assay can provide a measure of the number of receptors, and of their affinity (K_d) for the ligand. K_{off}, dissociation rate constant. K_{on}, association rate constant.

of radioactivity bound can be measured, and under appropriate conditions it provides a measure of the number of specific binding sites. Binding studies can also provide an estimate of *affinity*, a measure of how tightly the ligand binds to the receptor (Fig. 11–3b).

Such binding assays are easy to perform, usually far easier than assays of the biological response mediated by the receptor. Moreover, it is possible to test rapidly whether a wide variety of compounds are possible receptor agonists and antagonists by determining whether they can compete with the radioactive ligand for binding to the receptor (Fig. 11–4a). When the amount of bound ligand is plotted as a function of the concentration of the different competitors (A_1–A_4 in Fig. 11–4b), a family of curves is generated. The concentration ($K_{1/2}$) at which these compounds displace half the radioactive ligand is characteristic for a given receptor. In other words, a detailed pharmacological profile of the binding site can be generated readily, without the need for radioactive labeling of each compound to be tested. Such studies have allowed the precise pharmacological definition of various receptor subtypes, some of which are summarized in Table 11–2. It will be evident that the ligand for these experiments must be chosen with care. Using the neurotransmitter itself is generally inappropriate, since most transmitters will bind simultaneously to several different classes of binding site, and this will hopelessly confound attempts to define the pharmacology. However, it usually is possible to find a selective ligand that binds only to one or another subset of the receptors for a particular neurotransmitter. These kinds of receptor binding assays have been and continue to be widely used by the pharmaceutical industry to identify and characterize novel drugs that interact with specific neurotransmitter receptors.

It is essential, however, to keep in mind that *a binding site is not necessarily a physiological receptor*. Recall that neurotransmitters must bind to a variety of proteins including uptake systems and metabolic enzymes (Chapter 10). To determine whether a binding site is a real receptor, it is necessary to compare its pharmacology with that of the biological response mediated by the receptor. Only if the pharmacological profiles coincide can one be confident that the binding site and the receptor are the same. This can be illustrated by one of the earliest examples of a ligand-binding assay, the use of [^{3}H]-naloxone to quantify opiate receptors. Naloxone is well known as an opiate antagonist, and in the early 1970s several groups demonstrated that a specific binding site for [^{3}H]-naloxone is present in the brain. When the ability of various opiate agonists and antagonists to compete for naloxone binding was compared with their potencies in producing or antagonizing analgesia, it was found that their effective concentrations were very similar in the two assays (Fig. 11–4c). These find-

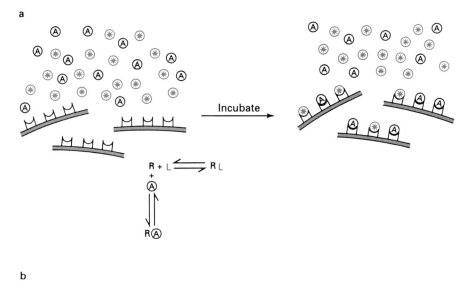

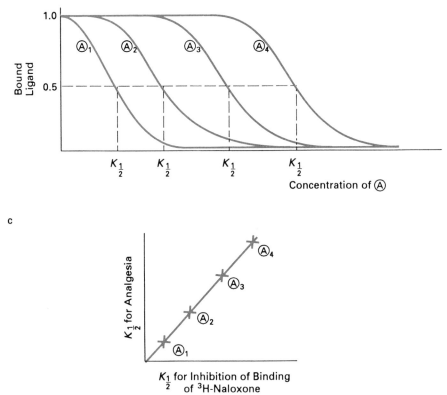

Figure 11–4. Ligand-binding assays can be used to determine the pharmacological profile of the receptor. *a*: The equilibrium between the ligand (L) and the receptor (R) can be disturbed by including in the assay a receptor agonist or antagonist (A). *b*: Plot of the amount of radioactive ligand bound at different concentrations of various agonists or antagonists (A_1–A_4). *c*: The pharmacological profile for inhibition of binding can be compared with the pharmacological profile of the same series of agonists and antagonists in some biological response mediated by the receptor. $K_{1/2}$, concentration of A required for half maximal inhibition of ligand binding.

ings strongly suggest that the [^{3}H]-naloxone binding sites in brain are indeed functional opiate receptors. Subsequently, competition for the binding of radioactive opiates was one of the assays used to identify and purify endogenous opiates, the enkephalins, as described in Chapter 10.

Pharmacological Diversity of Receptors Reflects Structural Diversity

What is the molecular underpinning for these pharmacologically distinct classes of receptor for a single neurotransmitter? Are there multiple receptor molecules, as we have seen for ion channels and neurotransmitter transporters, or can a single receptor molecule take on different pharmacological guises? These questions could be answered definitively only by isolating receptor molecules. It did not escape the attention of receptorologists that, in addition to providing an assay for receptors in their normal membrane-bound state, ligand binding might be used to measure numbers of receptor molecules during purification. Furthermore, appropriate ligands might be exploited not only for assay but also as reagents to be used in purification—as *affinity reagents*. Let us take as a classic example the first neurotransmitter receptor to be purified by methods based on these concepts, the nicotinic acetylcholine receptor and its associated ion channel. It was the first because it was the easiest; a high-affinity and highly selective ligand was available, and there was a rich source of receptor in the electric organs of certain eels and fish.

A *toxin that binds to nicotinic acetylcholine receptors.* Certain creatures appear to have been designed by evolution as gifts to neurobiologists. The story of the nicotinic acetylcholine receptor, like that of the ionic mechanism of the action potential, belongs to two groups of such animals, each with its unique specializations for survival. The first group is a family of snakes whose venoms contain toxins that bind with extremely high affinity and selectivity to the nicotinic acetylcholine receptor. These snakes paralyze and kill their prey by blocking neuromuscular transmission with the toxins. The most thoroughly characterized of these toxins is *α-bungarotoxin*, from the venom of the Taiwanese cobra *Bungarus multicinctus*. This toxin is a polypeptide of 74 amino acids, which binds to the nicotinic receptor with a dissociation constant in the range of 10^{-15} M (Fig. 11–5). Once it binds to the receptor the half-time for its dissociation is many days! This makes it an ideal reagent for receptor assay and affinity purification.

A *rich source of nicotinic acetylcholine receptors.* The second set of creatures that has contributed so greatly to our understanding of the nicotinic receptor are various species of the genus *Torpedo*, the electric rays, and the genus *Electrophorus*, the electric eels. The electric organs in these animals consist of modified muscle cells, which are flattened and organized in parallel arrays known as *electroplaques*. These cells have lost their contractile apparatus and have neuromuscular junctions that cover virtually the entire surface of one of the flattened faces of the cell, but not the other. The geometry of the electroplaque is such that voltage differences across the many cells add in series, producing a very large voltage that can stun prey.

The advantage of using the electric organ as a source of nicotinic receptor becomes obvious when we examine the density of the receptor in the membrane of the *Torpedo* electroplaque cells. Most receptors and ion channels are relatively rare membrane proteins. Typically, one or a few receptor molecules are found per square micron of membrane surface area. In contrast, the *Torpedo* electroplaque membrane is packed tightly with nicotinic receptor, to a density as high as 10,000 to 30,000 per square micron, and indeed there appears to be little room for any additional protein in the membrane! Thus the rays have done a significant part of the purification for us, by inserting the protein and very little else into a membrane that can be isolated with relative ease.

Structure of the nicotinic acetylcholine receptor. With this rich source of material and the rapid, sensitive, and specific α-bungarotoxin assay, large amounts of homogeneous nicotinic receptor can be obtained. Biochemical analysis demonstrates that the receptor is a large complex consisting of five subunits (Fig. 11–6). There are two α subunits of molecular weight (MW) approximately 40,000, and one each of a β (MW 48,000), γ (MW 58,000), and δ (MW 64,000) subunit. Each α subunit contains a site for binding acetylcholine (and α-bungarotoxin) (Fig. 11–6b). This is consistent with physiological data, which indicate that the binding of two acetylcholine molecules is necessary for the opening of the nicotinic receptor's associated ion channel.

cDNA clones encoding the various subunits of the nicotinic receptor were obtained from amino acid sequence information, as described previ-

$$\text{NAChR} + \alpha\text{-BT} \xrightarrow[k_{on}]{k_{off}} \text{NAChR} - \alpha\text{-BT}$$

$$K_d = \frac{k_{off}}{k_{on}} \approx 10^{-15} M$$

Figure 11–5. α-Bungarotoxin (α-BT) binds very tightly to the nicotinic acetylcholine receptor (NAChR). The affinity (K_d) of the toxin for the receptor is extremely high. K_{off}, dissociation rate constant. K_{on}, association rate constant.

ously for the sodium channel. Mutagenesis and heterologous expression experiments have provided a detailed picture of structure–function relationships in this receptor. The different subunits have substantial amino acid sequence homology with one another, which suggests that they may have evolved from a single ancestral protein. Each subunit has four hydrophobic domains that are predicted to be membrane-spanning sequences (Fig. 11–7). As we shall discuss below, much is now known about regions of the molecule that are involved in both ligand binding and ion conduction.

a

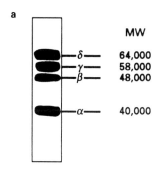

b

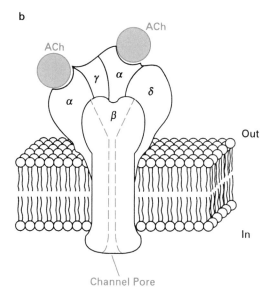

Figure 11–6. The nicotinic acetylcholine receptor from *Torpedo*. *a:* Polyacrylamide gel separation of the individual subunits of the purified nicotinic receptor. *b:* Cross-linking studies have demonstrated that the functional receptor molecule contains two α subunits, each with an acetylcholine (ACh) binding site, and one each of the β, γ, and δ subunits.

The important point we wish to make here is that when, considerably later, the muscarinic acetylcholine receptor from various sources was purified and cloned, its structure was found to be totally different from that of the nicotinic receptor. The muscarinic receptor has only a single kind of subunit, and the functional membrane receptor is probably an oligomer. The subunit molecular weight is 51,000, similar to that of the nicotinic receptor subunits, but a comparison of the amino acid sequences shows no relationship. From hydrophobicity measurements it is inferred that the muscarinic receptor has seven membrane-spanning domains, in contrast to the nicotinic receptor subunits, which are each thought to cross the membrane four times (Fig. 11–7).

Common Structural Motifs in Receptors: Receptor "Superfamilies"

It would appear that the nicotinic and muscarinic acetylcholine receptors have virtually nothing in common other than the fact that they bind and are activated by acetylcholine. They are present in different kinds of nerve, muscle, and gland cells (Fig. 11–2) and mediate very different physiological responses in terms of kinetics and mechanisms, and their amino acid

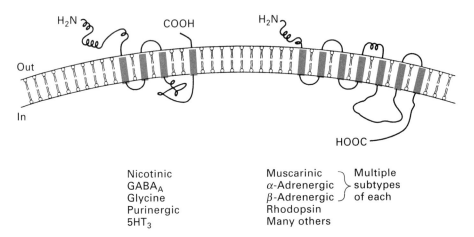

Nicotinic	Muscarinic	Multiple
GABA$_A$	α-Adrenergic	subtypes
Glycine	β-Adrenergic	of each
Purinergic	Rhodopsin	
5HT$_3$	Many others	

Figure 11–7. Topology of acetylcholine and other receptors. Hydrophobicity profiles predict that nicotinic acetylcholine receptor subunits, as well as those of the GABA$_A$, glycine, purinergic, and one subtype (5HT$_3$) of serotonin receptors, contain four membrane-spanning domains (*blue*). In contrast, muscarinic and related receptors are predicted to have seven membrane-spanning domains.

sequences and inferred structures show no similarities (Fig. 11–7). Because these discrepancies have been a disappointment to those biologists who seek unifying concepts in nature, it is all the more satisfying that unifying concepts have indeed emerged. Just as there are commonalities among the voltage-dependent ion channels (Chapters 3–7), there are indeed families of receptor molecules with common structural features. However, perhaps somewhat surprisingly, the family groupings are not based on the neurotransmitter that binds to the receptor; rather they reflect the *transduction mechanism*, the molecular mechanism that the receptor uses to translate the extracellular signal into a physiological response in the target cell. We shall now discuss one family, that of the *ligand-gated ion channels*, to which the nicotinic acetylcholine receptor belongs. We will describe the structural features that the family members share, as well as the transduction mechanism that they use to excite or inhibit a neuron. In the next chapter we shall describe other receptor families in which the transduction mechanisms are more complex. These include the family to which the muscarinic acetylcholine receptor belongs, the *G protein–coupled receptors*.

The Family of Directly Coupled Receptor–Ion Channel Complexes

The simplest way of transducing an extracellular signal into a change in excitability of the target neuron is by direct coupling of the neurotransmitter receptor to the ion channel whose activity it regulates. This is the mechanism used by the various ligand-gated ion channels. The ligand-binding site and the ion channel are part of the same molecule or macromolecular complex. Occupation of the receptor by the neurotransmitter leads to a conformational change that is passed along to the closely associated ion channel, and as a result channel properties are altered (Fig. 11–8). Note that in Figure 11–8 we show a channel that is closed in the resting state and that opens as a result of transmitter action, allowing the ion (X^+) to flow across the membrane. Although this is the way most of the known ligand-gated ion channel systems appear to function, in principle it is possible that a transmitter might close some channel that is open in the resting state.

An important feature of this general mechanism is that the modulation of ion channel properties is dependent on continued occupation of the receptor by the transmitter. The conformational change induced by receptor occupancy is readily reversible, and as soon as the receptor is no longer occupied by transmitter, the channel returns to its normal resting state (reverse arrow in Fig. 11–8). Accordingly, it might be expected that the ligand-gated ion channel systems would mediate rapid-onset and rap-idly reversible synaptic transmission, and this is indeed the case.

The muscle nicotinic acetylcholine receptor. It is now clear that the nicotinic acetylcholine receptor complex is one of these ligand-gated ion channels, in that it contains not only the acetylcholine-binding site but also the ion channel that is activated by acetylcholine binding. Most of the data that support this conclusion, including the amino acid sequence information from which the transmembrane topology has been inferred, come from work on the *Torpedo* and muscle nicotinic receptors. However, studies of a large family of neuronal nicotinic receptors place them in this same cat-egory of ligand-gated ion channels as well.

Biochemical evidence for direct receptor–channel coupling. How do we know that the receptor and ion channel of the ligand-gated systems are indeed part of the same macromolecular complex? Let us consider the evidence for the nicotinic acetylcholine receptor. First, recall from the discussion above that affinity chromatography, using a ligand that binds to the acetyl-choline-binding site, purifies a macromolecular complex consisting of four polypeptide subunits (Fig. 11–6). Early experiments to test the direct

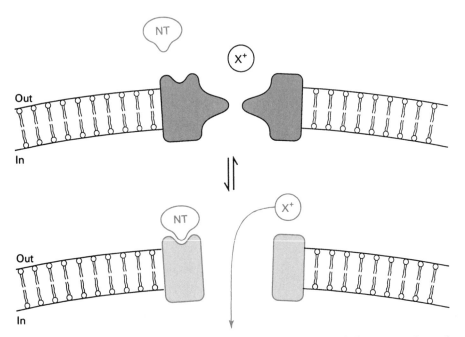

Figure 11–8. Direct receptor–channel coupling. In directly coupled receptor–channel systems the neurotransmitter (NT) binding site and the ion channel are intimately as-sociated in a single macromolecular complex. Contrast with Figures 12–2 and 12–6.

coupling hypothesis involved reconstitution of the purified complex into liposomes (phospholipid vesicles) and measurement of the transport of radioactive cations across the liposome membrane (Fig. 11–9). The phospholipid bilayer membrane of the liposome is impermeant to ions, and hence ion flux will occur only if there is an open ion channel in the mem-

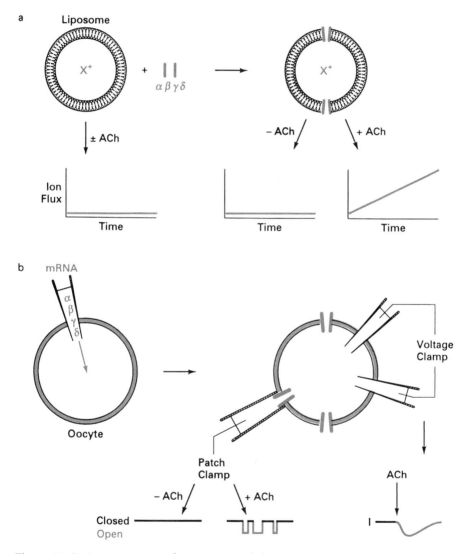

Figure 11–9. Reconstitution of receptor-coupled ion channel activity. *a*: Liposomes, spherical membrane vesicles made from artificial phospholipid, can be loaded with an ion (X^+). The flow of X^+ out of the liposome can be measured under various experimental conditions. *b*: Eric Barnard and Ricardo Miledi first demonstrated heterologous expression, in *Xenopus* oocytes, of messenger RNA for the nicotinic acetylcholine (ACh) receptor subunits (see Barnard et al., 1982).

brane. Experiments such as this demonstrate that the complex consisting of the α-, β-, γ-, and δ-protein subunits is sufficient to reconstitute acetylcholine-dependent ion flux (Fig. 11–9a). In other words, the acetylcholine-binding site and its associated ion channel copurify on the affinity column, indicating that they must be intimately associated.

Heterologous expression and site-directed mutagenesis. These data were confirmed and extended once the nucleotide sequences coding for the different subunits became available. A series of striking experiments have elucidated specific roles for each subunit and for particular amino acids in channel gating and conduction. These experiments involve injection of messenger RNA for the α, β, γ, and δ subunits into *Xenopus* oocytes, a heterologous expression system that we have met previously. The oocyte has no endogenous nicotinic acetylcholine receptor, and so the functional expression of exogenous messenger RNA can be detected readily by voltage clamp or single channel recording techniques.

Functional acetylcholine receptor/channels with properties identical to those in muscle can indeed be expressed following injection of messenger RNA for the α, β, γ, and δ subunits into oocytes (Fig. 11–9b). This confirms the conclusion from the biochemical reconstitution data that these subunits are sufficient to produce a complete functional receptor–channel complex. A similar approach, using messenger RNA for two subunits (α and β) of a receptor–channel complex that recognizes GABA, demonstrated that expression of the α and β subunits is sufficient to produce a GABA-activated chloride current. This kind of experiment in itself provides little new information—indeed, oocyte expression per se is little more than a sophisticated reconstitution system—but the heterologous expression of cloned subunits provides the opportunity to use mutational analysis to ask more detailed questions about structure–function relationships in the receptor–channel complex.

Early experiments of this sort took advantage of the fact that the nicotinic receptor/channels from mammalian muscle and *Torpedo* electric organ have similar but not identical gating properties (i.e., the channel mean open times differ significantly). By injecting messenger RNAs for the mammalian and *Torpedo* subunits in various combinations, it was found that substitution of the *Torpedo* δ subunit with that from muscle is sufficient to change the gating properties of a *Torpedo* receptor to those of a muscle receptor (Fig. 11–10). A similar approach demonstrated that differences in both gating and conduction between fetal and adult forms of the mammalian muscle receptor/channel can be accounted for by a developmentally regulated switch from the γ subunit, which is expressed in the fetus, to the closely related ϵ subunit that is expressed later in development. The major conclusions from these cleverly designed experiments were that the γ/ϵ subunits are important for determining the single channel conductance, and both these and the δ subunit are involved in determining the kinetics of channel gating.

Other experiments have focused on identifying particular amino acid sequences within each subunit that are important for the various functions of the receptor–channel complex. Chimeric subunits, consisting of various *Torpedo* sequences substituted in the mammalian subunits and vice versa, have demonstrated that the second membrane-spanning segment (called

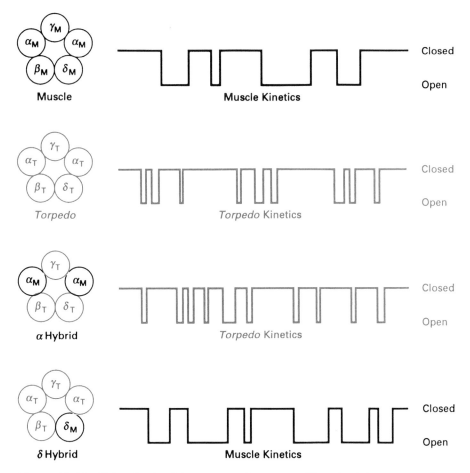

Figure 11–10. Chimeric nicotinic receptors in oocytes. The nicotinic receptors from muscle (*black*) and *Torpedo* (*blue*) display different opening and closing kinetics. Shosaku Numa and Bert Sakmann constructed chimeric receptors, which contain some muscle and some *Torpedo* subunits, by injecting the appropriate messenger RNAs into *Xenopus* oocytes (see Sakmann et al., 1985).

M2) forms part of the ion conduction pathway or pore. This has been confirmed by subsequent experiments, several of them being quite elegant. In one of them, the receptor was probed with a local anesthetic blocker that is known to permeate and block the channel pore. Mutagenesis showed that particular amino acids within the M2 segments of all the subunits interact with the blocker, and hence must line the pore. In another experiment that led to similar conclusions, each amino acid residue within M2 was replaced in turn with cysteine, and the resulting channels were probed with chemical reagents that can enter the pore and react covalently with cysteine residues to identify specific residues in M2 whose side chains are accessible to the pore. Such *cysteine scanning mutagenesis* has proven extremely useful for dissecting various structural features of ion channels and other proteins.

A powerful technique called *electron diffraction analysis* has provided new insight into the structure of the nicotinic acetylcholine receptor. The receptor is so tightly packed in *Torpedo* membranes that it forms a two-dimensional crystalline array, from which three-dimensional structural information can be obtained by electron microscopy. Using this innovative approach, Nigel Unwin has obtained images of the nicotinic receptor in both the closed and open states (Fig. 11–11). From these images, conformational changes in the channel protein can be inferred; these changes appear to be associated with channel gating.

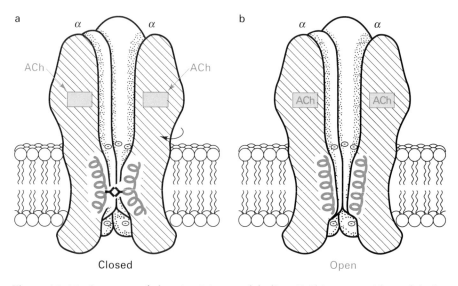

Figure 11–11. Structure of the nicotinic acetylcholine (ACh) receptor/channel in its closed (*left*) and open (*right*) states. These drawings by Nigel Unwin are based on electron diffraction analysis (modified from Unwin, 1993).

These various approaches have provided an increasingly detailed picture of the relationship between structure and function in the *Torpedo*/muscle nicotinic acetylcholine receptor/channel and, by analogy, in the other members of this receptor family. Most important in the present context, there is compelling evidence that the neurotransmitter binding site and the ion conduction pore are indeed part of the same macromolecular complex in this prototype member of the ligand-gated ion channel family.

Neuronal nicotinic acetylcholine receptors. Although the *Torpedo* and muscle nicotinic acetylcholine receptors have been most thoroughly studied and are best understood, it has been known for some time that nicotinic receptors are also present in the brain. This is not surprising in view of the well-established behavioral, cognitive, and addictive actions of nicotine. However, an understanding of neuronal nicotinic receptors was slower to develop because most of them are not sensitive to α-bungarotoxin, the tool that has proven so useful in characterizing *Torpedo* and muscle nicotinic receptors. Molecular cloning has established that at least two families of subunits, α and β, are found in neuronal nicotinic receptors (Table 11–3). There are a large number of distinct neuronal α-subunit genes (numbered $\alpha2$ through $\alpha10$) that exhibit substantial homology with the *Torpedo*/muscle α subunit (numbered $\alpha1$), and multiple β-subunit genes that do not resemble the *Torpedo*/muscle β (or anything else) and are often called *non-α* subunits. In some cases the functional receptor is formed by some combination of α and β subunits, whereas the $\alpha7$, $\alpha8$, and $\alpha9$ subunits each are capable of forming functional homomeric nicotinic receptor/channels. Once again we see that there is the potential for enormous diversity generated both by multiple gene products and the formation of heteromultimeric channels, and this diversity is reflected in the pharmacological and biophysical properties of both native and heterologously expressed neuronal nicotinic receptors (Table 11–3).

The GABA_A receptor. Among the other ligand-gated ion channel systems that have been well-characterized is the mammalian brain GABA$_A$ receptor. In fact, there are at least three classes of receptors for GABA: the

Table 11–3 Properties of Some Neuronal Nicotinic Receptors of Different Subunit Composition

Subunit Composition	Single Channel Conductance (pS)	EC$_{50}$ (μM) for Acetylcholine
$\alpha3\beta2$	15	350
$\alpha4\beta2$	20	0.7
$\alpha3\beta4$	22	30
$\alpha7$	45	110

Modified from McGehee and Role, 1995.

GABA$_B$ receptor, which is not directly coupled to its ion channel; the GABA$_C$ receptor, which appears to be restricted to visual pathways; and the GABA$_A$ receptor, on which we will focus here. This receptor was first purified using specific affinity reagents. Its subunit structure resembles that of the nicotinic acetylcholine receptor. The inhibitory action of GABA results from activation of a chloride channel that is directly coupled to the GABA$_A$ receptor (Fig. 11–12a; contrast this with the nicotinic receptors, which are coupled to cation channels that allow sodium and potassium to flow). In the previous chapter we referred to the fact that the receptor for GABA has a rich pharmacology, in that it is the site of action of a number of clinically important drugs, including the benzodiazepines such as Valium and Librium, which are used widely as antianxiety and relaxant drugs, and the barbiturates, which are important anticonvulsants and sedatives. These agents produce their clinical consequences by enhancing the effect of GABA on the chloride channel that is coupled directly to the receptor (Fig. 11–12b). GABA$_C$ receptors are also coupled to chloride channels, but do not respond to barbiturates and have a pharmacological profile distinct from that of GABA$_A$ receptors.

The GABA$_A$ receptor was purified to homogeneity by isolating proteins that bind to benzodiazepines through the technique of affinity chromatography. This purifies a complex with most of the pharmacological binding sites of the GABA$_A$ receptor in native neuronal membranes. The purified complex contains α (MW 53,000) and β (MW 57,000) subunits with the stoichiometry $\alpha_2-\beta_2$, as well as other subunits. Protein sequence information was used to clone cDNAs encoding the α and β subunits, and heterologous expression of these two subunits together produces GABA-activated chloride channels with most, but not all, of the properties of native GABA$_A$ receptors. Homology screening, using sequences from the cloned α and β subunits, resulted in the cloning of multiple subtypes of α and β subunits, as well as distinct γ, δ, and other subunits. The benzodiazepine binding site is only present in recombinant GABA$_A$ receptors when the γ subunit is expressed together with α and β, indicating that the fully functional receptor must contain at least three different kinds of subunits.

The combination of multiple subunit genes (at least 15), alternative splicing of messenger RNA, and the requirement for a heteromultimeric complex together give rise to impressive diversity in the family of GABA$_A$ receptors. Another striking finding is the similarity of GABA$_A$ and nicotinic acetylcholine receptors in their overall structural features. The number and distribution of predicted transmembrane domains are the same for all the subunits of the GABA$_A$ and nicotinic receptors, there is significant sequence homology in certain regions of the subunits, and the functional receptor/channel in both cases is a pentamer consisting of several different kinds of subunits.

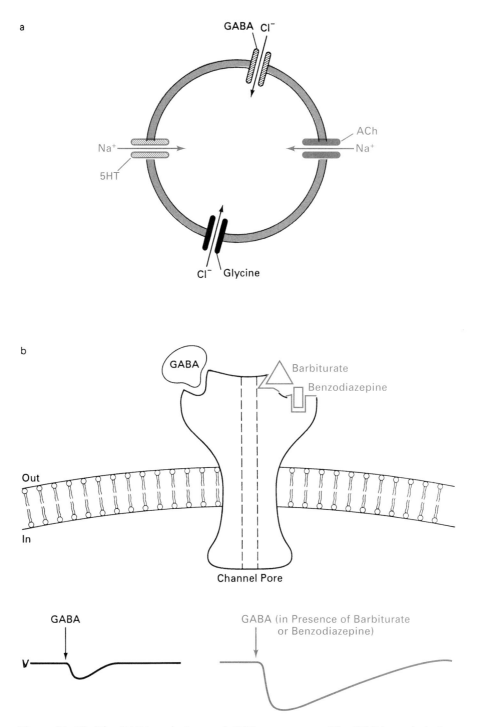

Figure 11–12. The GABA$_A$, glycine, and 5HT$_3$ receptors. *a*: The GABA$_A$ and glycine receptors are intimately coupled to channels selective for chloride ions. In contrast, the nicotinic acetylcholine (ACh) and 5HT$_3$ receptors are coupled to cation channels. *b*: The GABA$_A$ receptor–channel complex has binding sites for barbiturates and benzodiazepines, which can markedly enhance the hyperpolarizing response to GABA.

The glycine and 5-HT$_3$ *receptors.* In some parts of the central nervous system, in particular in the brain stem and spinal cord, glycine rather than GABA is the major inhibitory neurotransmitter. At these sites glycine functions just like GABA, by activating a receptor linked to a chloride channel (Fig. 11–12a). The convulsant drug strychnine blocks inhibition by selectively antagonizing glycine-mediated (but not GABA-mediated) inhibition, and strychnine has been used for assay and affinity purification of the glycine receptor. The receptor complex consists of α and β subunits, with molecular weights of about 48,000 and 58,000, respectively, and cross-linking studies suggest an overall pentameric structure with a molecular weight of about 260,000. Both the α and β subunits share substantial sequence homology and predicted structure with those for the corresponding subunits of the nicotinic and GABA$_A$ receptors, particularly in the putative membrane-spanning segments. Multiple genes and alternative splicing contribute to glycine receptor heterogeneity in the brain and spinal cord.

Serotonin (5-HT) is another neurotransmitter for which multiple classes of receptors exist. One of these classes, the so-called 5-HT$_3$ receptor, falls into the family of ligand-gated ion channels by virtue of its rapid onset and rapidly reversible electrical response, and its overall structural homology with other family members. Like the nicotinic receptor/channels, 5-HT$_3$ receptors are directly coupled to a cation channel (Fig. 11–12a). A remarkable experiment has confirmed the close relationship among the various ligand-gated receptor/channels and revealed that discrete structural domains of these proteins can function as independent functional units. A chimeric receptor–channel complex, formed from the amino terminal domain of the $\alpha7$ subunit of the neuronal nicotinic receptor and the transmembrane region and carboxyl terminal domain of the 5-HT$_3$ receptor, forms a functional receptor–channel complex that is activated by acetylcholine and other nicotinic agonists but has the permeation properties of 5-HT$_3$ channels.

The glutamate receptors. The receptors for glutamate are of particular interest, in part because glutamate is the major excitatory neurotransmitter in the mammalian brain, but also because glutamate receptors are widely believed to play an important role in some kinds of learning and memory (see Chapter 20). At least four classes of glutamate receptor are known, based on amino acid sequence, agonist pharmacology, and transduction mechanism (Table 11–4). One of these classes transduces its signal via an intracellular second messenger cascade; this *metabotropic* glutamate receptor will be discussed in the next chapter. The remaining three classes consist of ligand-gated ion channels, or *ionotropic* receptors. They are named after the agonists that activate them most effectively: (1) kainic acid (KA), (2) α-amino-3-hydroxy-5-methyl-4-isoxazole propionic acid (AMPA), and (3) N-methyl-D-aspartic acid (NMDA) (Fig. 11–13). The KA and AMPA receptors are closely related, whereas the NMDA receptors are distinct both functionally and structurally.

An essential difference lies in the properties of the different ion channels activated by the KA and AMPA receptors on the one hand and the NMDA receptors on the other (Fig. 11–14). The KA and AMPA receptors activate cation channels that allow sodium and potassium ions to flow. Near a neuron's resting potential the driving force for potassium is low and that for sodium is high, so activation of these channels leads to depolarization as a result of an inward sodium current (Fig. 11–14a). In contrast, NMDA receptors activate cation channels that allow not only sodium and potassium but also calcium ions to flow (Fig. 11–14b). It might be thought that activation of these channels would also cause a depolarization that would simply add to that produced by the KA and AMPA receptor channels. Near the resting potential, however, this does not occur because of an interesting property of the NMDA receptor channels—they are blocked by extracellular magnesium ions in a voltage-dependent manner.

The way the NMDA receptor/channel works is shown in Figure 11–14. When a neuron is near its resting potential, magnesium ions bind to the outside of the channel and effectively prevent the movement of other ions through the pore (Fig. 11–14a). When the cell is depolarized, however, the magnesium ions are driven out of the channel, allowing the other ions free access (Fig. 11–14b). The amount of current passing through NMDA receptor channels is therefore much greater at depolarized than at hyperpolarized membrane potentials. Thus, when the cell is depolarized in the presence of glutamate, calcium (as well as sodium) flows into the cell through the NMDA receptor channels (Fig. 11–14b).

Table 11–4 Four Kinds of Glutamate Receptor

Receptor Subtype	Cloned Subunits	Agonists
AMPA	GluR1–GluR4	AMPA, quisqualate
KA	GluR5–GluR7 KA1–KA2	KA, quisqualate
NMDA	NMDAR1 NMDAR2A–NMDAR2D	NMDA
Metabotropic	mGluR1–mGluR6	trans-ACPD, quisqualate

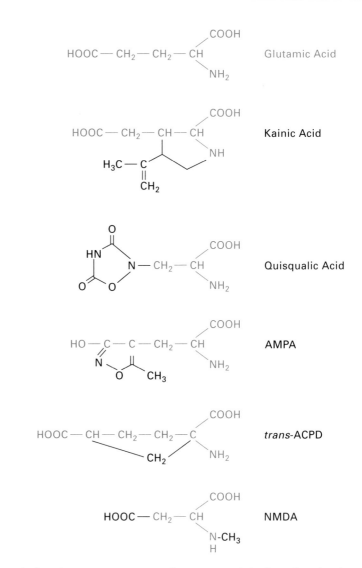

Figure 11–13. Ligands for glutamate receptors. The portion of the ligand molecule that resembles glutamate is shown in blue.

Figure 11–14. Different kinds of responses mediated by the glutamate (GLU) receptor subtypes. *a*: The response to a weak presynaptic stimulus is activation of only the KA/AMPA receptor subtypes. *b*: In contrast, a stronger stimulus causes ions to flow through both the KA/AMPA and NMDA receptor channels. Voltage-dependent Mg^{2+} block of the NMDA receptor channel was demonstrated by Philippe Ascher and colleagues (see Nowak et al., 1984) and by Mark Mayer and Gary Westbrook (see Mayer et al., 1984).

a   Weak stimulus activates only KA/AMPA receptor channels

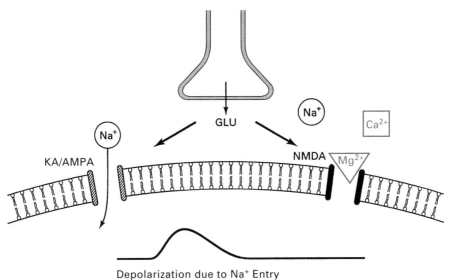

Depolarization due to Na⁺ Entry

b   Strong stimulus depolarizes sufficiently to relieve
    voltage-dependent magnesium block of NMDA receptor channels

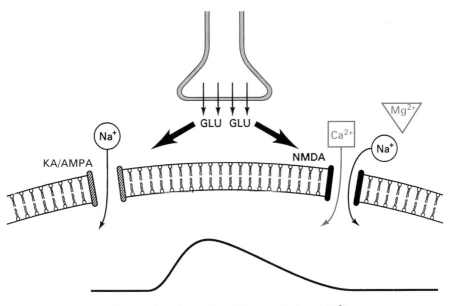

Larger depolarization with both Na⁺ and Ca²⁺ entry

The presence of several distinct receptor types coupled to different ion channels allows the target cell to respond differently to different intensities of synaptic stimulation. A moderate stimulus produces only a small depolarization, and no calcium entry, as a result of activation only of the KA/AMPA receptor channels. Although glutamate binds to the NMDA receptors, no current flows through the NMDA channels under these conditions. With more intense stimulation the depolarization becomes sufficient to relieve the magnesium block of the NMDA receptor channels, resulting in further depolarization and calcium entry.

Another important difference between the KA/AMPA and NMDA receptors is that the activity of the NMDA receptor is influenced by glycine, acting at a site distinct from that at which glutamate binds. In fact it is thought that glycine is necessary for the activation of NMDA receptors, making it a *coagonist* with glutamate. The extent to which regulated release of glycine occurs in higher brain regions (other than the brain stem and spinal cord) is not known, but clearly the involvement of glycine provides yet another means for fine tuning the activity of NMDA receptors.

The presence of the three pharmacologically and functionally distinct ionotropic glutamate receptor subtypes also allows a postsynaptic cell to respond differently to presynaptically released glutamate, depending on whether the target cell is actively firing action potentials. A moderate synaptic stimulus to a silent cell will activate AMPA and KA channels, but will not produce sufficient depolarization to activate the NMDA channels. In contrast, the same stimulus to an active postsynaptic neuron, whose membrane is of course relatively depolarized by the action potentials, allows calcium to enter through the NMDA receptor/channels because their magnesium block has been relieved by the depolarization. Similarly, glycine, perhaps released by other active neurons, will contribute to the regulation of NMDA receptor activity and hence of calcium entry. As we shall see in Chapter 20, it is believed that the calcium that enters through the NMDA receptor channels at glutamatergic synapses may contribute to long-lasting changes in the properties of the postsynaptic neurons.

Molecular structures of the glutamate receptors. The glutamate receptors have been hard to clone. The lack of a rich source or suitable ligands made purification of the receptor protein difficult, and no mutations were available in appropriate organisms for positional cloning, as was the case for potassium channels (see Chapter 5). The glutamate receptors finally fell to a cloning strategy called *expression cloning* (Fig. 11–15). This involves making a cDNA library from a tissue that expresses the receptor. Messenger RNA transcribed from these cDNAs is then injected into *Xenopus* oocytes, and the oocytes are tested for expression of a functional glutamate receptor. The cDNA library is then subdivided into several parts, and messenger RNA transcribed from each part is tested in the same way. The part that produces a functional receptor is then subdivided further, until ultimately a single cDNA clone encoding the functional receptor is obtained (Fig. 11–15). It is important to note that for expression cloning to work, it is essential that a functional receptor/channel be formed from a single type of subunit. Fortuitously, this turned out to be the case for the AMPA, NMDA, and metabotropic glutamate receptors, all of which were cloned in this way (Fig. 11–15). Once these initial clones were available, further cloning by sequence homology uncovered an enormous number of related subunits, including those of the KA receptors (Table 11–4).

Hydrophobicity plots predict four membrane-spanning segments in the subunits of the ionotropic glutamate receptors, but these subunits are about twice as large as those of the nicotinic, $GABA_A$, glycine, and $5-HT_3$ re-

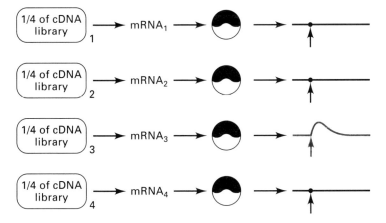

a   Make messenger RNA from cDNA library and test for expression of glutamate receptors

b   Fractionate the library and make messenger RNA from each part

c   Further fractionate fraction 3, and repeat until a single cDNA clone is isolated that produces a functional receptor

Figure 11–15. Expression cloning. When homology screening or positional cloning is not feasible, receptors and channels may be cloned by their functional expression in *Xenopus* oocytes.

ceptors, and clearly form a separate family (Fig. 11–16). They have a large extracellular amino-terminal domain that probably contributes to the ligand-binding site, and the region between membrane-spanning segments M1 and M3 may not span the membrane completely (that is, there is no fully membrane-spanning M2 segment), but rather may dip into the membrane and back out again to form a potassium channel–like pore domain (Fig. 11–16a). According to this model, the large loop between M3 and M4 is extracellular and may also participate in ligand binding, whereas it is thought to be intracellular in the other ligand-gated ion channels (Fig. 11–7). Cysteine scanning mutagenesis, similar to that used to deduce structural features of the nicotinic acetylcholine receptor, has confirmed this general model and provided some additional details of the structural design of the glutamate receptor/channel pore.

A glutamate-gated ion channel has been purified and cloned from a bacterium and has been named *GluR0*. Interestingly, the predicted extracellular domain of this protein exhibits amino acid sequence homology with the ligand-binding domains of the eukaryotic glutamate receptors,

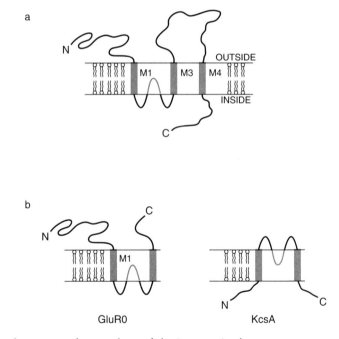

Figure 11–16. Predicted structures for members of the ionotropic glutamate receptor family. *a*: Transmembrane arrangement of the mammalian glutamate receptor subunits. *b*: A bacterial glutamate receptor subunit (GluR0) contains a potassium-selective ion channel and resembles an upside down KcsA potassium channel. Compare with the other ligand-gated ion channels in Figure 11–7.

whereas the pore region sequence is related to that of the bacterial potassium channel whose structure was elucidated by Roderick MacKinnon and colleagues (although it is "backward," with the potassium selectivity filter near the intracellular side of the pore; see Fig. 11–16b). When the function of this channel was examined in a heterologous expression system, it was found that the channel is indeed potassium-selective and is gated by glutamate. This intriguing finding provides evidence that the ligand-gated and voltage-gated ion channel families may have arisen from a common prokaryotic ancestor.

Molecular architecture of the postsynaptic membrane. How are the various glutamate receptors distributed and organized in the postsynaptic membrane of excitatory synapses in the central nervous system? Clues have emerged from the identification of synaptic proteins that associate tightly with one or more glutamate receptor subtypes, often via highly specific protein–protein interaction domains. One such domain that is critical for the molecular organization of both the presynaptic terminal and the postsynaptic membrane is called the *PDZ domain*, because it was first described in three related proteins with strikingly uninformative names: PSD-95, DLG, and Z01. The domain is about 80–100 amino acids long and is defined by the presence of multiple repeats of the sequence Gly-Leu-Gly-Phe within this stretch; it binds with nanomolar affinity to short peptide sequences in target proteins. Many synaptic proteins contain within their sequences multiple PDZ domains as well as other functional domains (Fig. 11–17), each of which may interact with a different target protein to help build a macromolecular complex.

How does one identify the proteins in such a complex? The *yeast two-hybrid screen*, a powerful technique that takes advantage of yeast genetics to identify proteins that interact with other proteins, has proven ex-

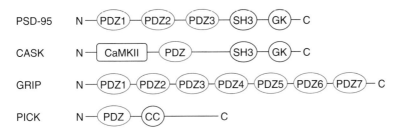

Figure 11–17. Molecular organization of some PDZ domain–containing proteins. Some proteins that participate in the organization of the postsynaptic membrane (see Fig. 11–19) may contain several distinct PDZ domains (*blue*) with different amino acid sequences.

tremely useful in this context. The two-hybrid screen is based on the fact that certain proteins called *transcription factors*, which regulate the synthesis of mRNA from DNA, have distinct DNA-binding and transcriptional activation domains (Fig. 11–18a). The two domains can be expressed as separate proteins in a yeast cell (Fig. 11–18b), but transcription of mRNA from the DNA cannot occur under these circumstances unless the two domains are brought together. One way this can occur is if the two separate domains are linked by the interaction domains of two other proteins, such as synaptic proteins (Fig. 11–18c). For example, part of a specific synaptic protein can be used as "bait" by linking it to the DNA-binding domain. A cDNA library is then made that encodes a large number of different proteins linked to the transcriptional activation domain. A few of these proteins may be "fish" proteins that will bind tightly to bait protein, whereas most of the proteins encoded by the cDNA library are unrelated and will not bind the bait. The cDNAs encoding "fish" can then be isolated readily, and in this way the yeast two-hybrid technique allows the identification of binding partners for any particular bait.

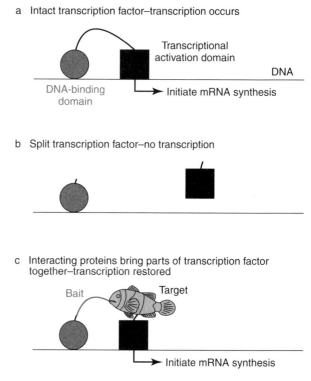

Figure 11–18. Drawing to illustrate the yeast two-hybrid screen. See text for details.

This approach has been used extensively with glutamate receptor channels and other synaptic proteins, and has provided evidence for a multicomponent scaffold of proteins (some with colorful names such as PICK, CASK, GRIP, GRASP, SHANK, and HOMER) that organizes the receptors and links them to the cytoskeleton and to various intracellular signaling pathways as well as to each other (Fig. 11–19; compare with the pictures of the postsynaptic membranes in Figs. 18–8 and 18–19). New components of these molecular assemblies are still being discovered including proteins such as Piccolo and Bassoon that help to define the presynaptic active zone. It is evident from studies of this sort that signaling at the synapse must involve the tightly coordinated activities of an astonishingly large complement of molecular components.

RNA *editing determines glutamate receptor/channel properties*. An unusual and striking finding for several of the AMPA receptor/channel subunits was that the sequence of their cDNA differs from that of their genomic DNA in the region of the pore domain. This is not due to an error in transcribing the genomic DNA into messenger RNA (from which the cDNA is derived). Rather, the DNA is transcribed faithfully, and the sequence difference arises from RNA editing—specifically in this case, the enzymatic deamidation of a specific adenosine to inosine in the messenger RNA. The consequence of this editing is that a codon (CAG) that formerly coded for a glutamine residue in the pore domain is changed to one (CIG) that codes for arginine, and this results in a dramatic change in the conduction properties of the channel. More recently, RNA editing has also been discovered in the

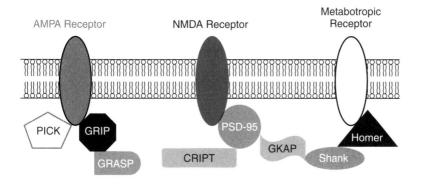

Figure 11–19. Molecular organization of the postsynaptic membrane at glutamatergic synapses. Protein–protein interactions, many of them identified by the yeast two-hybrid screen, link different kinds of glutamate receptors to one another and anchor them to the cytoskeleton. Compare with the organization of the neuromuscular junction illustrated in Figure 18–19.

messenger RNAs for some kinds of potassium channels. If RNA editing can be regulated, for example, in different cell types or at different developmental stages, this novel and intriguing mechanism could provide yet another way of generating diversity in the voltage-dependent and ligand-gated ion channels.

Summary

The question of how cells respond to signals from their environment is relevant to all aspects of cell biology. Thus it will come as no surprise that many of the signaling molecules discussed in Chapter 10 are not restricted to the nervous system but can act on many cell types. The common feature that allows neurons and other cells to respond to these extracellular signals is the presence of specific receptors in the plasma membrane that may be very similar in their structure and functional properties in different kinds of cells. It has been known for a long time from pharmacological studies that there may be several different kinds of receptors for individual neurotransmitters. This has important implications for the way information is processed in neuronal networks. This heterogeneity has been confirmed as the structures of many receptors have been elucidated. A gratifying picture has emerged from these structural studies: many receptors can be grouped into families based on structural, functional, and regulatory homologies that are far more extensive than had been appreciated previously.

Perhaps surprisingly, the family groupings reflect common receptor transduction mechanisms rather than common ligand-binding sites. One such family is that of the ligand-gated ion channels. The members of this family were first linked on the basis of a functional criterion—direct coupling between the receptor and the ion channel whose activity it regulates. Biochemical and molecular studies provide a structural basis for dividing these receptors into two subfamilies, one for the glutamate receptors and the other encompassing the other ligand-gated ion channels. The sequence homologies and remarkably similar predicted arrangement of transmembrane segments suggest that the various subunits of the different receptors within a subfamily may have evolved from a single ancestral subunit. Evolution has allowed the ligand specificity of the receptor site and the ion selectivity of the channel pore to diverge. However, the essential overall structural design of the ligand-gated receptor–channel complex has been preserved. We shall now consider the molecular details of other, more intricate, signal transduction pathways.

12

Receptors and Transduction Mechanisms II: Indirectly Coupled Receptor/Ion Channel Systems

The recognition of extracellular signals by specific receptors on the target cell is not the final step in intercellular communication. Cells must also possess mechanisms to *transduce* the extracellular signal, to convert it into some biological response that is characteristic of the particular target cell. In neurons, the biological response is often the modulation of the properties of one or more membrane ion channels. We have seen that in the ligand-gated ion channel family, the tasks of recognition and transduction reside in a single protein complex. Other families of receptors alter neuronal excitability through more complicated changes in the biochemistry of the cell (Fig. 12–1).

G Protein–Coupled Receptor/Ion Channel Systems

Most neurotransmitter receptors are not coupled directly to the ion channel whose activity they regulate. Among the indirectly coupled receptor/channel systems is a large (and ever-growing) family coupled via *guanyl nucleotide-binding proteins*, or *G proteins*. It can be seen from an examination of Table 12–1 that at first glance the various G protein–coupled receptors have little in common. This receptor family includes several peptide receptors, the muscarinic acetylcholine receptor subtypes, and receptors for most of the major classes of biogenic amines. It even contains, in addition to other sensory receptors, the visual pigment rhodopsin, which does not respond to a signaling molecule but can be thought of as a "receptor" for light (see Chapter 14). Note that cell surface receptors in yeast and in the slime mold *Dictyostelium*, cell types far removed from neurons, are included in the list, emphasizing the commonality of mechanisms in neurons and other kinds of cells.

Why would we possibly want to gather these diverse receptors in the same list? As in the example of the directly coupled receptor systems described in the last chapter, many of these are linked on the basis of a func-

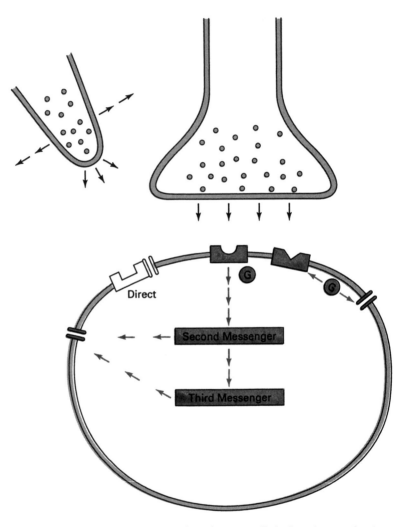

Figure 12–1. Intercellular communication. This chapter will deal with transduction mechanisms that are not mediated via direct receptor channel coupling, but rather involve either protein–protein interactions in the plane of the plasma membrane or intracellular messengers (*blue*). Guanyl nucleotide-binding proteins (G) play an essential role in these transduction mechanisms.

tional criterion, in this case, transduction of the extracellular signal via a G protein. As we will see later in this chapter, many receptors use G proteins to activate intracellular enzymes that produce second messengers. These are diffusible molecules that may influence a variety of cellular constituents, including ion channels. It is now realized that G proteins also interact directly with some ion channels to regulate their activities (Fig. 12–2), without the mediation of a second messenger. Such modulation of ion channel properties, via protein–protein interaction in the plane of the membrane, may be slower in onset and somewhat longer lasting than that mediated by the intramolecular conformational changes in the directly coupled systems (compare with Fig. 11–8).

Receptors coupled to G proteins belong to a family. Molecular cloning has made it clear that this grouping of receptors in Table 12–1 is indeed appropriate. The first members of the family to be sequenced were the opsin visual pigments. The most striking feature in the sequence was the presence of seven stretches, each of 20–28 hydrophobic amino acids, which were interpreted to represent membrane-spanning domains. This of course is very different from the four membrane-spanning regions characteristic of the directly coupled receptors (see Fig. 11–7). When one of the mammalian β-adrenergic receptors was subsequently cloned and sequenced, it was also found to have seven hydrophobic membrane-spanning domains and substantial amino acid homology with bovine opsin. This is also the case for the α-adrenergic receptors, although they differ markedly from the β receptors in their binding site pharmacology. We have already pointed out in Chapter 11 that the various muscarinic acetylcholine receptor subtypes also exhibit these structural features (see Fig. 11–7).

This structure has now been seen in the hundreds of other members of the G protein–coupled receptor family for which sequence information

Table 12–1 Some of the Many Receptors That Use G Proteins to Transduce Extracellular Signals

Substance K receptor
Yeast mating factor receptor
Slime mold cyclic AMP receptor
Luteinizing hormone-releasing hormone receptor
Muscarinic acetylcholine receptors
Adrenergic receptors
Purinergic receptor
Metabotropic glutamate receptors
Rhodopsin
Olfactory receptors

is available. What is most interesting is that the pattern is so consistent. New receptors whose transduction mechanism is not understood can be assigned with confidence to this family solely on the basis of their amino acid sequence. A good example of this is the receptor for substance K, one of several related peptides called the *tachykinins*. Among the biological actions of these peptides are important effects on sensory processing. Before its amino acid sequence was determined, the transduction mechanism for the actions of substance K was not known. However, the sequence showed the presence of seven membrane-spanning domains. This allowed the prediction that the receptor is coupled to a G protein. Similarly, the *metabotropic glutamate receptors*, which mediate slow responses to glutamate and are not directly coupled to ion channels like their ionotropic cousins described in Chapter 11, clearly fall into the family of G protein–coupled receptors (Table 12–1) on the basis of their molecular structures.

How do G proteins work? To discuss G protein modulation of ion channels we must first consider the structure of G proteins and some aspects of the molecular mechanism by which they act. G proteins are heterotrimers con-

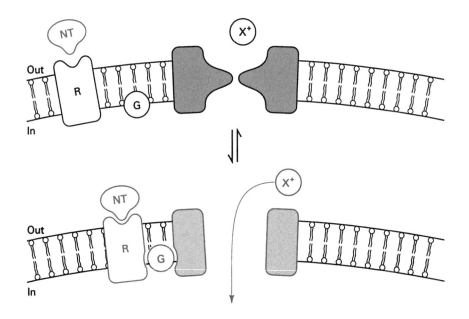

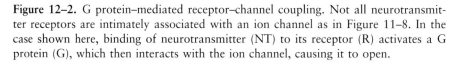

Figure 12–2. G protein–mediated receptor–channel coupling. Not all neurotransmitter receptors are intimately associated with an ion channel as in Figure 11–8. In the case shown here, binding of neurotransmitter (NT) to its receptor (R) activates a G protein (G), which then interacts with the ion channel, causing it to open.

sisting of one each of an α, β, and γ subunit (Fig. 12–3), and a large number of structurally and functionally distinct G proteins is known to exist. Molecular cloning has been used to define a number of subfamilies of α subunits, and multiple β and γ subunits also exist. Although the β and γ subunits can be dissociated from one another under denaturing conditions in a test tube, they remain together as a functional $\beta\gamma$ complex under physiological conditions. The $\beta\gamma$ complex was originally thought to subserve only the important but relatively humdrum function of anchoring the G protein to the plasma membrane, but as we shall see below, they do far more than that. The membrane anchoring is achieved via a post-translational modification that attaches an isoprenoid lipid group covalently to a cysteine residue at or near the carboxyl terminal of the γ subunit. The lipid moiety is extremely hydrophobic and interacts tightly with the plasma membrane (Fig. 12–3).

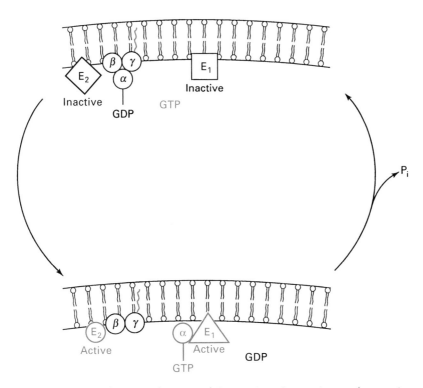

Figure 12–3. Mechanism of action of G proteins. G proteins are heterotrimers consisting of one each of an α, β, and γ subunit. They are anchored to the plasma membrane by a lipid group (*blue*) that is attached covalently to the γ subunit. In the presence of GTP, the α subunit dissociates from $\beta\gamma$, and both α and $\beta\gamma$ can influence the activities of other proteins (E_1 and E_2). A GTPase activity intrinsic to the α subunit completes the cycle. See the review by Neer (1995).

All of the known heterotrimeric G proteins operate via the same general mechanism illustrated in Figure 12–3. In its inactive state the G protein has GDP bound to a specific guanyl nucleotide-binding site on the α subunit. As it moves in the plane of the membrane, the G protein occasionally bumps into an appropriate agonist-occupied membrane receptor (or, in the case of the photoreceptor G protein transducin, a light-activated rhodopsin molecule). This receptor–G protein interaction allows GTP to displace GDP from the guanyl nucleotide-binding site. The displacement is accompanied by the dissociation of the α subunit from the $\beta\gamma$ complex, and both α and $\beta\gamma$ can then interact with and activate effector systems. The effector system might be an ion channel as in Figure 12–2, or some enzyme (denoted by E_1 and E_2 in Fig. 12–3). The α subunit carries an intrinsic GTPase activity, and so after some time the bound GTP is hydrolyzed to GDP. Following this hydrolysis the α subunit recombines with $\beta\gamma$, allowing the cycle to begin again (Fig. 12–3).

A variety of biochemical probes have been instrumental in proving the above sequence of events and in identifying and analyzing biological responses mediated by G proteins. These include several GTP analogs such as GTPγS and Gpp(NH)p (guanylylimidodiphosphate), which displace GDP from the guanyl nucleotide-binding site but are not hydrolyzed by the GTPase. These compounds act as essentially irreversible *activators* of the G proteins. In contrast, the GDP analog GDPβS, which binds very strongly to the binding site, maintains the G protein in the inactive GDP state, thus *inhibiting* G protein–mediated responses. Two bacterial toxins have also been extremely useful. *Cholera toxin* irreversibly activates some G proteins by causing ADP-ribose to be covalently attached to an arginine residue on the α subunit. *Pertussis toxin* irreversibly inhibits other G proteins by catalyzing the same reaction with their α subunits.

Some ion channels are modulated directly by G proteins. As we shall see later in this chapter, second messengers whose synthesis is controlled by G proteins influence the activity of many ion channels. Such indirect G protein involvement in ion channel modulation appears to be a rather ubiquitous phenomenon. Some ion channels, however, may interact directly with G proteins. That is, the effector system (E in Fig. 12–3) is not an enzyme, but is the ion channel protein itself (Fig. 12–2). The list of ion channels that are regulated directly by G proteins is growing steadily. We shall illustrate this mechanism by considering the inwardly rectifying potassium channel in the heart, whose activity is increased by acetylcholine acting at muscarinic receptors. This K_{ACh} channel is responsible for the slowing of the heart on stimulation of the vagus nerve, thus this story is of historical interest (see the Otto Loewi experiment described in Chapter 1), as well as being the first and most thoroughly characterized example of this kind of channel modulation.

A variety of evidence indicates that there is no second messenger involvement in the muscarinic activation of K_{ACh}. However, a role for a G protein was suggested by the finding that potassium current can be activated only when GTP and GTP analogs are added to the electrode in the whole-cell recording configuration (Fig. 12–4a). Furthermore, the channel can be activated in detached membrane patches by GTP applied to the cytoplasmic membrane surface (Fig. 12–4b). In addition, pretreatment with

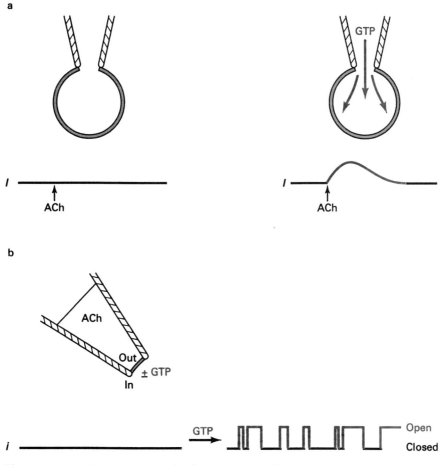

Figure 12–4. A G protein is involved in activation of a cardiac potassium channel by acetylcholine. Acetylcholine (ACh) binds to a muscarinic receptor and activates a potassium channel in cardiac muscle cells. This response, whether measured by whole-cell recording (*a*) or in a detached membrane patch (*b*), requires GTP (see Breitwieser and Szabo, 1985; Pfaffinger et al., 1985).

pertussis toxin prevents the activation of the potassium current by muscarinic agonists.

Purified G proteins that have been activated by prior treatment with GTP analogs can be applied directly to the cytoplasmic membrane surface of detached patches containing K_{ACh} channels (Fig. 12–5). This treatment activates the channel, confirming a direct interaction of the G protein with the channel or with some unknown regulatory protein that is very closely associated with the channel. In an extension of these experiments, isolated α subunits or $\beta\gamma$ complexes were applied to the inside of the patch, and it was found that $\beta\gamma$ can modulate channel activity. This was the first indication that $\beta\gamma$ (as well as α) can directly influence effector systems, and the list of effectors activated by $\beta\gamma$ continues to grow.

Inwardly rectifying potassium channels: yet another potassium channel family. The inwardly rectifying potassium channels like the K_{ACh} channel in the heart remained uncloned during the extensive homology screens that followed the initial characterization of *Shaker*. Like the glutamate receptor/channels described in the last chapter, they finally fell to an expression cloning approach, and subsequent homology screens have uncovered a large family of inward rectifiers that clearly is distinct from the other families of voltage-dependent potassium channels. The predicted structure of the inward rectifier potassium channels is interesting (see Fig. 7–11). They

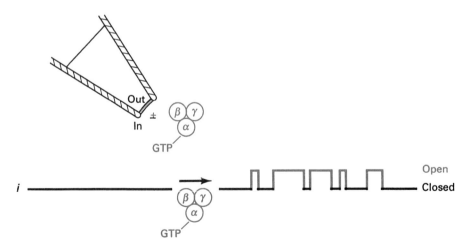

Figure 12–5. Purified G proteins can activate the cardiac muscarinic potassium channel. In detached membrane patches in which the endogenous G proteins have been previously inactivated by treatment with pertussis toxin, addition of an activated G protein can produce gating of the potassium channel (see Logothetis et al., 1987).

contain two putative membrane-spanning segments, flanking a pore do-main that is very similar in sequence to that of the voltage-dependent potas-sium channels. Interestingly, another inwardly rectifying potassium chan-nel, whose activity is inhibited by intracellular ATP (a K_{ATP} channel), appears to be modulated by G protein α subunits rather than by $\beta\gamma$. In view of the similarities between K_{ACh} and K_{ATP} channels, it appears that only subtle structural differences are sufficient to alter the specificity for G protein subunits.

Second Messenger–Coupled Receptor/Ion Channel Systems

The third category of receptor–channel coupling that we shall discuss is channel modulation via intracellular second messengers. In this case the receptor and channel are not part of a single macromolecular complex (Fig. 11–8), nor do they interact directly in the plane of the membrane (Fig. 12–2). Rather the receptor is coupled, via a G protein, to an enzyme, the activity of which is regulated by the occupation of the receptor by a neurotransmitter (Fig. 12–6). When the receptor is occupied by transmit-ter (the so-called first messenger), the enzyme is activated and can catalyze the formation of an intracellular second messenger (Fig. 12–6). The sec-ond messenger can then set in motion a sequence of events that ultimately influences the properties of, or *modulates*, an ion channel. Note that the channel properties do not immediately revert to the normal resting state when the transmitter dissociates from the receptor, as is the case for the directly coupled systems. Instead the channel modulation persists (in the example in Fig. 12–6, the channel remains open) until the actions of the second messenger are reversed. This may involve a sequence of molecular events, requiring seconds, minutes, or even hours. Thus second messenger coupling provides a mechanism for ion channel modulation that may be delayed in onset. In addition, it can long outlast the initial stimulus, the occupation of receptor by neurotransmitter.

Several other features of this general scheme deserve mention. First, we have already mentioned that most second messenger pathways involve G protein–activated enzymes. Accordingly, second messenger–mediated re-ceptor–channel coupling might be thought of as just a special case of G protein coupling, but in fact the temporal and molecular complexities in-troduced by having a second messenger mediate the response justify a sep-arate category for this coupling mechanism. A second important feature is that amplification can occur at each step of what may be a multistep second messenger cascade (Fig. 12–7), so that the activity of many target ion channels may be modulated by the occupation of a relatively small number of receptors. A corollary of this is that activation of a second messenger system may produce coordinated changes in the activity of more than one kind of ion channel in the cell membrane (Fig. 12–7; see also Chapter 13). Furthermore, while tuning the activity of ion channels, a second messenger can also influence other cellular processes that have nothing to do with ion fluxes. Clearly these features are not generally characteristic of directly coupled systems.

Different Kinds of Second Messengers

A comprehensive treatment of the vast field comprising second messenger systems is far beyond the scope of this book; indeed whole books have been written about individual second messengers. Therefore, at the risk of omitting some that are favorites of our readers, we will confine ourselves in this and the next chapter to a summary of a few intracellular signaling

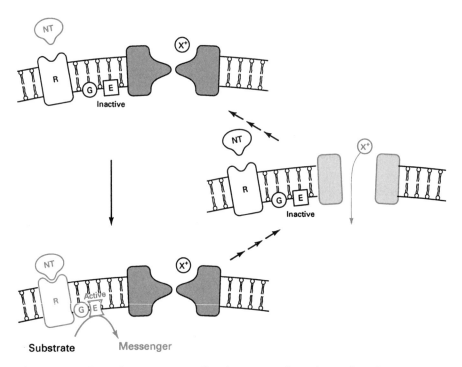

Figure 12–6. Second messenger–mediated receptor–channel coupling. In some cases neither the neurotransmitter receptor (R) nor the G protein (G) interacts directly with the ion channel. In these cases an intracellular second messenger influences ion channel activity. Contrast with Figures 11–8 and 12–2. E, enzyme regulated by G protein.

pathways that are known to play important roles in the modulation of neuronal excitability. In this chapter we will present an overview of the biochemistry of second messenger production and mechanism of action. Specific experimental examples that illustrate the role of each pathway in neuromodulatory phenomena will be given in the next chapter.

The specific pathways that we will discuss in detail include

1. the adenylate cyclase/cyclic AMP–dependent protein kinase system;
2. the guanylate cyclase/cyclic GMP–dependent protein kinase system; and
3. the phospholipase-mediated turnover of membrane phospholipids, which can lead to the production of the three distinct second messengers: inositol trisphosphate (IP$_3$), diacylglycerol (DAG), and arachidonic acid.

Before we discuss these, however, let us consider the general question of how changes in ion channel properties mediated by second messengers might be identified. Changes that last for a long time are, of course, strong candidates, but this criterion is not an unequivocal one. However, the cell-attached mode of the patch clamp technique does provide a convincing test for second messenger–mediated alteration of ion channel properties, independent of what the second messenger might be (Fig. 12–8).

The gigaohm seal between a patch electrode and the plasma membrane prevents the movement of neurotransmitter (and other) molecules between

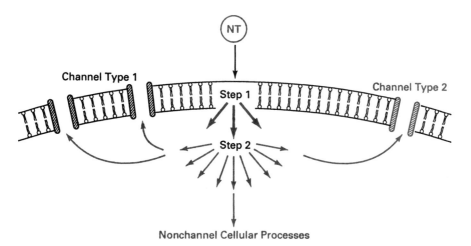

Figure 12–7. Amplification in second messenger cascades. With second messenger coupling the binding of a single neurotransmitter (NT) can activate many channels of a given class, activate several classes of channels, and affect other cellular processes not associated with ion channels.

the extracellular bathing medium and the inside of the electrode. Accordingly, transmitters placed in the bathing medium cannot have access to receptors within the patch electrode (Fig. 12–8, top). Therefore, directly coupled ion channels within the patch (black in Fig. 12–8) cannot be activated by a transmitter outside the patch electrode. If the transmitter activates ion channels within the patch, it must do so by binding to receptors out-

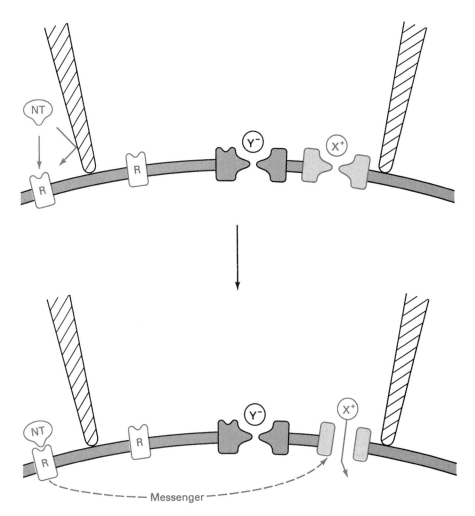

Figure 12–8. A test for second messenger mediation of neurotransmitter effects on ion channels. A neurotransmitter (NT) applied outside a patch electrode does not have access to receptors (R) within the patch. Accordingly, it can affect ion channels within the patch only by interacting with some receptor outside the patch. These receptors can communicate with channels inside the patch only by means of some diffusible intracellular messenger.

side the electrode. The only way these receptors can communicate with the channels in the patch is via some diffusible intracellular messenger (Fig. 12–8, bottom). An important feature of this general test for second messenger modulation is that it requires no a priori assumptions about the identity of the particular second messenger involved.

The adenylate cyclase/cyclic AMP–dependent protein kinase system. Cyclic AMP was first described by Earl Sutherland and colleagues as the second messenger mediating hormonally stimulated glycogen breakdown in the liver. A surprisingly long time elapsed before it was accepted as the intermediary in some neurotransmitter responses in nerve cells, but many such cyclic AMP–mediated responses have now been described. The major components of this system are illustrated in Figure 12–9a. Cyclic AMP is synthesized from ATP by the enzyme *adenylate cyclase*, which is coupled to a variety of different receptors via a specific G protein. The second messenger then activates the *cyclic AMP–dependent protein kinase*, which is a tetrameric complex of two each of two kinds of subunit. The holoenzyme complex is completely inactive. Binding of cyclic AMP to the *regulatory subunits* causes them to dissociate from the *catalytic subunits*. The free catalytic subunits are active (Fig. 12–9b), and can catalyze the transfer of the terminal phosphate from ATP to the hydroxyl groups of serine or threonine residues in the target protein to produce a phosphoprotein. This system is turned off by two kinds of enzymes: *phosphodiesterases*, which break down the cyclic AMP, and *phosphoprotein phosphatases*, which dephosphorylate the substrate proteins (Fig. 12–9a).

As we shall see below and in subsequent chapters, phosphorylation (and dephosphorylation) of enzymes, ion channels, or other proteins can lead to large changes in their functional properties. The way in which a particular cell responds to an elevation of cyclic AMP will thus depend on its particular spectrum of cell-specific substrate proteins that can be phosphorylated by the cyclic AMP–dependent protein kinase. Some specific examples of different cyclic AMP–mediated modulations in nerve and muscle cells are presented in Chapter 13. It was thought for a long time that all actions of cyclic AMP in eukaryotic cells are mediated by the cyclic AMP–dependent protein kinase as described above. However, it is now known that cyclic AMP interacts directly with some ion channels and activates them independently of kinase activation. This will be covered in Chapter 14, when we discuss sensory neurons in olfactory epithelia.

The guanylate cyclase/cyclic GMP–dependent protein kinase system. The basic components of the cyclic GMP signaling system (Figs. 12–10a and 12–11) are, to a considerable extent, similar to those for cyclic AMP. Some ex-

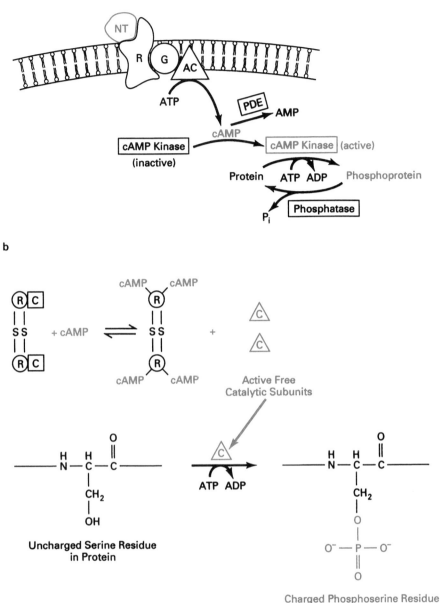

Figure 12–9. The adenylate cyclase/cyclic AMP–dependent protein kinase system. *a*: Cyclic AMP (cAMP) is synthesized from ATP by the enzyme adenylate cyclase (AC), and broken down by a phosphodiesterase (PDE). It activates a cyclic AMP–dependent protein kinase (cAMP kinase). G, G protein; NT, neurotransmitter; R, receptor. *b*: The cyclic AMP–dependent protein kinase is an inactive holoenzyme consisting of two regulatory (R) and two catalytic (C) subunits. Cyclic AMP binds to the regulatory subunits, releasing the catalytic subunits that are now active and can catalyze serine (or threonine) phosphorylation of target proteins.

tracellular ligands are known to elevate intracellular cyclic GMP levels, but the coupling mechanisms between the membrane receptor for the ligand and the guanylate cyclase (which is often a soluble enzyme) are less well understood than for the cyclic AMP system. In the case of *atrial natriuretic factor* (ANF), a peptide hormone, the amino acid sequence of its receptor contains a guanylate cyclase catalytic domain on the intracellular side (Fig. 12–10a).

Glutamate acting via NMDA receptors can also activate guanylate cyclase and increase intracellular cyclic GMP, but the coupling to guanylate cyclase is much less direct than in the case of ANF (Fig. 12–10b). Calcium that enters through the NMDA receptor/channels (see Chapter 11) acti-

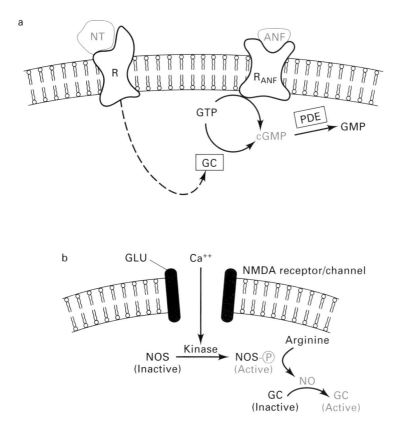

Figure 12–10. Production of cyclic GMP. *a*: The enzyme guanylate cyclase (GC) produces cyclic GMP (cGMP) from GTP. GC may be coupled directly to some receptors such as that for atrial natriuretic factor (ANF) (R_{ANF}). NT, neurotransmitter; R, receptor. *b*: GC can be stimulated indirectly by glutamate (GLU), acting via NMDA receptors and Ca^{2+}/Cam kinase II to produce the gas nitric oxide (NO). NOS, nitric oxide synthase.

vates a calcium/calmodulin-dependent protein kinase (Chapter 9) that in turn can phosphorylate and activate an enzyme called *nitric oxide synthase* (NOS). The NOS catalyzes the biosynthesis of the gas *nitric oxide* (NO) from the common amino acid arginine, and NO is an important biological messenger molecule. Among the targets that it stimulates is guanylate cyclase (Fig. 12–10b), by binding with high affinity to iron in the heme group that is a cofactor of this enzyme. Because NO is a gas that can diffuse readily across cell membranes, its actions may not be restricted to the cell in which it is generated. For example, one model for a long-term change in synaptic function involves diffusion of NO from the postsynaptic cell in which it is formed, to presynaptic terminals in which it may influence neurotransmitter release.

Having gone to all this trouble to produce cyclic GMP, how does the neuron make use of it? Like cyclic AMP, cyclic GMP can interact directly with ion channels, for example, the light-dependent ion channel in vertebrate photoreceptors (Chapter 14). However, many or most of the actions of cyclic GMP are mediated by a cyclic GMP–dependent protein kinase (Fig. 12–11a), which is a dimeric protein with two identical subunits linked

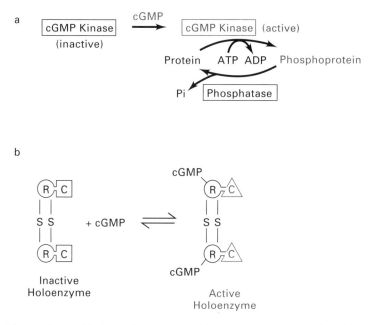

Figure 12–11. The cyclic GMP–dependent protein kinase system. *a*: Cyclic GMP (cGMP) can activate a cyclic GMP–dependent protein kinase. *b*: The cyclic GMP–dependent protein kinase is an inactive holoenzyme, and the regulatory (R) and catalytic (C) domains reside on a single subunit.

by disulfide bridges (Fig. 12–11b). Each subunit contains a cyclic GMP–binding domain, whose amino acid sequence is homologous to the cyclic AMP–binding region of the cyclic AMP–dependent protein kinase regulatory subunit. Similarly the catalytic domain in each subunit is homologous to the cyclic AMP–dependent kinase catalytic subunit. However, there is no subunit dissociation involved in the activation of the cyclic GMP–dependent kinase. Instead, cyclic GMP binding induces a conformational change that exposes and activates the catalytic domain (Fig. 12–11b). The role of the cyclic GMP system in neuromodulatory phenomena is less well understood than that of cyclic AMP, but there are now several examples of ion channel modulation in nerve cells that clearly are mediated by cyclic GMP–dependent protein phosphorylation.

Turnover of membrane phospholipids. Lowell and Mabel Hokin first demonstrated in 1952 that acetylcholine and other neurotransmitters and hormones can stimulate the breakdown and resynthesis (*turnover*) of the minor membrane phospholipid *phosphatidylinositol* (PI). Almost 25 years passed, however, before it was widely recognized that PI (and other phospholipids) might participate in signal transduction, and recent years have seen rapid, indeed explosive, growth in this field. This may be contrasted with the cyclic nucleotides, which were discovered later but very quickly became established as important second messenger molecules. Why was the PI story so long in developing? It is interesting to speculate that it might have been because lipid biochemistry is so difficult. Only a small, brave band of biochemists was prepared to struggle with these complex, water-insoluble phospholipids, whereas the majority extracted and discarded the lipid from their preparations as quickly as possible so it would not interfere with their study of proteins. In any event, the latent period is now behind us, and there is ample evidence that speaks to the fundamental importance of phospholipid metabolism in signal transduction in neurons as well as other kinds of cells.

A critical breakthrough came with the demonstration that the phospholipid species whose metabolism is stimulated by agonists is not PI itself but rather its doubly phosphorylated derivative, *phosphatidylinositol-4,5-bisphosphate* (PIP$_2$). As shown in Figure 12–12a, many receptors are coupled (via a G protein) to the membrane enzyme *phospholipase C* (PLC). This acts as a phosphodiesterase to split PIP$_2$ into two products, the water-soluble *inositol-1,4,5-trisphosphate* (IP$_3$), and *diacylglycerol* (DAG), which remains in the membrane. *Arachidonic acid* (AA), which is usually the fatty acid present in the 2 position of the glycerol backbone of PIP$_2$ (see Fig. 12–12b), can be released from DAG through the action of another membrane phospholipase, *phospholipase A$_2$* (PLA$_2$), which may also release AA directly from PIP$_2$. All three of these products—IP$_3$, DAG, and AA—are important second messengers.

The mechanisms by which these three second messengers work are summarized in Figure 12–13. The IP$_3$ diffuses in the cytoplasm and binds to specific receptors on the endoplasmic reticulum (see below). This binding opens a calcium channel in the endoplasmic reticulum membrane, and as a result, calcium ions are released into the cytoplasm from storage sites in the lumen of the endoplasmic reticulum (Fig. 12–13a). As we shall dis-

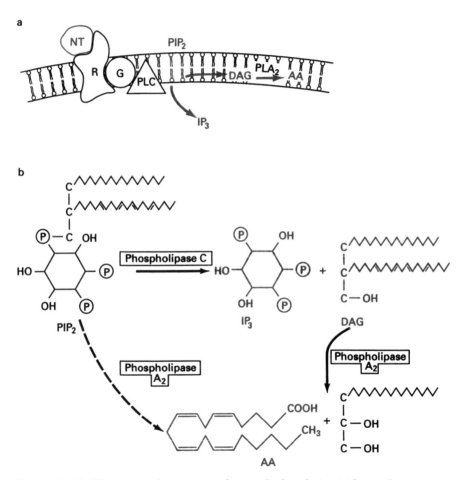

Figure 12–12. Three second messengers from polyphosphoinositides. *a*: Some neurotransmitter (NT) receptors (R) are coupled (via a G protein [G]) to the enzyme phospholipase C (PLC). b: The chemical structures of the second messenger molecules derived from the breakdown of the polyphosphoinositides (see review by Berridge, 1997). AA, arachidonic acid; DAG, diacylglycerol; IP$_3$, inositol trisphosphate; PIP$_2$, phosphatidylinositol-4,5-bisphosphate; PLA$_2$, phospholipase A$_2$.

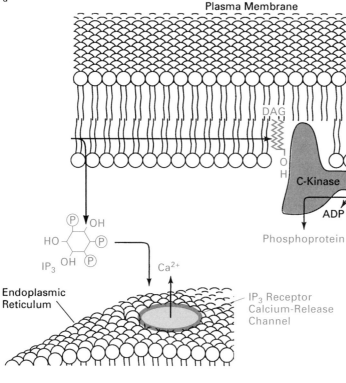

a

Plasma Membrane

DAG

O
H

C-Kinase

Protein

ADP   ATP

Phosphoprotein

P OH

HO

P

IP₃   OH   P

Ca²⁺

Endoplasmic
Reticulum

IP₃ Receptor
Calcium-Release
Channel

b

Lipoxygenase
Pathway

Leukotrienes

AA

COOH

CH₃

Cyclooxygenase
Pathway

Prostaglandins

Activate
Protein Kinase C
Directly

Activate
Ion Channels
Directly

Figure 12–13. Mechanisms of action of the phospholipid-derived second messengers. *a*: Diacylglycerol (DAG) activates a protein kinase called protein kinase C (PKC or C kinase). Inositol trisphosphate (IP₃) opens calcium channels in the endoplasmic reticulum (see reviews by Berridge, 1997; and Divecha and Irvine, 1995; drawing modified from Berridge, 1997). *b*: Arachidonic acid (AA) may directly activate PKC or some ion channels. It can also be metabolized to the leukotrienes and the prostaglandins.

cuss below, the elevated cytoplasmic calcium can influence ion channel activity and a myriad of other cellular functions.

The DAG, in contrast, remains associated with the membrane. An increase in DAG results in a translocation from cytoplasm to membrane of *protein kinase* C (often called PKC), another member in the family of protein kinases that catalyze the phosphorylation of serine and threonine residues in substrate proteins (some of which are ion channels). Protein kinase C becomes active only when it associates with the membrane and binds DAG (Fig. 12–13a). A specific example of neuromodulation mediated by protein kinase C can be found in Figure 13–6.

In the test tube, protein kinase C can be activated by the addition of DAG together with phosphatidylserine, the latter apparently serving as a substitute for the cell membrane. In addition, a series of compounds called *phorbol esters*, first characterized as tumor-promoting agents, are useful pharmacological tools that can substitute for DAG in activating protein kinase C, both in the test tube and when applied to intact cells. PIP_2 may not be the most important source of DAG; PIP_2 is only a minor component of the plasma membrane, and the amounts of DAG produced in response to an agonist are often too large to be accounted for solely by PIP_2 breakdown. However, some agonists activate a *phospholipase D* (again via a G protein), which catalyzes the release of phosphatidic acid from *phosphatidylcholine*, the major membrane phospholipid. The phosphatidic acid can then be metabolized further to DAG. This pathway provides a mechanism for producing DAG and activating protein kinase C without concomitant activation of the IP_3 calcium release system.

The actions of AA, the third second messenger product of phospholipid turnover, are less well understood. Arachidonic acid can be metabolized via several different pathways, each of which gives rise to biologically active products including the prostaglandins and the leukotrienes (Fig. 12–13b). In addition, AA can act as an activator of one form of protein kinase C in the brain.

The complexity of lipid signaling is in fact even greater than indicated above. It is now known that a phosphatidylinositol-1,4,5-trisphosphate (PIP_3) can be produced in cell membranes via the action of an enzyme called *PI-3 kinase*, and this may also be involved in the modulation of membrane ion channels. In addition, receptor-mediated hydrolysis of a complex membrane lipid called *sphingomyelin* produces several products that may act as intracellular messengers. Undoubtedly there are surprises still to be uncovered in this area.

Down-regulation of G protein–coupled receptors. We have mentioned briefly that many neurotransmitters are subject to *down-regulation*, also often called *desensitization*. These terms refer to a progressive decrease in the response to a neurotransmitter during maintained exposure or multiple exposures of the cell to the same transmitter. In some cases desensitization results from receptor *internalization*, the removal of receptors from the plasma membrane by the pinching off and internalization of membrane vesicles that contain receptor molecules (Fig. 12–14a). This agonist-dependent process is best understood for certain growth factor receptors and may be important for regulating β-adrenergic receptors as well. Internalization may result in degradation of the receptors within the cell, although in at least some cases the internalized receptors can be recycled back to the plasma membrane (Fig. 12–14a).

Several members of the G protein–coupled receptor family can also be down-regulated by phosphorylation. Photoreceptors contain an enzyme called *rhodopsin kinase*, which specifically phosphorylates light-activated rhodopsin and decreases its sensitivity to light (Fig. 12–14b). The agonist-occupied β-adrenergic receptor can be phosphorylated and down-regulated by the cyclic AMP–dependent protein kinase as well as by a more specific β-adrenergic receptor kinase (βARK; see Fig. 12–14b). There are a number of serine and threonine residues that are potential sites for phosphorylation near the carboxyl terminal of the G protein–coupled receptors (on the cytoplasmic side of the membrane). These residues and adjacent amino acid sequences are well conserved in other members of this receptor family, and some of them are also down-regulated by phosphorylation. Phosphorylation by several different protein kinases is also involved in desensitization of at least one member of the ligand-gated receptor/channel family, the nicotinic acetylcholine receptor, and thus this mechanism may be widespread.

Features of G protein signaling—a reprise. Modulation of neuronal properties by G proteins, either via direct interaction with ion channels or via second messenger systems, is ubiquitous. Thus it is worth summarizing here some of the key features that are characteristic of G protein signaling. First, it provides a wide temporal range for physiological responses, ranging from tens of milliseconds for direct ion channel modulation to seconds or even minutes for second messenger–mediated responses. A second important feature is that G protein signaling often involves enzymatic cascades that can vastly amplify the response to just a small amount of neurotransmitter or other first messenger. Finally, because a second messenger system may influence several different kinds of ion channels or other effector systems, G protein signaling may allow for the coordinate modulation of multiple effectors to produce a coherent cellular response.

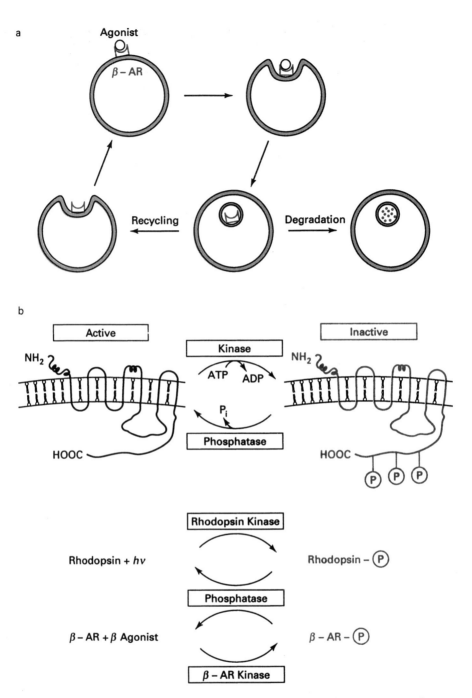

Figure 12–14. Receptor down-regulation. *a*: Agonist-occupied receptors may be internalized by endocytosis, and either recycled to the cell surface or degraded. *b*: Members of the G protein–coupled receptor family, such as rhodopsin or the β-adrenergic receptor (β-AR), may also be down-regulated by phosphorylation. These down-regulations can be reversed by phosphoprotein phosphatases. *hν*, photon of light.

306

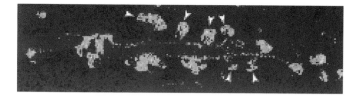

PLATE 1. Pseudo-color representation of dendritic spine movements such as those in Figure 1–5. Areas of greatest movement are red while those that do not move are dark. Note that the spine heads (*arrows*) are highly dynamic, whereas the dendritic shaft is not. From an experiment by Martijn Roelandse and Andrew Matus.

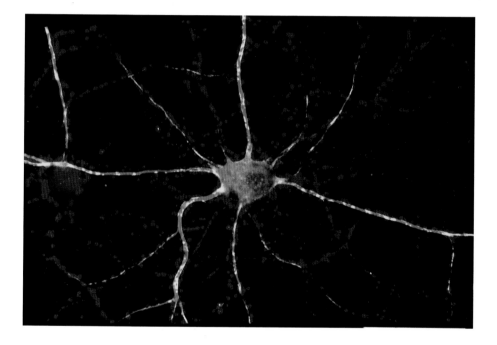

PLATE 2. Synaptic inputs on a cultured hippocampal neuron (courtesy of Pietro De Camilli). See also Figure 1-9.

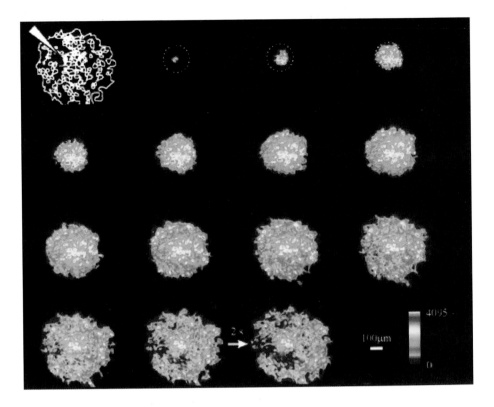

PLATE 3. Pseudo-color image to show the spread of calcium waves through a network of astrocytes in cell culture. Compare with Figure 2–2. From an experiment by Phil Haydon and collaborators.

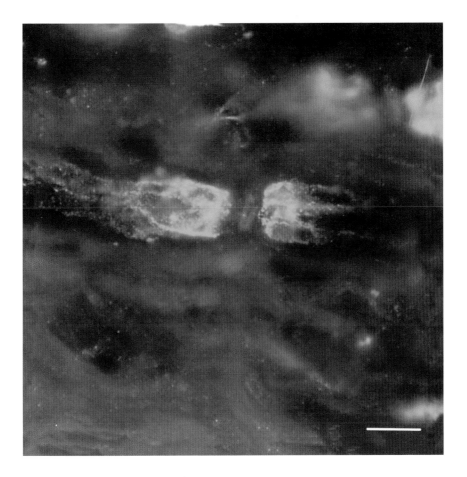

PLATE 4. Distribution of ion channels in myelinated axons. Sodium channels (*red*) are concentrated at the node of Ranvier, whereas potassium channels (*green*) are in the juxtaparanodal region. From experiments by Matt Rasband, Jim Trimmer, and colleagues.

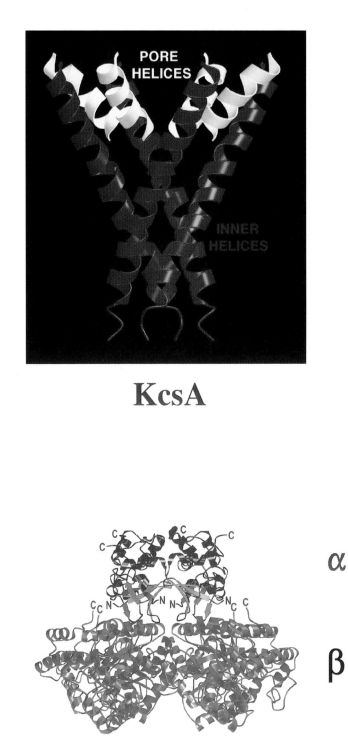

PLATE 5. Structures of potassium channel subunits from X-ray crystallography. Top, ribbon diagram to illustrate the "inverted teepee" structure formed by the helices of the bacterial KcsA potassium channel. Modified from Doyle et al., 1998. See also Figure 5–13. Bottom, ribbon diagram to illustrate the structure of part of the cytoplasmic domain of a voltage-dependent potassium channel α subunit (*red*), bound to its β subunit (*blue*). Modified from Gulbis et al., 2000. See also Figure 7–14.

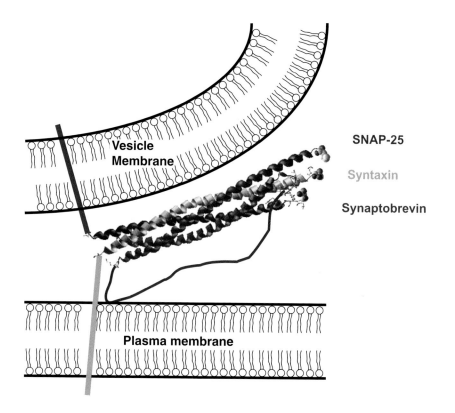

SNAP-25

Syntaxin

Synaptobrevin

Vesicle Membrane

Plasma membrane

PLATE 6. Structure of the SNARE complex. The interactions of synaptobrevin, syntaxin, and SNAP-25 have been determined by X-ray crystallography. Locations of the vesicle and plasma membranes and the transmembrane regions of the proteins are drawn in for clarity (Sutton et al., 1998).

Stimulation

67 ms

200 ms

333 ms

467 ms

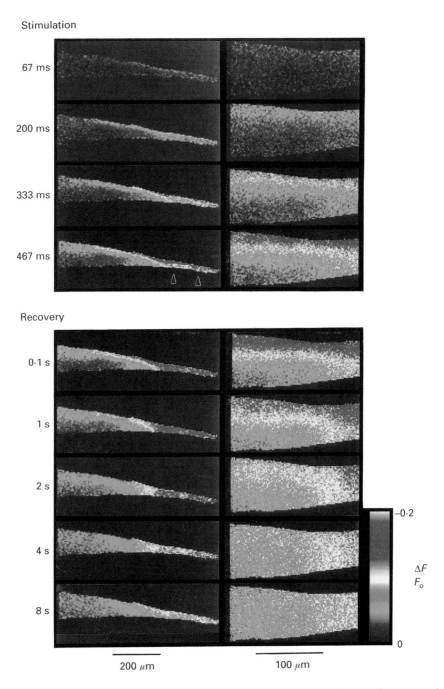

Recovery

0·1 s

1 s

2 s

4 s

8 s

−0·2

$\dfrac{\Delta F}{F_o}$

0

200 μm

100 μm

PLATE 7. Video images of the levels of intracellular calcium in the squid presynaptic terminal, during and after stimulation. Calcium was measured using the calcium indicator fura-2, with high levels of calcium shown in red and low levels in blue. Active zones are at the top of the terminal, which is shown at low power (*left*) and high power (*right*) (Smith et al., 1993; see also Fig. 9–6).

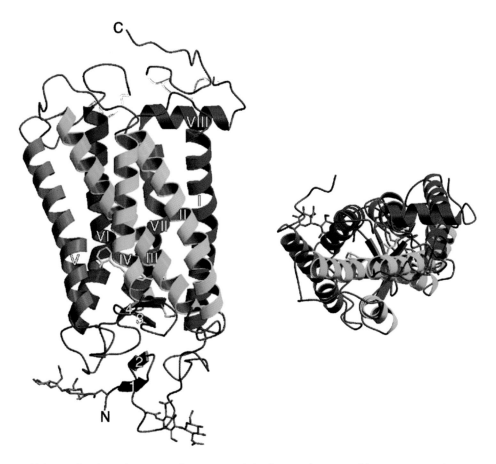

PLATE 8. The three-dimensional structure of rhodopsin, determined by X-ray crystallography. *Left:* Organization of the transmembrane regions viewed from the plane of the membrane. *Right:* A view of the protein from the cytoplasmic side of the membrane (Palczewski et al., 2000).

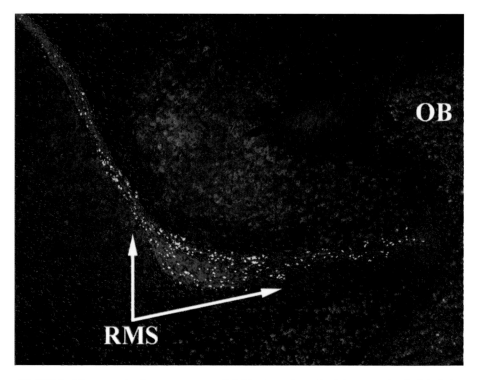

PLATE 9. The rostral migratory stream (RMS). A section of adult mouse brain labeled with bromodeoxyuridine (*green*) to show newly formed neurons migrating towards the olfactory bulb (OB). Dyes have also been used to show mature neurons (*red*) and the rostral migratory stream (RMS, *blue*) (van der Kooy and Weiss, 2000). See also Figure 15–6.

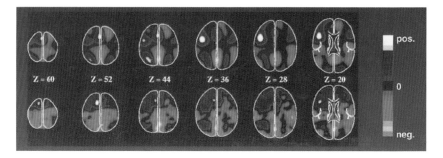

PLATE 10. Images of regional blood flow in different parts of the human brain. The bright colors indicate areas of high blood flow that reflects enhanced neuronal activity. From an experiment by Marcus Raichle and colleagues (Raichle, 1998).

Calcium Signaling

Free cytoplasmic calcium plays a ubiquitous role in neuronal signal transduction processes. Its concentration is some four or five orders of magnitude lower than that in the extracellular space or in intracellular calcium
storage sites, and is tightly regulated by a variety of pumps and binding
proteins. One important source of cytoplasmic calcium is entry across the
plasma membrane through voltage-dependent calcium channels; another
is release from storage sites in the endoplasmic reticulum, particularly under the influence of IP_3.

Intracellular calcium-release channels. How is IP_3 able to cause calcium release from the endoplasmic reticulum stores (Fig. 12–13)? It does so by
binding to an *IP_3 receptor*, a ligand-gated ion channel located in the membrane of the endoplasmic reticulum. The IP_3 receptor/channels are formed
as tetramers of large (about 300 kDa) protein subunits, each of which can
be divided into three domains (Fig. 12–15a): a ligand-binding domain, a
modulation/transduction domain, and a channel domain that includes six
membrane-spanning segments and a pore region related to that in the voltage-dependent ion channels (see Chapters 3–7). The IP_3-gated ion channel formed from these subunits can be observed by reconstituting endoplasmic reticulum membranes into artificial phospholipid bilayers (Fig.
12–15b) or by patch clamping isolated nuclei (the endoplasmic reticulum
is continuous with the nuclear membrane). They are cation-selective channels that resemble in many ways plasma membrane ion channels (Fig.
12–15b).

Neurons and other cells also contain an endoplasmic reticulum calcium-release channel, called the *ryanodine receptor*, that is opened by elevated cytoplasmic calcium. Thus calcium that enters the cell via plasma
membrane voltage-dependent calcium channels can activate the ryanodine
receptor/channel and cause a regenerative release of calcium. It is also possible that calcium released into the cytoplasm through IP_3 receptor/chan-
nels can activate nearby ryanodine receptor/channels, hence giving rise to
complex patterns of intracellular calcium signaling. The subunits of the
ryanodine receptor are similar in overall structure to those of the IP_3 receptor (Fig. 12–15a) but are almost twice as large. There are multiple sites
for phosphorylation, by a variety of protein kinases, in both the IP_3 and
ryanodine receptors, and they appear to be modulated in complex ways.

Calcium as a second messenger. Calcium plays a central role in the activity
of all cells. In nerve cells and other cells that possess calcium channels in
their plasma membranes, we have seen that calcium can act as a charge

carrier to modulate beating or bursting activity, action potential shape, and other aspects of electrical activity.

Charge transfer, however, may be among the more banal of calcium's many functions (Fig. 12–16). Its entry across the plasma membrane or release from intracellular stores produces such diverse effects as (1) triggering of secretion, (2) muscle contraction, and (3) activation of protein kinases, other enzymes, and calcium-dependent ion channels. Changes in intracellular calcium can be induced directly by certain neurotransmitters, such as those linked to formation of IP$_3$, or others that activate calcium-permeable ion channels such as the NMDA receptor channel (see Chapter 11). Let us not forget, however, that changes in this second messenger also occur as a *direct result of neuronal activity*. Calcium entry through voltage-dependent calcium channels results in transduction of an electrical signal—a change in voltage—into a chemical signal.

a

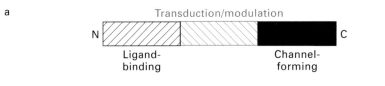

b   Control

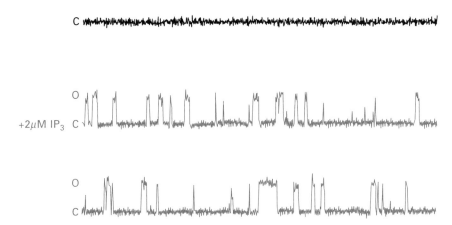

Figure 12–15. Calcium-release channels. *a*: Structural domains of the IP$_3$ and ryanodine receptors (modified from Furuichi et al., 1994). *b*: An example of an IP$_3$ receptor/channel reconstituted in an artificial bilayer membrane. The channel is closed (C) and opens (O) only in the presence of IP$_3$ (from an experiment by Barbara Ehrlich and colleagues).

The intracellular calcium signal is received and decoded by calcium-binding proteins including the ubiquitous small protein *calmodulin*, which we discussed in Chapter 9. Calcium binding induces a large conformational change in calmodulin, exposing a hydrophobic domain that can interact with a large variety of effector proteins (Fig. 12–16). Among these are a variety of ion channels (see Chapter 13), and at least four different types of calcium/calmodulin-dependent protein kinase. One of these kinases, the *multifunctional calcium/calmodulin-dependent protein kinase* (Ca^{2+}/Cam kinase II; see Chapter 9), is present at high concentration in both presynaptic terminals and postsynaptic densities and in fact comprises as much as 1% of total brain protein. Like the cyclic AMP–dependent protein kinase, this enzyme acts on a wide range of substrates, among them NOS (Fig. 12–10b) and other proteins that may be involved in synaptic transmission. We described in Chapter 9 the modulation of neurotransmitter release at the squid giant synapse by Ca^{2+}/Cam kinase II in the presynaptic terminal, and its high concentration in postsynaptic densities has led to speculation about its role in receptor and/or ion channel modulation. One feature of this enzyme is that, like many other kinases, it can undergo autophosphorylation. That is, it phosphorylates itself in a calcium/calmodulin-dependent manner. Particularly intriguing is the fact that once several of the subunits are phosphorylated, the enzyme becomes

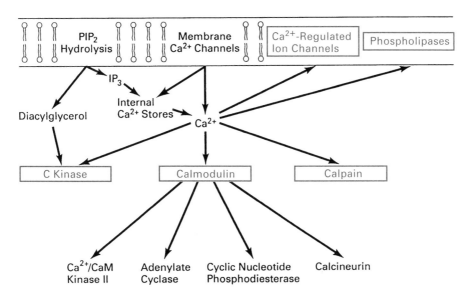

Figure 12–16. Some actions of intracellular calcium ions. Calcium can interact directly with several membrane and cytoplasmic proteins and regulate their properties. Among its cytoplasmic binding proteins is calmodulin, which in its calcium-bound form regulates the activities of many enzymes. (Modified from Kennedy, 1989.)

active independent of calcium/calmodulin (Fig. 9–12). Thus a transient calcium signal can produce long-lasting activation of this kinase, a finding that has led to hypotheses that the enzyme acts as a "calcium switch" to produce long-lasting changes in neuronal properties of the sort discussed in Chapter 20.

Calmodulin as an auxiliary subunit of ion channels. Another feature of calcium signaling deserves mention here. It has been known for many years that calcium can influence the activity of some ion channels, such as the calcium-dependent potassium channels that we have discussed in several different contexts and will meet again in later chapters. More recently it has become evident that at least some of these actions of calcium on ion channel properties are mediated by channel-associated calmodulin. For example, the activities of several different classes of calcium-permeant channels (among them voltage-dependent calcium channels, NMDA receptor/channels, and the cyclic nucleotide-gated channels in sensory receptor neurons that we shall discuss in Chapter 14) are inhibited by calcium, acting via calmodulin that is bound constitutively to the channel (Fig. 12–17, left). In contrast, the intermediate (IK) and small (SK) conductance calcium-dependent potassium channels described in Chapter 7 are activated by calcium, via constitutively bound calmodulin (Fig.12–17, right). The emerging theme is that calmodulin, in addition to its many other cellular roles, can act as an ion channel auxiliary subunit that mediates feedback inhibition of calcium entry.

Interactions and commonalities among second messenger systems. The diversity in second messenger systems does not (yet) approach that of the first messengers—the extracellular signaling molecules—or their membrane receptors. However, there is considerable complexity in second messenger systems because the different second messenger systems can interact at various levels. For example, G proteins may participate in the formation of several different second messengers. In addition, one second messenger may influence the activities of enzymes that are involved in the turning on or off of another messenger pathway. To give just several examples, there are calcium/calmodulin-dependent cyclic AMP phosphodiesterases and phosphoprotein phosphatases, and calcium can both stimulate and inhibit adenylate cyclases. In the face of this complexity it is gratifying to find common features among these pathways. Most second messengers are generated via G protein–mediated enzymatic reactions, and most use protein phosphorylation as their final common mechanism for producing a biological response. Nevertheless, one must always take into account the interactions among second messenger systems in drawing conclusions about their roles in physiological responses. We shall elaborate on this theme in our discussion of transduction in specialized nerve cells and mechanisms of modulation of neuronal electrical behavior in subsequent chapters.

Receptors Linked to Tyrosine Kinases

Some receptor families transduce their signals through pathways other than those we have described thus far. The *receptor tyrosine kinases* are a specialized class of protein kinases that phosphorylate proteins exclusively on tyrosine residues. In contrast to the other protein kinases we have discussed, the activity of the receptor tyrosine kinases is not regulated by intracellular second messenger molecules. Instead the enzymatic activity resides in an intracellular catalytic domain, which is part of the membrane receptors for certain growth factors (Fig. 12–18). In other words, the growth factor receptors themselves are tyrosine kinases, which are activated directly by the binding of the growth factor. Once activated, these

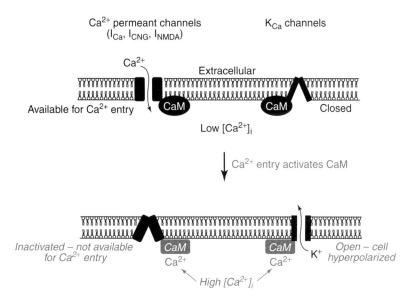

Figure 12–17. Calmodulin confers calcium sensitivity on certain ion channels. Calmodulin binds to some channels that allow calcium entry (*top left*). The entering calcium then activates the channel-bound calmodulin, causing channel inactivation and feedback inhibition of calcium entry (*bottom left*). In contrast, calmodulin bound to IK and SK calcium-dependent potassium channels (*top right*) mediates channel opening in the presence of calcium, resulting in membrane hyperpolarization and again feedback inhibition of calcium entry (*bottom right*). (Modified from Levitan, 1999.)

kinases phosphorylate themselves as well as other substrates, which include ion channels. Among the growth factors that act via such receptors are *epidermal growth factor* (EGF) and *nerve growth factor* (NGF) and related *neurotrophic factors*. As we shall see in later chapters, neurotrophic factors play a crucial role in neuronal differentiation during development of the nervous system, and they can also modulate neuronal excitability and synaptic transmission in the mature nervous system. It is known from site-directed mutagenesis experiments that the stimulation of tyrosine kinase activity is essential for the biological actions of growth factors that act through tyrosine kinase-linked receptors.

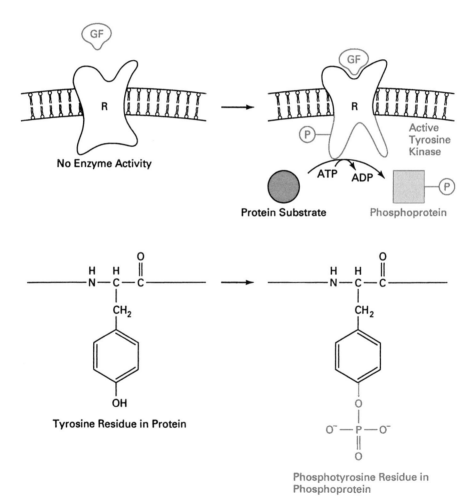

Figure 12–18. Receptors linked to tyrosine kinases. The receptors (R) for a number of growth factors (GF) contain an intracellular domain that can catalyze the phosphorylation of proteins on tyrosine residues. This tyrosine kinase activity is observed only when the receptor is occupied by the growth factor.

Other Receptor Families

Although we have focused our attention on the G protein–coupled receptor family in the discussion of second messengers, it is important to realize that there are other receptor families whose activity can also influence the same second messenger pathways. For example, some growth factor receptors, structurally unrelated to the G protein-coupled family, also stimulate the IP_3/DAG pathway directly. In addition, the receptor for one peptide hormone, atrial natriuretic factor, contains a cytoplasmic domain that is a guanylate cyclase (Fig. 12–10a). This may be the forerunner of an entirely new class of membrane receptors.

The fact that we have not dealt with other receptors in as much depth as the directly coupled or G protein–coupled families should not be taken to imply that other receptor systems are any less important. Rather, it reflects the breadth of the field and the fact that more is known about how these two families regulate neuronal excitability. We have also chosen the directly coupled and G protein–coupled receptors as examples of receptor families in which the relationship between structure and function is beginning to be understood. Other families are indeed known, and we can be confident that there are even more out there waiting to be discovered in the future.

What Determines the Biological Response

Where does the specificity lie in the response of a target cell to a particular extracellular signal? This is a dilemma that has been with us since it was realized that cyclic AMP can mediate different biological responses in different kinds of cells. In the particular case of cyclic AMP, some answers are beginning to emerge. It is now known that neurons and other cells contain a class of proteins, known as *cyclic AMP–dependent protein kinase anchoring proteins* (AKAPs), that bind to the regulatory subunit of the kinase. Different AKAPs have unique targeting domains that localize the AKAP–kinase complex to discrete cellular compartments adjacent to specific substrate proteins. Thus the specificity of the response to cyclic AMP in a particular cell or region of a cell may depend on the particular AKAPs present in that cell. It is also known that some protein kinases may bind directly to a particular ion channel, without an anchoring protein as an intermediary.

The question of specificity has become even more pressing with the recognition that G proteins are involved in the production of a wide variety of responses. We are still without a complete understanding of this issue of response specificity, but important clues have emerged from experiments in which receptors have been expressed in cell types in which they are not normally found. These receptors can couple to the host cell's endogenous transduction mechanisms, and activation by agonist then produces a biological response that is characteristic of the host cell rather than of the exogenous receptor and its ligand. For example, serotonin receptors, which may be coupled to ion channels in the nerve cells from which they are isolated, can cause malignant transformation when they are expressed in fibroblasts and activated by serotonin. Similarly, changes typical of the response to sperm can be evoked by serotonin when one of its receptors is expressed in eggs. These experiments tell us that the specificity resides in the target cell and in the particular biological response system(s) that the cell makes available to interact with the receptor and transduction mechanism.

Summary

Extracellular signals must be recognized by the target cell and transduced into an appropriate biological response. Signal recognition is accomplished by the specific membrane receptors that are coupled to different kinds of transduction mechanisms, which in nerve cells usually regulate the activity of ion channels. The simplest receptor–ion channel coupling system, discussed in the previous chapter, consists of the ligand-binding site and channel within a single protein molecule or macromolecular complex. A coupling mechanism of intermediate complexity involves protein–protein interactions, between a G protein and ion channel, in the plane of the plasma membrane. Finally, many ion channels are coupled to receptors via diffusible intracellular second messengers. The purpose of this diversity in the categories of receptor–channel coupling may be to provide a wide temporal range in the responses of neurons to neurotransmitters, hormones, and sensory stimuli.

Diversity also exists within the category of second messenger–mediated coupling. There are a variety of second messenger systems that at first glance appear to bear little relationship to one another. However, several of these share a common final mechanism of action on response systems, namely protein phosphorylation via one of several second messenger-dependent protein kinases. As we shall see in Chapter 13, modulation of neuronal excitability by protein phosphorylation often involves direct phosphorylation of the ion channel protein itself or of some closely associated regulatory component.

13

Neuromodulation: Mechanisms of Induced Changes in the Electrical Behavior of Nerve Cells

*A*ll neurons are not created equal. Even neighboring nerve cells may be distinct in their electrical properties and exhibit very different patterns of endogenous electrical activity. As we know from the discussion in Part II of this book, these diverse patterns of activity reflect the complement of ion channels that are active under a given set of conditions. The fundamental issue that we address now is the fact that these patterns of electrical activity are not fixed, but are subject to modulation resulting from synaptic or hormonal stimulation. Neurons may undergo long-lasting changes in the shape and amplitude of their action potentials, in the temporal pattern of action potential firing, and in the ways they respond to synaptic stimulation (Fig. 13–1). Such modulation of neuronal electrical properties, mediated by transduction mechanisms, some of which are described in Chapters 11 and 12, not only allow the nervous system to adapt its output in the face of a continually changing environment but also are the basis for many long-lasting changes in behavior. Because neuromodulation underlies the choice of different patterns of behavior at different times, it is of critical importance for the proper functioning of the nervous system.

In this chapter we will discuss several examples of neuromodulation that are understood, at least partly, in terms of their biochemical mechanisms and physiological consequences. The theme here, as it has been in a number of previous chapters, is one of diversity. Different kinds of ion channels may be modulated in different cells, and a variety of molecular mechanisms are employed to effect the modulation. Accordingly, we have chosen to present several examples of modulatory phenomena, in different organisms, to provide a feel for the diversity. We shall also take a historical perspective, beginning with some early examples of neuromodulation to illustrate the experimental approaches that have been taken and the general lessons that have been learned. Among these lessons is the finding that direct phosphorylation of ion channels is a mechanism mediating many, although by no means all, neuromodulatory events.

Modulation of the Size and Shape of Action Potentials

When we discussed the ionic mechanisms of the action potential in Part II, we emphasized that the action potential is an all-or-none phenomenon, the amplitude of which is invariant because it depends only on the sodium concentration gradient. Although this is essentially correct for the special case of the squid giant axon, it is an oversimplification for most nerve cells. We know now that in many neuronal somata there is a calcium current that contributes to the depolarizing phase of the action potential and a series of different potassium currents that participate in repolarization and help to determine action potential shape. We also know that many of

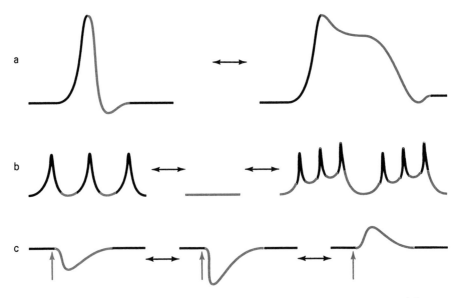

Figure 13–1. Modulation of neuronal membrane properties. Common modulatory changes in neuronal membrane properties include (*a*) changes in the amplitude and/or duration of action potentials, (*b*) changes in endogenous firing patterns between beating (*left*), silent (*middle*), and bursting (*right*) modes, and (*c*) changes in the efficacy of synaptic inputs.

these currents can be modulated, leading to changes in the size and shape of action potentials. An important functional consequence of such changes is the modulation of transmitter release triggered by the action potentials when they invade presynaptic terminals.

Dorsal root ganglion neurons. One of the earliest examples of modulation of action potential duration was in neurons of the chick *dorsal root ganglion* (DRG), a way station in the pathway through which sensory information from the periphery reaches the spinal cord. A variety of neurotransmitters can cause a narrowing of action potentials in DRG neurons (Fig. 13–2a). Among the transmitters that produce this effect are the peptides enkephalin and somatostatin, as well as serotonin, GABA, and norepinephrine. In principle, there are two possible ways such a shortening could come about. There might be an increase in the potassium currents that are responsible for spike repolarization; alternatively, or in addition, the transmitters might directly decrease the calcium or sodium currents that underlie the depolarizing phase of the spike. Voltage clamp experiments strongly support

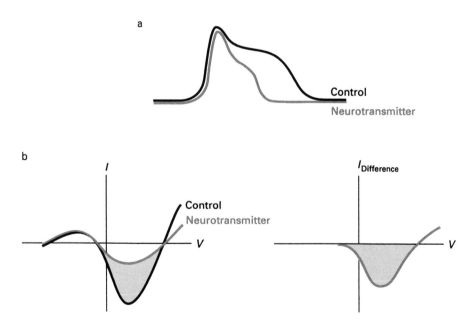

Figure 13–2. Modulation of action potential duration in dorsal root ganglion neurons. *a*: As first demonstrated by Dunlap and Fischbach (1978), a variety of neurotransmitters can cause a shortening of the action potential in dorsal root ganglion neurons. *b*: Voltage clamp analysis indicates that this results from a decrease in inward current. At the right the difference current elicited by the neurotransmitter is plotted. *I*, current; *V*, voltage.

the latter explanation. As shown in Figure 13–2b, the various transmitters cause a decrease in a current with a voltage dependence expected for a calcium current (compare with Fig. 7–1c).

What is the molecular mechanism mediating this shortening of action potentials in DRG neurons? Intracellular application of GDPβS, or pretreatment of the DRG neurons with pertussis toxin, can block the actions of norepinephrine or GABA. In addition, application of a diacylglycerol (DAG) activator of protein kinase C can decrease the calcium current in these neurons, and a protein kinase C inhibitor can block the transmitter-induced spike shortening. Taken together, these results suggest that a G protein–mediated activation of phospholipase C, with the ensuing release of DAG and activation of protein kinase C (see Chapter 12), is responsible for the decrease in calcium current and shortening of the action potential. The physiological consequence of this shortening is likely to be a decrease in transmitter release at the DRG neuron terminals and an attenuation of the amount of sensory information that is allowed to reach the spinal cord. This is of particular interest in the case of enkephalin. An enkephalin-induced decrease in action potential duration, with a consequent decrement in release of the pain pathway sensory transmitter, substance P, from DRG neurons, might account for some of the analgesic actions of enkephalin and other opiate agonists.

Cardiac myocytes. Another of the earliest, and probably most thoroughly understood, examples of modulation of action potential duration is the spike prolongation evoked by β-adrenergic agonists in cardiac cells. We do recognize that cardiac muscle cells are not, strictly speaking, neurons. However, we may define them as honorary neurons because there are so many parallels between cardiac and nerve cells with respect to mechanisms of electrical signaling and its modulation. The resemblance between neurons and other types of cells, which we have emphasized throughout, is nowhere more evident than it is here.

The fundamental mechanism of the cardiac action potential and its modulation are well understood. The action potential is predominantly a calcium spike, and it can be prolonged dramatically by treatment with noradrenaline or other β-adrenergic agonists (Fig. 13–3a). This prolongation, together with a series of other biochemical and electrophysiological changes, contributes to the multifaceted consequences of β-adrenergic stimulation that include changes in the rate and force of contraction of the heart. β-adrenergic receptor antagonists (commonly known as β *blockers*) have long been used widely as drugs to treat a variety of cardiovascular syndromes.

As in the case of the DRG neurons discussed above, a priori it seems

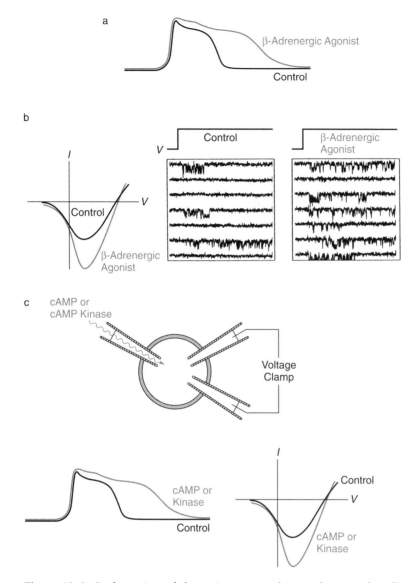

Figure 13–3. Prolongation of the action potential in cardiac muscle cells. *a*: Studies from the laboratories of Harald Reuter, Richard Tsien, and Wolfgang Trautwein have shown that β-adrenergic agonists increase the duration of the cardiac action potential. *b*: This is due to an increase in calcium current (*left*), resulting from an increase in the activity of voltage-dependent calcium channels (*right*). *c*: Intracellular injection of cyclic AMP or cyclic AMP–dependent protein kinase elicits the same changes (see Tsien, 1987 and Levitan, 1999). *I*, current; *V*, voltage.

possible that changes in either inward or outward currents (or both) could account for the modulation of action potential duration. Voltage clamp experiments demonstrate that the ionic mechanism of the change in spike duration is an increase in the calcium current, which is responsible for the plateau phase of the depolarization (Fig. 13–3b; compare with Fig. 13–2b). Single channel analysis confirms that β-adrenergic stimulation produces an increase in the activity of calcium channels (Fig. 13–3b), which leads in turn to spike broadening. All of these effects can be mimicked by the intracellular injection of cyclic AMP or the extracellular application of membrane-permeant cyclic AMP analogs, as well as by the injection of the active catalytic subunit of the cyclic AMP–dependent protein kinase (Fig. 13–3c). Clearly, cyclic AMP–dependent protein phosphorylation mediates this example of modulation of action potential duration. Later in this chapter we shall consider the experimental evidence that the phosphorylatable regulatory protein is actually the ion channel protein itself.

The theme of diversity, to which we referred at the beginning of this chapter, will already be evident in these first two classical examples of modulation of action potential shape. Both involve changes in calcium current, but in one case the current is decreased whereas in the other it is enhanced. Furthermore, entirely separate transduction mechanisms mediate the modulatory responses. Now we shall introduce another level of complexity as we move on to discuss an example from the *Aplysia* nervous system, in which action potential amplitude and duration can be regulated by several different ion currents and/or several different transduction mechanisms within an individual neuron.

Aplysia bag cell neurons. The bag cell neurons are two clusters of homogeneous neurosecretory neurons associated with the *Aplysia* abdominal ganglion (Fig. 13–4). As we will discuss in Chapter 19, the bag cell neurons synthesize and release several neuroactive peptides that trigger a series of events necessary for reproduction. Secretion of the peptides is evoked by a long-lasting discharge called an *afterdischarge* (see Fig. 19–10), during which both the amplitude and duration of the action potentials are enhanced. We shall consider here the mechanisms involved in this modulation of action potential size and shape.

Because all the bag cell neurons in an intact cluster are coupled to one another via electrical synapses, it is impossible to voltage clamp the cells to examine their electrical properties. However, the neurons retain many of their morphological and electrical characteristics when they are isolated in primary cell culture, and this preparation has been exploited to investigate neuromodulatory phenomena. Although such isolated neurons generally exhibit no spontaneous electrical activity, they can be induced to fire action potentials in response to depolarizing current pulses. Both the amplitude and duration of these action potentials are enhanced when cyclic AMP levels in the cell are increased (Fig. 13–5a). This can be effected by treatment with a peptide transmitter synthesized and released by the bag cell neurons themselves (see Chapter 19) or by membrane-permeant cyclic AMP analogs. The modulation of the action potential by cyclic AMP, which presumably acts as an intracellular second messenger for the peptide, is mimicked by the injection of the catalytic subunit of cyclic AMP–dependent protein kinase (Fig. 13–5a) and blocked by injection of a protein kinase inhibitor.

What ion current is modulated by cyclic AMP–dependent protein phosphorylation to produce these changes in the action potential in the bag cell neurons? Again, both calcium and potassium currents are a priori candidates, and one could not predict the answer based on the examples we have examined thus far. Voltage clamp experiments (Fig. 13–5b) have demonstrated that the answer in this case is potassium. The bag cell neurons have several components of delayed rectifier potassium current involved

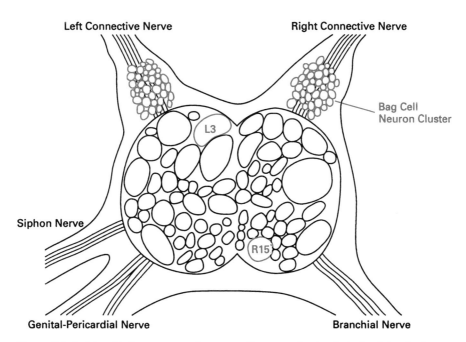

Figure 13–4. Identified neurons and groups of neurons in the *Aplysia* abdominal ganglion. Drawing, after one by Eric Kandel and colleagues (Kandel, 1976), of the dorsal surface of the *Aplysia* abdominal ganglion. The bag cell neuron clusters and several identified neuronal cell bodies described in this and other chapters are shown in blue.

in spike repolarization. Decreases in these potassium currents lead to the marked prolongation of the action potential following treatment with cyclic AMP.

Cyclic AMP is not the only second messenger that modulates the action potential in bag cell neurons. Treatment of isolated neurons with phorbol ester activators of protein kinase C causes an increase in action potential amplitude, in this case with little or no change in the duration (Fig. 13–6a). This effect can be mimicked by direct intracellular injection of protein kinase C (Fig. 13–6a) and blocked by protein kinase C inhibitors. In contrast to the actions of cyclic AMP, phorbol esters do *not* alter voltage-dependent potassium currents in the bag cell neurons. Instead, the increase in action potential amplitude can be accounted for by an increase in the calcium current, which is a major contributor to the rising phase of the spike (Fig. 13–6b). When the microscopic mechanism of this change is examined by single channel analysis, it can be seen that the enhancement of the whole-cell calcium current by activators of protein kinase C involves the recruitment of a novel calcium channel. In control neurons the calcium current is carried by a class of voltage-dependent calcium

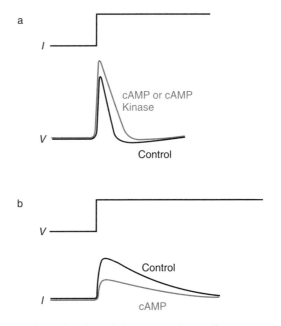

Figure 13–5. Changes in action potential amplitude and duration in bag cell neurons. *a:* The amplitude and duration of action potentials (*V*), evoked by a depolarizing current (*I*) pulse, change when the cell is injected with cyclic AMP analogs or the catalytic subunit of the cyclic AMP–dependent protein kinase. *b:* Spike modulation is accompanied by changes in the kinetics and amplitude of the delayed rectifying potassium current (see Loechner and Kaczmarek, 1990).

channels with a single channel conductance of about 12 pS. After exposure of the neurons to phorbol ester or diacylglycerol these channels are
still present. In addition, there is a new 24 pS calcium channel that is never
seen in control cells (Fig. 13–6b). Although the possibility that the small
channels are converted into large ones cannot be ruled out entirely, this

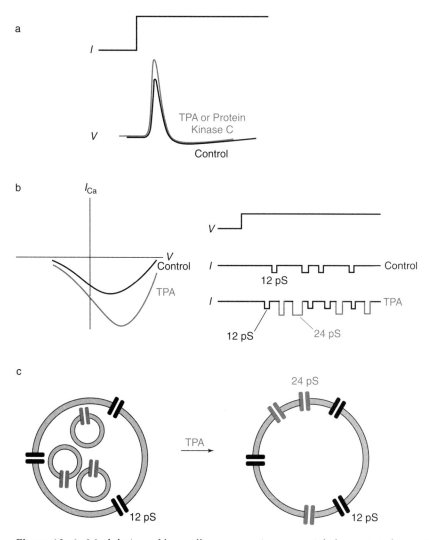

Figure 13–6. Modulation of bag cell neuron action potentials by protein kinase C. *a*:
Protein kinase C injection or phorbol ester (TPA) treatment increases the amplitude
but not the duration of the action potential. *b*: TPA increases voltage-dependent calcium current (I_{Ca}) (*left*). This is due to the recruitment of a novel calcium channel,
which is not seen in the absence of TPA (*right*). *c*: The possible recruitment of new
calcium channels from intracellular vesicles is illustrated (see DeRiemer et al., 1985;
Strong et al., 1987).

seems unlikely because the smaller conductance channels are seen with about the same frequency in control and phorbol ester–treated bag cell neurons. Furthermore, the two channels exhibit different spatial distributions over the neuronal membrane surface. Images made using the fura-2 technique to measure the distribution and levels of intracellular calcium (see Chapter 9) reveal new sites of calcium entry following activation of protein kinase C. One interesting possibility is that protein kinase C may trigger the recruitment of the 24 pS channel to the plasma membrane from intracellular vesicles (Fig. 13–6c).

Modulation of action potential size and shape: are there any rules? We could go on to provide other examples of modulation of the amplitude and duration of action potentials in neurons and other excitable cells, but those described above are among the best understood and suffice for the messages we wish to convey here. The first is that this kind of modulation is ubiquitous, and can be seen in many different types of nerve and muscle cells. On reflection this is not surprising. Such changes in action potentials will result in changes in the amount of calcium entering the cell, and we have seen that calcium is of central importance to many cell functions, including secretion of neurotransmitters and hormones. The second message is that different cells choose different mechanisms to modulate their action potentials. The cyclic AMP, diacylglycerol, and other second messenger systems may be involved, sometimes cooperating and sometimes opposing each other's actions in a single cell. Finally, changes in the action potential can result from modulation of either calcium channels or of several distinct potassium channels, and it is not unusual for more than one kind of channel to be modulated in a single cell. The one feature that appears to be common to many of these systems is that the modulations involve protein phosphorylation. We shall see now that this diversity of mechanisms is also characteristic of modulation of intrinsic neuronal excitability and of action potential firing patterns.

Modulation of Intrinsic Neuronal Excitability and Spontaneous Discharge

The intrinsic electrical activity of a neuron can be examined by isolating it from hormonal or synaptic inputs from other cells. This can be achieved by physically removing the cell from the nervous system and placing it alone in a tissue culture dish or by using pharmacological treatments to block intercellular interactions. When this is done it becomes evident that some neurons display no spontaneous electrical activity, whereas others fire action potentials at more or less regular intervals (see Fig. 3–12). We shall see now that the nervous system uses biochemical modulatory mechanisms to alter in various ways these patterns of intrinsic excitability.

Modulation of bursting in Aplysia *neuron* R15. Bursting activity, the grouping of action potentials in bursts separated by periodic hyperpolarizations known as *interbursts*, is widespread in nervous systems. As we mentioned in Chapter 3, bursting is used to drive rhythmic behaviors, as well as to increase the efficiency of secretion of peptide hormones. Although in some cases bursting activity is an emergent property of a multineuronal network (see Chapter 19), certain neurons generate bursts endogenously in the absence of synaptic or hormonal input. The archetypal endogenous burster is *Aplysia* neuron R15 (see Figs. 3–12c and 13–4). The activity of R15 can be modulated for long periods of time by synaptic stimulation, or by the application of a number of different hormones or neurotransmitters. This is illustrated most dramatically by the fact that even though R15 is an endogenous burster, it is under tonic synaptic inhibition and only rarely is permitted to burst in the intact animal.

We shall consider here one well-understood example of modulation of bursting activity, the regulation of the activity of neuron R15 by serotonin. Serotonin application alters the activity of R15 in complex ways (Fig. 13–7a). An increase in the amplitude and duration of the interburst hyperpolarization is observed, and occasionally this can become so pronounced that bursting is inhibited completely. At the same time, the frequency of firing of action potentials within the burst is increased. Voltage clamp analysis reveals the ionic mechanisms that underlie these changes (Fig. 13–7b). Serotonin causes an increase in an inwardly rectifying potassium current and also increases a calcium current that contributes to the negative slope region of the steady-state current–voltage relationship. It might be thought that simultaneous increases in two opposing currents, one an inward depolarizing current and the other an outward hyperpolarizing current, might simply cancel each other out. However, note that both currents are voltage dependent and are active in very different membrane voltage ranges (Fig. 13–7b). The inwardly rectifying potassium current is activated during the interburst hyperpolarization, and its enhancement by serotonin thus leads to a more pronounced interburst. In contrast, the calcium current is active only at more depolarized voltages, and, accordingly, its enhancement by serotonin provides more depolarizing drive and an increase in spike frequency during the burst. The net effect of these concerted changes in two ionic currents is a more vigorous burst, which modulates the release of R15's neurosecretory peptide. This peptide is involved in regulation of water balance in *Aplysia*, and thus modulation of the bursting activity of R15 plays an essential role in the animal's osmoregulation.

Both of these actions of serotonin are mediated by cyclic AMP and cyclic AMP–dependent protein phosphorylation. The neuropeptide egg-laying hormone (ELH; see Fig. 8–6), which is released from the bag cell neurons during their afterdischarge, increases these same currents in neuron R15 (see Fig. 19–10a) via cyclic AMP. Thus two distinct first messengers, serotonin and ELH, acting via a single second messenger, cyclic AMP, have *divergent* actions on two different ion channels (Fig. 13–8a). Furthermore, calcium also modulates the activity of these same two ion channels, and cyclic GMP regulates the calcium (but not the potassium) channel. In other words, there are also *convergent* actions of several different second messenger systems on a single class of ion channel (Fig.

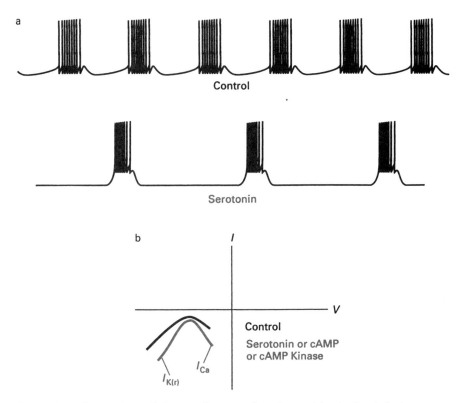

Figure 13–7. Serotonin modulates endogenous bursting activity in the *Aplysia* neuron R15. *a*: Serotonin causes an increase in the amplitude and duration of the interburst hyperpolarization as well as an increase in the frequency of action potentials during the burst in neuron R15. *b*: These changes result from increases in two voltage-dependent currents, an inwardly rectifying potassium current ($I_{K(r)}$) and a calcium current (I_{Ca}) (see Levitan and Levitan, 1988).

13–8b). These findings, in neuron R15 and the bag cell neurons, are re-capitulated in other neurons in creatures ranging from flies to humans. They emphasize that an understanding of how various modulatory systems *interact* is essential for a complete description of the regulation of neuronal firing patterns.

Activity-dependent modulation of neuronal excitability. An example of longer-term modulation of intrinsic neuronal excitability, mediated by yet another mechanism, comes from studies of pyramidal neurons in the rat visual cor-

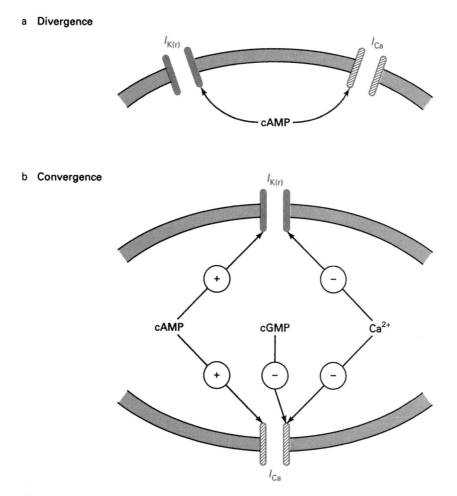

Figure 13–8. Divergence and convergence in second messenger actions. *a*: Cyclic AMP can have divergent actions on at least two different ion channels in neuron R15. *b*: The actions of several second messengers may converge on a single ion channel. The + and − symbols indicate activation and inhibition, respectively. I_{Ca}, calcium channel; $I_{K(r)}$, inwardly rectifying potassium channel.

tex. When the spontaneous electrical activity of these neurons is inhibited for a day or more, for example, by treatment with the sodium channel blocker tetrodotoxin, the neurons subsequently exhibit a decreased threshold and fire action potentials more robustly in response to the injection of depolarizing current (Fig. 13–9a). Voltage clamp analysis shows that calcium currents are not altered, but sodium current is increased (Fig. 13–9b) and a delayed rectifier potassium current is decreased by this treatment. Thus here again we see divergent effects on two different ion channels, both of which contribute to the increase in neuronal excitability.

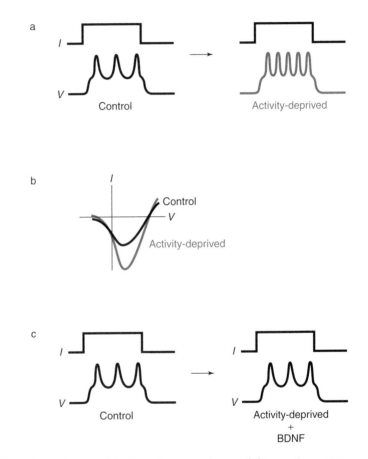

Figure 13–9. Activity-dependent modulation of neuronal excitability. *a:* Long-term (24–48 hr) blockade of neuronal activity leads to an increase in excitability after the blockade is removed. *b:* This modulation results in part from an increase in the voltage-dependent sodium current. *c:* Brain-derived neurotrophic factor (BDNF) treatment during the blockade prevents the modulation of excitability. *I,* current; *V,* voltage. (From experiments by Gina Turrigiano, Sacha Nelson, and colleagues.) See Desai et al., 1999a and b.

What is the molecular mechanism of this activity-dependent modulation of intrinsic excitability? It appears that a protein known as *brain-derived neurotrophic factor* (BDNF) plays a critical role. This protein is a member of the *neurotrophin* family of growth factors, which are important for the survival of neurons during development and for their maintenance in the adult (see Chapter 16). Brain-derived neurotrophic factor can also enhance synaptic transmission in the mammalian brain, and its actions appear to be necessary for some forms of learning (see Chapter 20). When activity blockade in the cortical pyramidal neurons is carried out in the presence of BDNF, the increase in intrinsic excitability does not occur (Fig. 13–9c). This suggests that the reduced activity increases the excitability of the cortical neurons by reducing the release of endogenous BDNF or a related factor. Because the receptor for BDNF (see Chapter 16) is a receptor tyrosine kinase (Fig. 12–18), it seems likely that phosphorylation is involved in some way in this long-term modulation of sodium and potassium currents.

Modulation of Synaptic Efficacy

It is widely believed that modulation of chemical synaptic efficacy may underlie many important behavioral phenomena, including learning and memory. Modulation of electrical synapses is also important, but it has been less thoroughly investigated and we will consider it only briefly at the end of this chapter. It is now evident that a change in the properties of ion channels can alter synaptic efficacy, without changing action potential amplitude and duration or spontaneous neuronal activity. We shall discuss these ideas in more detail in the context of behavior in Chapter 20, and will restrict ourselves here to a brief description of several examples that tie together changes in neuronal excitability and synaptic responsiveness.

Of bullfrogs and rats. A subtle action of a transmitter on neuronal excitability has been described in at least two kinds of vertebrate neurons: the large B cells of the bullfrog sympathetic ganglion and rat hippocampal pyramidal cells. In each of these cell types a neurotransmitter alters neuronal excitability by inhibiting a voltage-dependent potassium current that is not active at the resting potential. In the sympathetic ganglion neurons a potassium current called the *M current* (I_M) can be inhibited by a variety of neurotransmitters, including the peptides substance P and luteinizing hormone-releasing hormone (LHRH), and muscarinic cholinergic agonists. It is, in fact, inhibition of the M current by LHRH that is responsible for the late slow excitatory postsynaptic potential (EPSP) that we discussed in Chapter 10 (see Fig. 10–12). Because the M current is not very active at hyperpolarized potentials, application of one of these agonists has only a small effect on the cell's resting potential. However, the response to a depolarizing stimulus, for example, an excitatory synaptic potential, will be very much enhanced because the M current is not available to oppose the depolarization (Fig. 13–10a). Note the similarity of this effect, evoked acutely by application of a neurotransmitter, to the longer-term changes produced by activity blockade (Fig. 13–9).

A similar phenomenon is observed in hippocampal pyramidal neurons, in which norepinephrine blocks a calcium-dependent potassium current, thought to be carried by the SK class of calcium-dependent potassium channel, that is responsible for the afterhyperpolarization (AHP) that follows an action potential. This current (I_{AHP}) is not active at rest when calcium levels are low, and thus norepinephrine has little or no effect on the cell's resting potential. However, a depolarizing stimulus that produces ac-

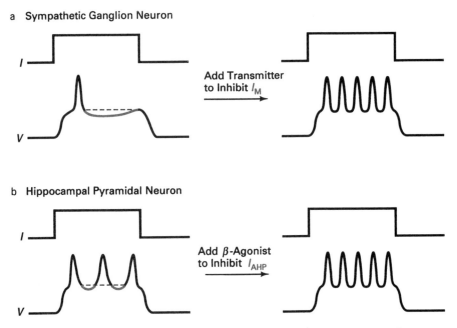

Figure 13–10. Modulation of responses to stimuli in vertebrate neurons. *a*: In experiments with sympathetic ganglion neurons of the bullfrog, addition of a transmitter that blocks the M potassium current (I_M) alters the cell's response to depolarizing stimuli. *b*: Similarly, norepinephrine modulates the response of rat hippocampal pyramidal neurons to depolarizing stimuli. I_{AHP} refers to the current responsible for the spike afterhyperpolarization in these neurons (see Jones and Adams, 1987).

tion potentials will be more effective in the presence of norepinephrine (Fig. 13–10b), because the calcium-dependent AHP, which normally follows the action potentials and dampens the excitatory response, has been suppressed.

These few examples suffice to emphasize that the action of one transmitter may be modulated profoundly by that of another. Although the effects of a single transmitter on resting membrane properties may appear to be minor, its true influence on the properties of a neuron may be evident only when it is coupled with stimulation of another synaptic or hormonal input.

Phosphorylation and Dephosphorylation of Ion Channels: A Common Mechanism in Neuromodulation

Many of the modulatory phenomena that we have discussed above occur through actions of protein kinases and phosphoprotein phosphatases. One question that immediately arises concerns the identity of the proteins that are phosphorylated by the kinases. By analogy to alterations in the activities of some enzymes, which are known to result from direct phosphorylation of the enzyme molecules themselves, it seems possible that ion channels are targets for protein kinases and phosphatases, and that direct phosphorylation of ion channel proteins alters their functional properties. However, the experiments described above do not speak to this question. They involve injecting a kinase (or kinase inhibitor) into the cell, and subsequently measuring membrane properties. Such experiments demonstrate clearly that phosphorylation is both necessary and sufficient for the modulatory responses. However, it is conceivable that the phosphorylation target is some nonchannel membrane protein, or even a cytoplasmic protein, whose phosphorylation sets in motion a sequence of events that culminates in ion channel modulation, without phosphorylation of the channel protein itself.

This issue has been put to rest convincingly by the demonstration that many ion channel proteins are substrates for protein kinases and phosphatases. Although undoubtedly other phosphorylated proteins may interact with and influence the activity of ion channels, channel phosphorylation and dephosphorylation can modulate channel function. Several different experimental approaches, combining biochemistry and molecular biology with physiological measurements, have led to this conclusion. We shall now present some representative examples of these approaches to illustrate the widespread occurrence and diverse consequences of ion channel phosphorylation.

Phosphorylation modulates channel activity in detached membrane patches. One experimental approach that can be used to explore this question is to investigate channel modulation in detached membrane patches. As detailed in Chapter 4, one of the modes of patch recording is the *inside-out* patch, in which the former cytoplasmic surface of the patch membrane is exposed to the bathing medium (see Fig. 4–2). If one suspects that a channel under study might be modulated by phosphorylation, it is a simple matter to add a protein kinase, together with the magnesium ions and ATP that are necessary for phosphorylation, while observing channel activity (Fig. 13–11a). This was first done for two molluscan channels: a serotonin-

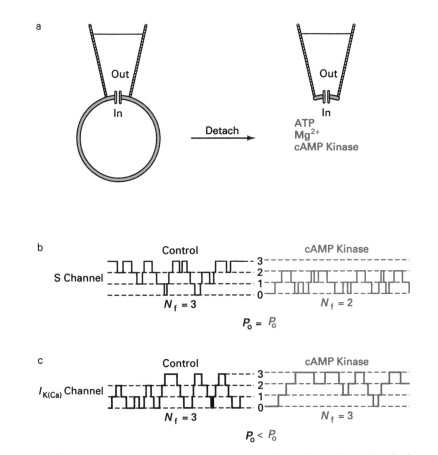

Figure 13–11. Phosphorylation modulates the activity of ion channels in detached membrane patches. *a*: Experimental configuration for testing the effects of a protein kinase on channel activity. *b*: Steven Siegelbaum and Eric Kandel found that the cyclic AMP–dependent protein kinase changes the number (N_f) of functional S potassium channels in detached patches from *Aplysia* sensory neurons. *c*: This kinase also can increase the open probability (P_o) of calcium-dependent potassium ($I_{K(Ca)}$) channels from *Helix* neurons. These findings are reviewed by Levitan (1994).

sensitive (S) potassium channel in *Aplysia* sensory neurons (Fig. 13–11b) and a calcium-dependent potassium channel in neurons from the garden snail *Helix* (Fig. 13–11c). In both cases addition of the catalytic subunit of the cyclic AMP–dependent protein kinase modulates the channel activity, as had been suspected from previous experiments involving intracellular injections of the kinase. Note that these two types of channel are modulated in different directions by the same kinase, consistent with the diversity observed in the whole cell experiments. Furthermore, the kinase induces a decrease in the number (N_f) of functional S channels, but does not alter the open probability (P_o) of those channels that are functional. In contrast, it is the open probability of the calcium-dependent potassium channels that is increased by the kinase without any change in the number of functional channels. These experiments, which have now been done with many other kinds of channels, demonstrate that the phosphorylation target cannot be a cytoplasmic protein, but must be some channel regulatory component that comes away with the membrane patch when it is detached from the cell. It might be the ion channel itself, but it might also be some cytoskeletal component or other element, which scanning electron micrographs have shown to be associated with these detached patches.

Phosphorylation modulates the activity of reconstituted ion channels. A complementary approach to the detached patch experiment is to examine the modulation of single ion channels reconstituted into artificial phospholipid bilayers. This is similar to the reconstitution of acetylcholine-dependent ion flux in liposomes, which we discussed in Chapter 11 (see Fig. 11–9), but the experimental conditions are designed to allow single channel openings and closings to be observed. One way of doing this is to make plasma membrane vesicles from the cells under investigation and allow them to fuse with a bilayer that occludes a small hole in a partition separating two aqueous solutions (Fig. 13–12a). When a vesicle fuses, it dumps its membrane proteins into the bilayer, and if an ion channel is among these proteins, it is possible to measure single channel currents using relatively simple electronics. Figure 13–12b illustrates the modulation, by cyclic AMP–dependent protein kinase, of a calcium-dependent potassium channel extracted from a snail neuron and fused into a bilayer. Such reconstitution experiments allow the fundamental conclusion that, for at least some ion channels, the phosphorylation site is part of either the ion channel protein itself or of some regulatory element that is so intimately associated with the ion channel that it swims with it in the bilayer.

Phosphorylation modulates the activity of purified ion channels. This approach has been extended in a particularly elegant way by examining the activity of ion channels that are reconstituted after they have been purified to ho-a

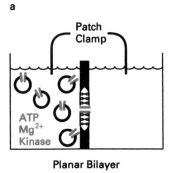

b $I_{K (Ca)}$ Channel

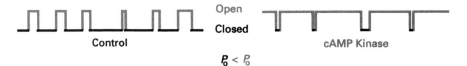

$P_o < P_o$

c Purified I_{Ca} Channel subunits

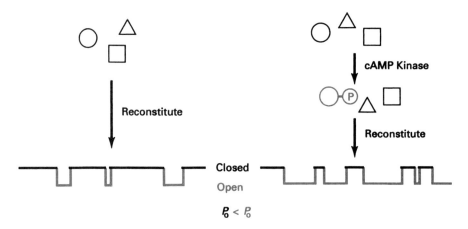

$P_o < P_o$

Figure 13–12. Phosphorylation modulates the activity of reconstituted ion channels. *a*: Configuration for ion channel reconstitution. *b*: The cyclic AMP–dependent protein kinase increases the activity of calcium-dependent potassium ($I_{K(Ca)}$) channels from *Helix* neurons in a bilayer. *c*: Phosphorylation modulates a purified reconstituted calcium (I_{Ca}) channel (summarized in Levitan, 1994). P_o, open probability.

mogeneity. One example of this is a voltage-dependent calcium channel from skeletal muscle, which was first purified on the basis of its ability to bind certain *dihydropyridines*, which are calcium channel modulators. The complex consists of several subunits (see Fig. 7–4), at least two of which are substrates for the cyclic AMP–dependent protein kinase. Calcium channel activity can be reconstituted in artificial bilayers from these purified subunits. The gating of the channel is very different if the subunits are phosphorylated in the test tube prior to reconstitution (Fig. 13–12c).

Phosphorylation modulates the activity of cloned ion channels. An obvious extension of these increasingly reductionist approaches is to examine the effects of phosphorylation on cloned ion channels whose ability to undergo phosphorylation has been altered by molecular engineering. Heterologous expression of cloned channels, combined with site-directed mutagenesis, has enabled the identification of specific amino acid residues whose phosphorylation influences channel function in very specific ways. This approach has been used for many members of the voltage-dependent and ligand-gated ion channel families, including the intracellular calcium-release channels we discussed in the last chapter. We shall take as examples two kinds of channels whose phosphorylation has been studied thoroughly, glutamate receptor/channels of the AMPA/kainate variety and rat brain sodium channels.

From studies of the type discussed earlier in this chapter, it is known that responses of some neurons to the neurotransmitter glutamate can be modulated by protein phosphorylation. The molecular basis of this neuromodulation can be investigated using cloned receptors. When a cloned glutamate receptor subunit is expressed in a non-neuronal mammalian cell line, functional receptors are inserted into the plasma membrane, and inward sodium currents can be evoked by treatment with glutamate or other agonists (Fig. 13–13a, left). These currents are increased when the cyclic AMP–dependent protein kinase is introduced into the cells (Fig. 13–13a, right). Protein kinases will not recognize and phosphorylate all serine, threonine, and tyrosine residues equally well. Instead, a particular protein kinase prefers phosphorylatable residues that lie within a particular consensus sequence that is different for different kinases. For example, the cyclic AMP–dependent protein kinase prefers to phosphorylate serine or threonine residues that are adjacent to several basic amino acids (arginines or lysines); the glutamate receptor subunit whose activity is illustrated in Figure 13–13 contains such a consensus serine residue. When this serine is mutated to an alanine and the resulting mutant receptor subunits are expressed, the cyclic AMP–dependent protein kinase can no longer influence the glutamate-evoked current (Fig. 13–13b). This is the most direct demonstration that phosphorylation of the ion channel protein itself is responsible for modulation of channel properties. Similar findings have been made for other AMPA, kainic acid (KA), and NMDA receptor subunits. It is now known that other protein kinases can phosphorylate different serines, threonines, and tyrosines that lie within distinct consensus sequences in these receptors, with diverse consequences for channel activity.

Similar kinds of experiments have been done with cloned sodium channels. We saw in Chapter 5 that the sodium channel α subunit is a large protein, and examination of its sequence reveals multiple consensus sequences for several kinds of protein kinases including the cyclic AMP–dependent protein kinase and protein kinase C. Early biochemical experiments had shown that the purified α subunit is an excellent substrate for

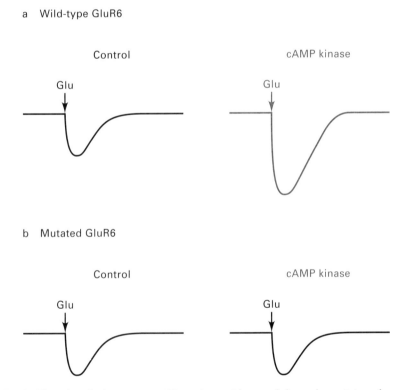

Figure 13–13. Phosphorylation at a specific serine residue modulates the activity of a cloned glutamate receptor/channel. *a*: Heterologous expression of the kainic acid (KA) receptor subunit GluR6 (see Table 11–4) produces glutamate-evoked currents, which are enhanced when the active catalytic subunit of cyclic AMP–dependent protein kinase is introduced into the cells. *b*: Mutation of a specific serine residue in GluR6 to alanine eliminates the effect of the kinase (from an experiment by Richard Huganir and colleagues; Raymond et al., 1993).

both of these protein kinases in the test tube. When tissue culture cells are transfected with cDNA encoding the α subunit, channel currents evoked by membrane depolarization are transient, reflecting channel inactivation (Fig. 13–14a; compare with Fig. 4–9). Following treatment with phorbol ester or diacylglycerol activators of protein kinase C, or injection of active protein kinase C into the cell, inactivation is much decreased (Fig. 13–14b). Such removal of inactivation will of course prolong the sodium current and profoundly influence the shape of the action potential. The intracellular loop between the third and fourth homologous domains of the α subunit contains a serine residue that lies within a good consensus sequence for phosphorylation by protein kinase C. When this serine is mutated to alanine, the inactivation of the resulting mutant channel cannot

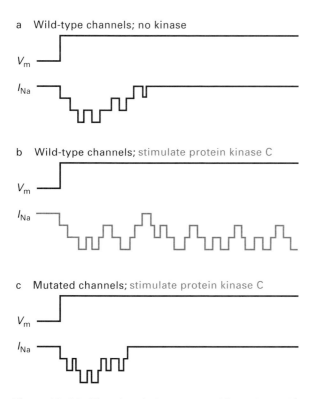

a   Wild-type channels; no kinase

V_m

I_{Na}

b   Wild-type channels; stimulate protein kinase C

V_m

I_{Na}

c   Mutated channels; stimulate protein kinase C

V_m

I_{Na}

Figure 13–14. Phosphorylation at a specific serine residue modulates sodium channel inactivation. *a*: Cloned sodium channels expressed heterologously in a mammalian cell line activate and then inactivate quickly during a prolonged depolarization. I_{Na}, sodium current; V_m, voltage. *b*: Stimulation of protein kinase C slows inactivation. *c*: Mutation of a specific serine residue in the intracellular loop between the third and fourth homologous domains abolishes the effect of protein kinase C (from experiments by William Catterall and colleagues (West et al., 1991)).

be modulated by protein kinase C (Fig. 13–14c). Recall that other experiments had also implicated this intracellular loop in the process of sodium channel inactivation (see Fig. 5–7).

It is also of interest to consider the specificity of ion channel modulation by protein phosphorylation. Again the cloned sodium channel provides an instructive example. Another protein kinase, the cyclic AMP–dependent protein kinase, also modulates sodium channels, but it produces a decrease in the peak sodium current without any change in channel inactivation. Mutagenesis demonstrates that this modulation results from phosphorylation of a serine residue in another part of the α subunit, remote from the loop between the third and fourth homologous domains. Thus activation of different second messenger pathways in neurons may influence the activity of the same ion channel, but in very different ways (see Fig. 13–8).

A role for protein phosphatases. Findings such as these emphasize that the participation of multiple intracellular signaling pathways can confer enormous complexity on the modulation of neuronal electrical activity. The complexity becomes even greater when one considers the involvement of the phosphoprotein phosphatases that remove phosphate groups from proteins. Although until recently the role of phosphatases was largely neglected, it is now evident that they comprise a large and diverse family of enzymes that themselves are subject to regulation. The availability of potent and specific phosphatase inhibitors has led to the demonstration that phosphatases are an important regulatory target in controlling the activity of ion channels as well as of fundamental physiological processes such as neurotransmitter release.

Summary

Different neurons exhibit different patterns of endogenous electrical activity: some cells are normally electrically silent, others may fire action potentials in an irregular manner, and still others display regular and often complex firing patterns. These patterns of activity are not fixed, but are subject to modulation by stimuli from the neuron's environment. Such neuromodulation underlies short- and long-term changes in nervous system function and thus is of fundamental importance for the survival of the organism.

The mechanisms of neuromodulation are also diverse. We have discussed modulation of action potential amplitude and duration, neuronal firing patterns, and responses to synaptic input. These modulations often involve changes in the properties of one or another membrane ion channel, but the identity of the ion channel whose activity is modulated may be different from one neuron to the next, or even within the same neuron in response to different modulatory stimuli. We have therefore presented a number of examples of modulation, to provide a sense of the diversity evident in this rapidly changing field. One feature common to many of these examples is regulation via protein phosphorylation. In many cases, phosphorylation of the ion channel protein itself on specific amino acid residues underlies the modulation of neuronal electrical properties.

14

Sensory Receptors

*A*lthough most neurons receive input from other neurons, the business of the brain is to act on information from the outside world. Specialized cells have evolved for the receipt of such information. These include cells that are responsible for sight, hearing, touch, taste, and smell, as well as those that signal to the brain the state of internal organs. Most external and internal stimuli are received by three classes of sensory cells: (*1*) those that respond to mechanical stimulation, (*2*) those that are influenced by light, and (*3*) those that sense changes in their chemical environment. In addition, some cells respond to other signals such as changes in temperature. In all cases, the stimulus alters the activity of ion channels, sometimes through the agency of second messengers. Sensory cells therefore provide clear examples of the principles encountered in previous chapters. We will now discuss briefly a few of the varied transduction mechanisms that have been found in each of the major classes of sensory cells.

Receptor Potentials

First let us consider in general terms the kind of output signal that these specialized sensory receptors send to the central nervous system. Some sensory cells are true neurons, with axons that travel from the sense organ to other parts of the nervous system. An external stimulus produces a depolarization or hyperpolarization of the membrane that is known as the *receptor potential*. As is shown in Figure 14–1, the time course and amplitude of the receptor potential generally mirror those of the stimulus. If

341

a depolarizing receptor potential is large enough to exceed the action potential threshold, the neuron will fire action potentials at a frequency that reflects the size of the stimulus. Thus we can see that information about stimulus strength is now encoded in action potential frequency. At the first synapse made by the sensory receptor neuron, the action potential frequency will determine the amount of transmitter released, and this in turn will control the magnitude of the depolarizing postsynaptic response. The latter will of course be translated back into a particular firing frequency in the postsynaptic cell.

Other sensory cells do not have axons. Although action potentials can sometimes be evoked in such cells, a sensory stimulus normally causes a depolarizing or hyperpolarizing receptor potential that does not cause firing. Instead, the change in membrane potential alters the rate of neurotransmitter release onto a postsynaptic neuron, and action potential frequency coding enters the picture only after this first synapse. As we shall see later, the classic example of this is the hyperpolarization of vertebrate photoreceptors in response to light.

Mechanoreceptors

Many sensory cells that respond to physical movement, termed *mechanoreceptors*, are found in or under the skin. These are true neurons, with their cell bodies in the dorsal root ganglion. Recall that we have already con-

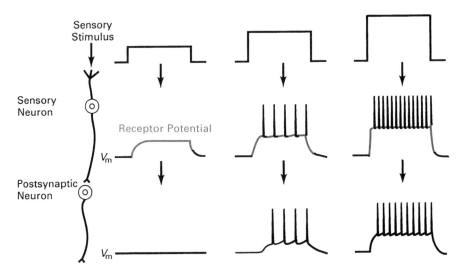

Figure 14–1. Receptor potentials and frequency coding. The size of a sensory stimulus determines the size of the receptor potential. This, in turn, is encoded in the frequency of firing of the sensory cell and/or its postsynaptic neuron. V_M, voltage.

sidered the excitability of dorsal root ganglion neurons in the previous chapter. The business end of these mechanoreceptors is at the peripheral endings of their axons in the skin. Figure 14–2 shows that the morphology of such endings is exceedingly varied. One type of mechanoreceptor ending, located deep below the surface, is the *Pacinian corpuscle*, which consists of the bare ending of an axon, surrounded by "onion skin" layers of connective tissue. *Meissner corpuscles* and *Ruffini endings* are found

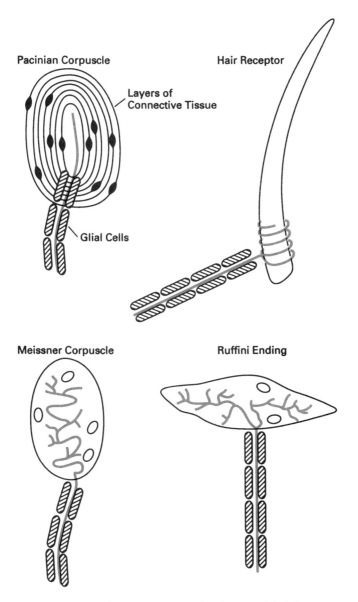

Figure 14–2. Mechanoreceptors in the skin (modified from Martin, 1981).

closer to the surface of the skin and consist of more elaborate branchings of a nerve fiber, also enclosed in connective tissue. Other receptors comprise bare nerve fibers wrapped around the base of a hair follicle. Although in Figure 14–1 we suggested that frequency of firing generally mirrors the amplitude of a sensory stimulus, this is complicated by the fact that many sensory cells adapt their response to a maintained stimulus. This is particularly true of these different types of mechanoreceptors, whose electrical responses differ in that some fire only transiently when pressure is applied to the skin whereas others fire persistently throughout a maintained tactile stimulus. These and other receptors account for some of the varied sensations of touch and pressure on the skin. Mechanoreceptors are also found in many other parts of the body. For example, Golgi tendon organs and muscle spindles are found in joints and muscles, and provide information on the position and length of muscles.

The means by which a mechanical movement is transduced into the pattern of firing of the axon of a mechanoreceptor is not yet known. It is worth mentioning, however, that many cells possess *stretch-activated* ion channels that are normally closed, but are induced to open when physical pressure is applied to the plasma membrane. Such pressure probably distorts some direct link between the channel and a component of the cytoskeleton. Stretch-activated channels are found in a diverse group of cells and their function is not known. It is possible, however, that such channels underlie the transduction of movement into the electrical impulses of mechanoreceptors.

Hair cells of the cochlea. *Hair cells* respond to a specialized form of mechanical stimulation and are found in the inner ear of vertebrates. (These cells are entirely unrelated to the cells that innervate hair follicles as in Fig. 14–2). They are found both in the vestibular organs and in the *cochlea*. In the former they are responsible for transducing information about gravity and movements of the head whereas in the cochlea, hair cells are the sensory cells of the auditory system. What is particularly interesting about these cells that are responsible for hearing is that they must not only provide the brain with information about the intensity of a sound but must also respond selectively to different frequencies of sound waves.

Figure 14–3 shows a typical hair cell. It is elongated in shape with a distinctive arrangement of hairs, termed *cilia*, located at one end. The cilia are of two types. Most, but not all, hair cells have one long *kinocilium*, which, in an electron microscope, closely resembles moving cilia such as those in a sperm tail. Its structure is maintained by microtubules that extend the length of the kinocilium, with two central microtubules surrounded by a ring of nine others (Fig. 14–4a). Some hair cells, however, such as

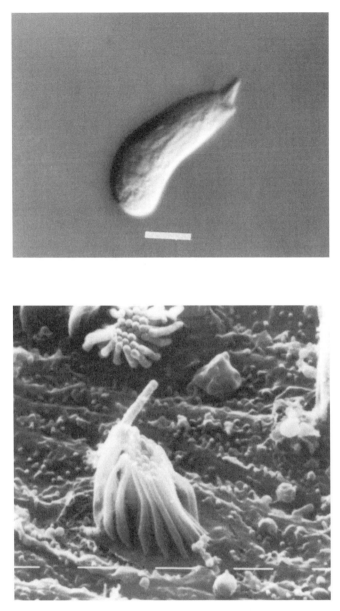

Figure 14–3. Hair cells. *Top*: Micrograph of a single hair cell isolated from the saccule of a toadfish. The tuft of cilia is at upper end of the cell (scale bar = 8 μm). *Bottom*: Scanning electron micrograph shows the cilia of such cells in more detail (scale bars = 1 μm) (courtesy of Dr. Antoinette Steinacker).

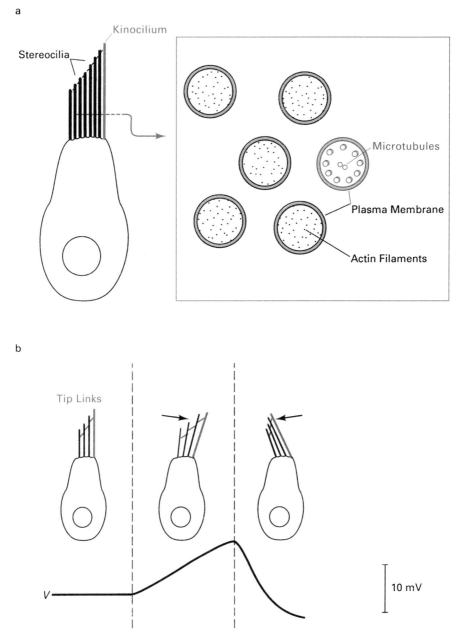

a

Kinocilium

Stereocilia

Microtubules

Plasma Membrane

Actin Filaments

b

Tip Links

V

10 mV

Figure 14–4. Hair cell cilia. *a*: Each hair cell has a single kinocilium and many stereocilia. *b*: Movement of the hair bundle toward the kinocilium depolarizes the cell. Movement in the opposite direction produces a hyperpolarization.

those in the mammalian cochlea, seem to do quite well without a kinocilium. The remaining 30–100 cilia, which are present in all hair cells and are
of varying lengths, are termed *stereocilia*. These do not contain microtubules
but are filled with filaments of actin and proteins that cross-link actin filaments. The entire collection of cilia is termed the *hair bundle*.

There is another important structural feature of the hair bundle in sensory hair cells. Each of the cilia is connected to an adjacent cilium by a
very fine filament, termed a *tip link*. As the name implies, these filaments
join the tip of one cilium to that of the next (Fig. 14–4b). The point at
which tip links are anchored to the membrane of a cilium is believed to
be the site at which the ion channels responsible for sensory transduction
are located.

Physical movements of the hair bundle cause a rapid change in the
membrane potential of a hair cell. When the bundle is moved toward the
kinocilium, the membrane depolarizes by 10–20 mV. In contrast, displacement of the bundle away from the kinocilium hyperpolarizes the cell
(Fig. 14–4b). The changes in membrane potential are caused by the opening and closing of channels located in the plasma membrane of the stereocilia themselves. It is the mechanical force that pulls or pushes on the tip
link filament that is thought to lead to the opening or closing of the channels. These channels are relatively nonselective for cations such as sodium,
potassium, and calcium ions. The response of the channels following mechanical displacement of the cilia occurs extremely rapidly, within 20–100
μsec. This means that opening of the channels is probably linked directly
to mechanical deformation of the cilia, rather than through a second messenger system. The mechanism of the mechanical coupling to channels is
not yet known. As we shall now describe, however, a striking feature of
the response of hair cells in the cochlea is that their responses are specifically tuned to different frequencies of sound.

Hair cells are tuned by position in the cochlea and by electrical resonance. Figure
14–5 shows that different cells respond optimally to different sound frequencies. This is illustrated by the *tuning curves* for several different hair
cells, which represent the intensity of sound of different frequencies that
must be applied to produce a fixed change in membrane potential. A major factor that determines the tuning curve for an individual cell is its position in the cochlea. The cell bodies of hair cells, together with their supporting cells, form a sheet of cells in the cochlea. The tips of the hair
bundles are normally in contact with a stiff, carbohydrate-containing sheet,
known as the *tectorial membrane*, that lies over the layer of cell bodies.
Vibrations caused by sound waves entering the cochlea set up lateral movement of the tectorial membrane relative to the underlying cells. This in

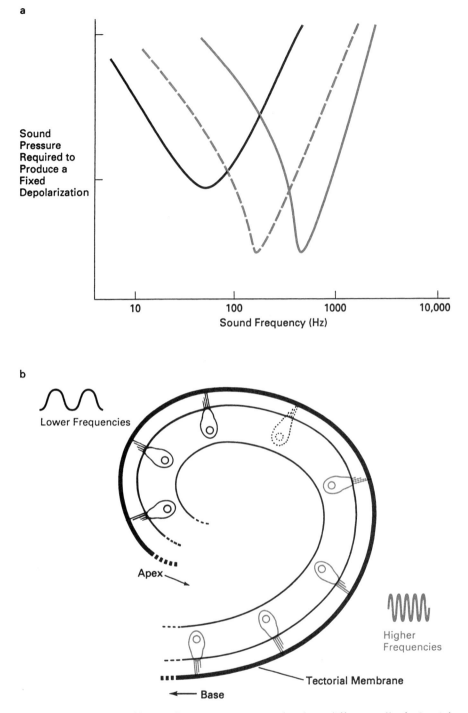

Figure 14–5. Tuning of hair cells. *a*: Tuning curves for three different cells. *b*: Spatial localization of cells with different frequency responses along the cochlea.

turn bends the hair bundles and transforms the mechanical vibration into an electrical oscillation of the membrane potential in the hair cells.

The mammalian cochlea is an elongated structure, folded into a spiral that resembles the shell of a snail (Fig. 14–5b). The sheets of hair cells extend from the base of the spiral to its apex. This mechanical design for the cochlea, coupled with the fact that changes in the thickness of the tectorial membrane occur along its length, provides a mechanism for the selective response of hair cells to different frequencies of sound. As was first suggested by the German physicist Helmholtz more than a hundred years ago and elaborated by Georg von Bekesy in the 1950s, low-frequency sounds cause the greatest vibrations to occur at the apex of the cochlea. In contrast, high-frequency sounds maximally deflect the hair bundles in cells at the base. The frequency to which a hair cell responds optimally is therefore determined by its physical position along the coiled cochlea.

In birds, and in amphibians such as bullfrogs and turtles, another mechanism for tuning has been discovered. The membrane potential of hair cells in these animals undergoes spontaneous oscillations or can be induced to oscillate after a transient depolarization (Fig. 14–6a). Although the frequency of oscillation can be increased or decreased by applying depolarizing or hyperpolarizing current, each cell has a characteristic frequency at which it oscillates around its resting potential. The characteristic frequency of different hair cells varies from tens to many hundreds of cycles per second. When a cell is stimulated with sound waves at its characteristic frequency, a maximal fluctuation of the membrane potential is evoked (Fig. 14–6b). Higher or lower frequency sounds are much less effective. The oscillations can largely be explained by the activity of only two types of ion channels: calcium channels and calcium-activated potassium channels. The opening of calcium channels causes the depolarizing phase of an oscillation. As calcium enters the cell, calcium-dependent potassium channels begin to activate. When a sufficient number of these have been opened, the membrane hyperpolarizes and calcium entry decreases. As intracellular calcium falls, the potassium channels close, and calcium channels again activate, renewing the cycle.

How is tuning to different frequencies achieved? Calcium current does not differ much from one hair cell to the next. In contrast, the rate at which the calcium-dependent potassium current activates varies enormously between cells (Fig. 14–7). It is these differences in the kinetics of potassium current that account for the fact that hair cells have different characteristic frequencies of oscillation. A particularly intriguing question that has yet to be answered is what determines the kinetics of the potassium channel in different cells. As we saw for the Shaker potassium channel in Chapter 5, alternative splicing of RNA from the *Slo* potassium channel gene (which encodes large-conductance calcium-activated potassium channels) produces a variety of channel proteins that differ in their kinetic properties. Moreover, β subunits of these channels also modify the rates of opening and closing of these channels. Gradients of different isoforms of the Slo channel and of β subunits have been found to exist in the cochlea of both higher and lower vertebrates, and are likely to account for the differences in the electrical properties of high-frequency and low-frequency hair cells. Such tuning of individual hair cells by electrical resonance accounts for the selective response of cells in the lower range of auditory frequencies, in species such as birds and amphibians. Although it is more

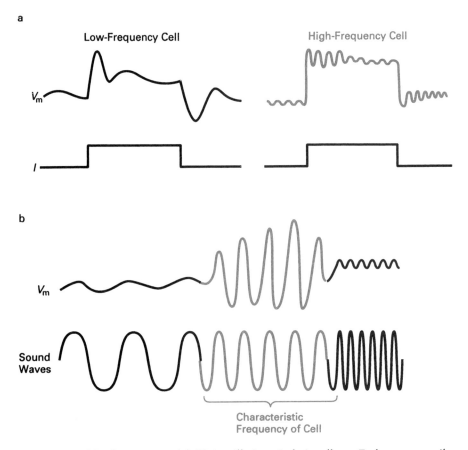

Figure 14–6. Membrane potential (V_M)oscillations in hair cells. *a*: Endogenous oscillations and oscillations evoked by depolarizing currents (*I*) were revealed in recordings by Fettiplace and colleagues. *b*: Sound waves at the characteristic frequency of a cell cause the largest fluctuation in membrane potential. Experiments of this kind, using mechanical displacement of the hair bundles as a stimulus, have also been carried out by Lewis and Hudspeth (1983).

difficult to record from hair cells in mammals, there is at present no evidence that such tuning occurs in mammalian species. It would be surprising, however, if electrical tuning of cells to specific frequencies of stimulation did not occur, at some level, in many nervous systems.

Outer Hair Cells Provide Mechanical Tuning

There are two types of hair cells in the mammalian cochlea. *Inner hair cells* are the actual sensory receptors that transmit information to the brain. There are about 4000 such inner hair cells in a human cochlea. Along the length of the cochlea, lying parallel to this row of inner hair cells, are found three rows of *outer hair cells* (Fig. 14–8a). The properties of these outer hair cells are entirely distinct from those of the inner hair cells. For example, rather than sending information toward the brain, they receive inputs from auditory nuclei in the brain stem. The most striking feature of the outer hair cells is, however, their response to rapid electrical simulation.

In contrast to most other cells, including the inner hair cells, the plasma membrane of outer hair cells is kept relatively rigid by a *cortical cytoskeleton* that lines the inside of the membrane. When viewed with the freeze fracture technique (see Fig. 8–2), the membrane itself is found have a very dense array of intramembranous particles. In response to electrical stimulation or to application of acetylcholine, this membrane contracts, producing a shortening of the cell (Fig. 14–8b). While at first glance this response appears to resemble that of a muscle cell, there is one key difference: changes in the length of an outer hair cell occur extremely rap-

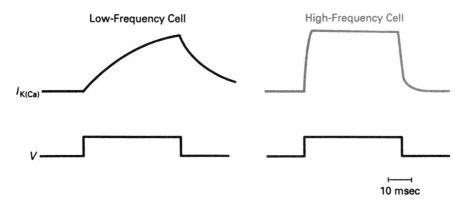

Figure 14–7. Calcium-dependent potassium current ($I_{K(Ca)}$) in hair cells. Voltage clamp recordings by Art and Fettiplace (1987) found rapidly activating currents in cells with high-frequency responses.

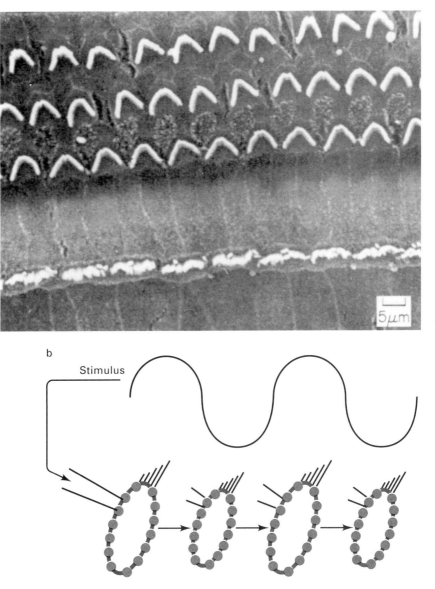

Figure 14–8. Outer hair cells. *a*: Electron micrograph showing a top view of three rows of outer hair cells and one row of inner hair cells. The stereocilia on the outer hair cells are arranged in a V-shape on each cell, while those on the inner hair cells are arranged in a straight line (from Pickles, 1988). *b*: Alternate contraction and relaxation of an isolated hair cell in response to a sinusoidal stimulus applied through a patch pipette. The putative contractile protein in the plasma membrane is shown in blue.

352

idly in response to changes in voltage. Thus the contractions of such a cell can follow stimulation at frequencies of 3000–8000 Hz or higher. The speed of this response entirely rules out a contractile mechanism such as that found in muscle cells.

A protein called *prestin*, which is evolutionarily related to proteins that transport anions across membranes, is found at a very high density in the lateral wall of the outer hair cells, but is absent from the nonmotile inner hair cells (Fig. 14–9). This protein may therefore be a key component of the contractile apparatus of outer hair cells. The ability of the outer hair cells to generate very rapid contractions is believed to produce movements of the membrane in which the hairs are embedded, providing further tuning of the membrane to different frequencies of sound. Information about this tuning, however, is relayed to the central nervous system by the less numerous inner hair cells.

Photoreceptors

The way that visual stimuli are translated into electrical activity of a photo-receptor cell in the retina is better understood than any other sensory event. The process termed *phototransduction* actually occurs in a variety of cells. For example, birds possess *extraretinal receptors*, which are found in the pineal gland within the brain itself. These allow a bird to sense changes in the light of its environment even in the absence of a functioning retina. In the retina of vertebrates there exist two cell types, the *rods* and the *cones*, which have different sensitivities and respond to different frequencies of light. The cone cells can further be subdivided into cells that preferentially sense different colors. It is rods, however, from a variety of species, that have been the favored cell type for studying visual transduction.

Rods, rhodopsin, and cyclic GMP. Figure 14–10 shows the structure of a rod photoreceptor. The cell has two parts. The rod *outer segment* is elongated and contains a stack of flattened discs made from internal membranes. This is connected by a thin bridge to the remainder of the cell, the *inner segment*, which contains the nucleus, the mitochondria, and the presynaptic terminal that synapses onto other neurons in the retina. It is the outer segment that is the business end for visual transduction. Within the internal membranous discs is found the light-sensitive protein *rhodopsin*. This is made up of an *opsin* protein, bound to a light-sensitive molecule, or *chromophore*, termed *retinal*. As was mentioned in Chapter 12, rhodopsin belongs to the family of G protein–coupled receptors, and it is the first protein of this family to have its three-dimensional structure de-

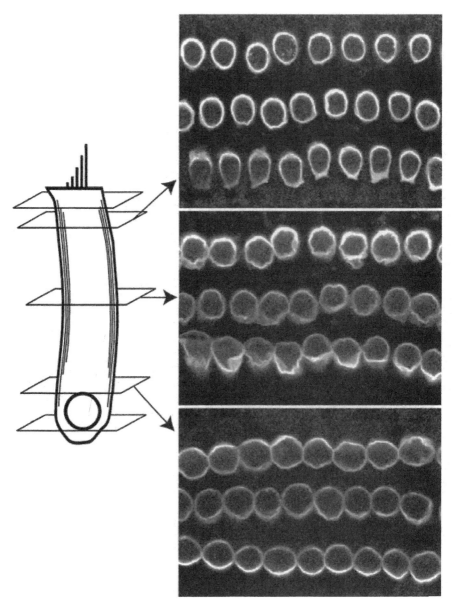

Figure 14–9. Location of prestin in outer hair cells. Outer hair cells were stained by Belyantseva et al. (2000) using an antibody against the prestin protein. Greatest levels are found in the lateral wall.

termined by electron microscopy and by X-ray crystallography (Plate 8). The chromophore molecule retinal may exist in a number of different forms, of which 11-*cis*-retinal and all-*trans*-retinal are the two major isomers (Fig. 14–11). On its own, neither opsin nor retinal absorbs visible light. In combination, however, absorption of a photon of light causes an isomerization of retinal from the 11-*cis* form to the all-*trans* form.

This light-dependent isomerization of retinal then causes a structural rearrangement of the protein. Rhodopsin that has been activated in this way is termed *meta*-rhodopsin. For all of the subsequent steps in visual transduction, it is useful to think of this molecule as analogous to a receptor that has just bound its neurotransmitter. In fact, the structure of the opsin protein is very similar to that of neurotransmitter receptors such

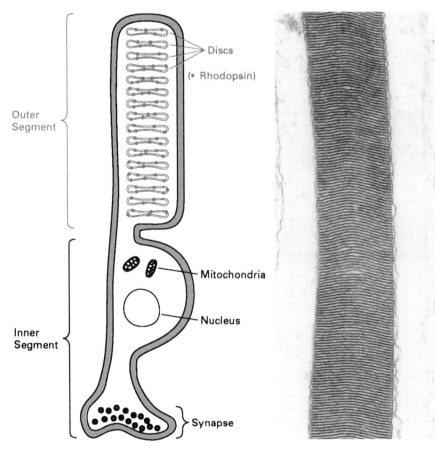

Figure 14–10. A photoreceptor. The drawing (*left*) is of an entire rod photoreceptor. The micrograph (*right*) shows only the outer segment of a salamander cone (courtesy of Dr. John E. Dowling).

as the β-adrenergic receptors. Recall that receptors such as the β-adrenergic receptor act through GTP-binding proteins. Not surprisingly, therefore, the steps that follow the production of *meta*-rhodopsin involve the production of a second messenger through the agency of a GTP-binding protein called *transducin* (G_T).

When *meta*-rhodopsin binds to transducin, GDP is replaced by GTP, and the $α_T$ subunit of transducin is liberated from its complex with the $βγ$ subunits. The target of the newly liberated $α_T$ is an enzyme in the membranous discs, a *phosphodiesterase*, that cleaves the second messenger cyclic GMP to 5'-GMP. Even in the dark, the levels of cyclic GMP in the outer segments are maintained by a balance between its rate of synthesis through guanylate cyclase and degradation by the phosphodiesterase. The action of $α_T$, formed after exposure to light, is to stimulate the phosphodiesterase, producing a drop in the levels of cyclic GMP. This drop occurs within about 100 msec of the onset of a light flash, sufficiently fast to account for a visual response. In many respects, photoreceptors are built backward. When excited by light, they respond by dropping, rather than raising, their concentration of the second messenger cyclic GMP. As we shall see, this results in the closure of channels that are normally kept open by this molecule. The channel closure in turn causes a hyperpolarization of the cell and a *reduction* in the rate of transmitter release at the terminal.

This cascade of reactions that follows the formation of *meta*-rhodopsin produces a very significant amplification of the signal generated by light.

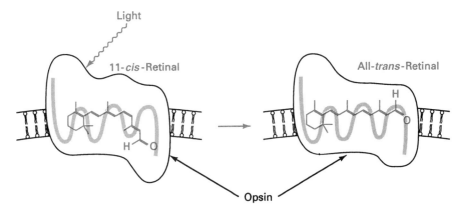

Figure 14–11. Rhodopsin is made up of an opsin protein, bound to the light-sensitive molecule retinal. The light-induced isomerization of retinal was discovered by George Wald.

It has been estimated that a single molecule of *meta*-rhodopsin, which is formed by the action of a single photon of light, diffuses in the membrane and activates several hundred transducin molecules before it is rendered inactive (see below). The subsequent stimulation of the phosphodiesterase by α_T provides further amplification such that a single photon of light can lead to the destruction of more than 10^5 molecules of cyclic GMP.

Cyclic GMP–gated channels. How is the change in cyclic GMP levels translated into an electrical response in the photoreceptor? To understand this we must first consider the electrical properties of a rod at rest in the dark. The dominant type of ion channel in the plasma membrane of the outer segments is a species of channel that allows sodium and calcium to enter the cell. Because of the abundance of sodium ions in the extracellular fluid, the major ion that enters the outer segments through these channels is sodium. The opening and closing of these channels is not very dependent on membrane potential. From our discussion of ion channels, we know that a cell with a preponderance of such sodium channels would be expected to have a very positive resting potential. The effect of the rod sodium channels is counterbalanced, however, by potassium channels. The interesting thing about these potassium channels is that they are found in a very different part of the cell, the membrane of the inner segment that includes the nucleus and synaptic terminal. Because there is good electrical continuity between the inner and outer segments, the mean membrane potential is kept fairly negative as a result of the open potassium channels. This spatial distribution of channels, however, creates a circulating current, termed the *dark current*, which flows in through the outer segment sodium channels, through the bridge into the inner segment, and out through the potassium channels (Fig. 14–12).

The effect of shining light on a rod is to shut down many of the sodium channels in the outer segment. This produces a marked decrease in the dark current (Fig. 14–12). As a result the potassium channels, which remain open in the inner segment, hyperpolarize the cell toward E_K, reducing the spontaneous release of neurotransmitter from the synaptic terminal. The closure of the sodium channels can be attributed directly to the drop in cyclic GMP in the cytoplasm of the outer segment.

Although in Chapter 12 we stated that second messengers such as cyclic AMP and cyclic GMP frequently act by engaging the services of a protein kinase, this is not the case in the rod outer segment. Instead, it appears that the sodium channels bind cyclic GMP directly, and remain open only when cyclic GMP is bound. This can be demonstrated by making an inside-out patch recording on membrane from the outer segments. When

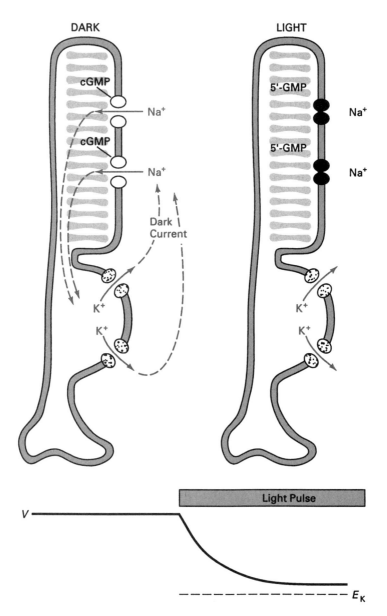

Figure 14–12. The dark current. In the dark, current flows through sodium channels in the outer segment of a rod photoreceptor. A pulse of light closes these channels, resulting in hyperpolarization of the rod. E_K, potassium equilibrium potentials.

cyclic GMP is added to the cytoplasmic face of the patch, a large increase in conductance, attributable to the opening of the sodium channels, can be measured (Fig. 14–13a). This occurs in the absence of ATP, which would be required for the activity of any protein kinase.

One interesting feature of these sodium channels is that, under normal conditions, the conductance of a single channel is extremely low. We stated earlier that the conductance of open channels in biological membranes typically ranges from about 5 to 400 pS. In contrast, the conductance of these rod channels is only about 0.1 pS. This is, in fact, too low to resolve individual openings and closings of the channel using patch clamp equipment, and this value for the conductance had to be obtained by another technique (known as *noise analysis*). An explanation for the low conductance is that the channels are partially blocked by calcium and magnesium ions, which are normally present in physiological solutions. The persistent barrage of these ions into the mouth of the channel produces a "flickering" block, effectively reducing the amount of current that is measured when the channel is open. This block is relieved when calcium and magnesium are omitted from the solutions, and individual opening and closing of the channel, which now has a conductance of ~25 pS, can be measured (Fig. 14–13b).

This channel has been purified and its gene has been cloned. The channel is a tetramer composed of at least two proteins, the α and β subunits. Surprisingly, each of these turns out to be a close relative of the Shaker family of potassium channels that we encountered in Chapter 5. Even though the channel cannot be activated by voltage in the absence of cyclic GMP, it retains an S4 region that resembles the voltage sensor of the potassium channels (Fig. 14–14). Moreover, the pore region also closely resembles that of the potassium channels. This pore region, however, lacks two amino acids, a tyrosine and a glycine, that are essential for providing selectivity in the potassium channels. As a result, the pore of the photoreceptor channels is relatively nonselective for cations, and, under physiological conditions, most of the current through the channel is carried by sodium ions. Binding of cyclic GMP to the channel occurs near the carboxyl terminus (Fig. 14–14), at a sequence that closely resembles the cyclic nucleotide binding domains in the cyclic AMP– and cyclic GMP–dependent protein kinases. Binding of cyclic GMP at these sites, however, leads to direct activation of the channel rather than triggering an enzymic reaction. As we shall see later in this chapter, other members of this family of cyclic nucleotide-gated channels also play key roles in the transduction of senses other than vision. Moreover, some of these channels are also found in cells other than sensory cells.

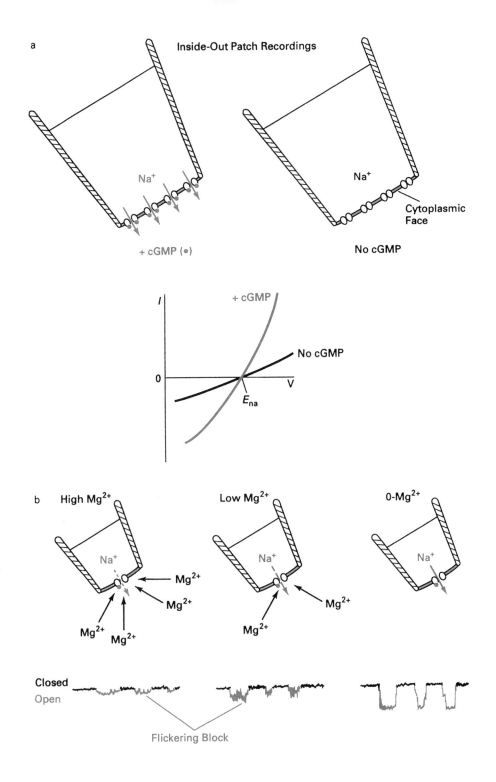

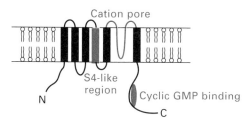

Figure 14–14. Presumed membrane organization of the cyclic GMP–gated cation channel. Compare with that of the Shaker potassium channels (see Fig. 5–8).

Terminating the light response. The analogies between visual transduction and neurotransmitter action can be taken further, when one considers how the response to a flash of light is terminated. In Chapter 12 we saw that rhodopsin can be phosphorylated by a rhodopsin kinase that resembles β-ARK, the kinase that phosphorylates the β-adrenergic receptor, leading to its down-regulation. Rhodopsin kinase preferentially phosphorylates *meta*-rhodopsin. This phosphorylation promotes the binding of *meta*-rhodopsin to *arrestin*, a 43 kDa protein whose function is to prevent the *meta*-rhodopsin from activating further transducin molecules, thereby terminating the light response. After phosphorylation, the all-*trans*-retinal dissociates from rhodopsin, leaving the opsin protein, which must bind another 11-*cis*-retinal before it can again be activated by light.

Figure 14–15 shows a simplified scheme representing the cyclic reactions that we have covered. Many features of visual transduction have yet to be explained. For example, calcium ions can also enter through the outer segment cation channels, and changes in intracellular calcium play an important role in adaptation of the rods to bright light. Furthermore, some invertebrate photoreceptors use mechanisms that differ from the vertebrate cascade. Although the transduction mechanism in these cells is not fully understood, light stimulates the formation of inositol triphosphate (IP$_3$) (see Chapter 12), which, through the release of calcium, regulates the response to light. Again, this emphasizes the similarity of visual transduction to neurotransmitter action.

Before we leave the topic of photoreceptors, it should be mentioned

---

Figure 14–13. Cyclic GMP opens sodium channels. *a:* When cyclic GMP (cGMP) is added to the cytoplasmic face of an inside-out patch of membrane from a rod photoreceptor, the I–V curve changes to reflect an increase in sodium conductance. This finding was obtained by Evgeniy Fesenko and colleagues. *b:* Flickering block of the cyclic GMP–regulated channel is relieved when divalent cations are omitted from the recording solutions (Haynes et al., 1986).

that the structure of the outer segments is a dynamic one. Cells in the epithelium that overlie the tips of the outer segments continually engulf and
digest these outermost tips, together with the enclosed rhodopsin-
containing discs. New membranous discs containing the transduction machinery are continually being assembled near the base of the segment to
replace the degraded discs (Fig. 14–16). The turnover of discs can be rapid,
with many discs being replaced within 1 hr. It may be that, for reasons
we do not understand, "newer" means "better" for the function of the
components in visual transduction.

Chemoreceptors

The olfactory system. The task of a *chemoreceptor* cell is to signal to the
nervous system a change in its chemical environment. Major use of
chemoreceptors is made in those parts of the body specialized for taste
(the *gustatory* sense) and smell (*olfaction*). The latter sense is particularly
remarkable in the specificity with which it can distinguish different odorant molecules. Figure 14–17a shows the structures of three molecules that,

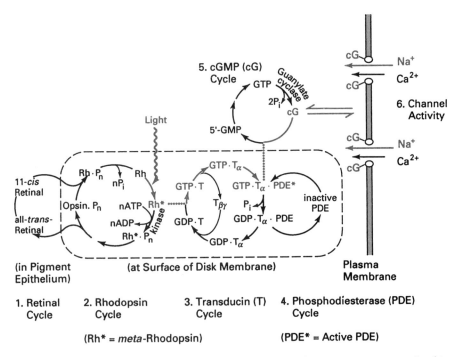

Figure 14–15. Cyclic reactions in visual transduction. The active messengers in this
simplified scheme are highlighted in blue (adapted from Lamb, 1986).

at first glance, appear generally similar in shape and size. The sensations that they elicit, however, leave no doubt that they stimulate different patterns of activity in neurons of the olfactory system.

Figure 14–17b shows the anatomy of olfactory chemoreceptors in a vertebrate. These are neurons that are aligned in sheets within the nasal epithelium. Their axons travel to the brain where they synapse within the olfactory bulb. Each receptor neuron has a dendrite that extends toward a layer of mucus lining the nasal cavity. There it forms a dendritic "knob" from which fine cilia extend into the mucus. It is this part of the cell that responds to odorant molecules that are borne in with the air circulating over the mucus.

It is perhaps not surprising that the response of the olfactory system to odorants results from a process directly analogous to neurotransmission. After all, odorants are simply chemicals that must interact with receptors on the sensory cells. Nevertheless, the olfactory system has to be able to respond appropriately to a vast number of possible odorants. It is estimated that we can distinguish between 5000 different odorants in the environment and can detect considerably more. To accomplish this, evo-

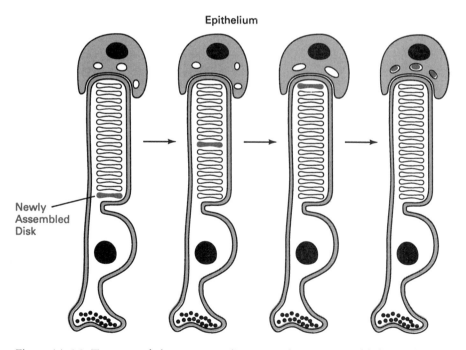

Figure 14–16. Turnover of photoreceptor discs. New discs are assembled near the base of the outer segment and travel to the tip of the cell where they are degraded.

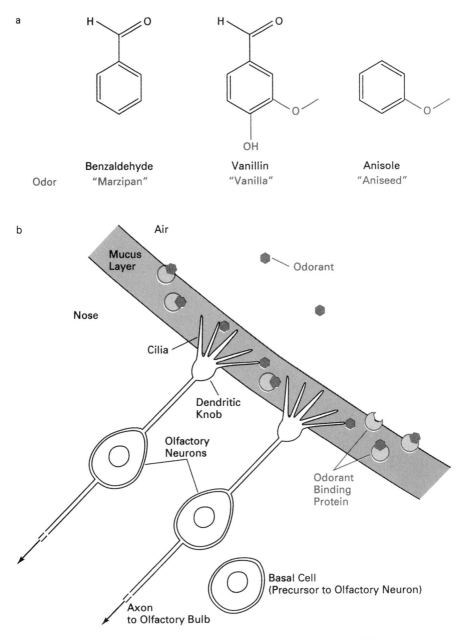

Figure 14–17. Olfaction. *a*: Three aromatic compounds with very different odors. *b*: Transport of odorants to olfactory neurons.

lution has provided a very large number of different receptor molecules, the *olfactory receptor* proteins.

Like rhodopsin in the visual system, olfactory receptor proteins, termed *ORs*, have seven hydrophobic membrane-spanning domains and are members of the G protein–coupled receptor family that we discussed in Chapter 12. Most tissues and parts of the brain need only a relatively small number of such receptors to allow them to respond appropriately to hormones and neurotransmitters. There are, however, as many as 1000 different olfactory receptor proteins, each encoded by its own gene. The information that is used to encode these olfactory proteins takes up approximately 1% of the genome of vertebrates. There is sufficient similarity in the amino acid sequence of different olfactory receptors to define them as a family of closely related proteins. Because some family members are more closely related than others, it is also possible to assign each member of this enormous family to one of a number of specific subfamilies. Despite these similarities however, there are several regions within the protein that are highly diverse in their sequence in different family members. The greatest diversity is found in the third, fourth, and fifth membrane-spanning domains (Fig. 14–18). It is these regions that are believed to bind specific odorant molecules.

The olfactory receptors are distributed among the olfactory sensory neurons, such that each individual sensory cell appears to express only

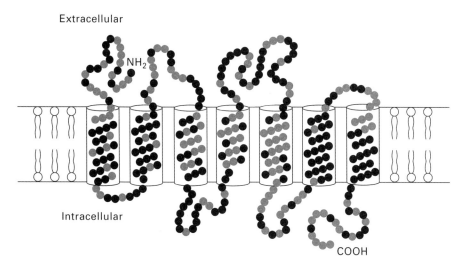

Figure 14–18. An odorant receptor protein. Individual amino acids are shown as circles. Residues that show the greatest variability between different odorant receptor proteins are shown in blue (modified from Ressler et al., 1994).

one, or a very small number, of the olfactory receptors. It has been possible to express the genes for some of the receptors in non-neuronal cells, and also in olfactory neurons, to test their response to odorants. It appears that the response of each receptor is rather specific. For example, one receptor, OR-I7, recognizes octanal, but is much less sensitive to the closely related molecule, heptanal, and is completely insensitive to most other odorants. Thus it is possible that, in the olfactory epithelium, a very low concentration of a specific odorant may activate one, and only one, specific receptor. Higher concentrations of odorants, however, probably activate several different receptors. The nature of the odor is thus encoded by the particular combination of sensory neurons that are activated by the odorant.

There are clear parallels between the activation of chemoreceptor cells and photoreceptors. Just as transducin is specific to photoreceptors, there exists a GTP-binding protein, termed G_{olf}, which is specific to the olfactory neurons. For olfaction, however, cyclic GMP appears not be involved. Instead, exposure to many odorants results in the activation of adenylate cyclase and the production of cyclic AMP or in the formation of inositol trisphosphate, a product of the activation of phospholipase C (see Fig. 12–12). The elevation of cyclic AMP levels activates a cation channel in the plasma membrane and this, in turn, produces an electrical response that, like that of rods, is relatively slow, with inward currents developing over several hundred milliseconds following application of odorants. This cation channel in olfactory cells closely resembles the cation channel in photoreceptors (Fig. 14–14) and is a member of the same channel family. Thus opening of the channel is achieved by the binding of cyclic AMP directly to the channel protein. The olfactory channel differs from that in rods, however, in that it can be opened by both cyclic AMP and by cyclic GMP; that in rods is highly specific for cyclic GMP.

Another point of similarity between olfactory and visual transduction is found in the way that the light-sensitive substance retinal and the odorant molecules are brought to the receptor cells. In the visual system, retinal is synthesized from the related molecule retinol, a highly lipophilic molecule. This is transported to the retina in a form that is bound to a carrier protein termed *retinol-binding protein*. This protein is closely related in its structure to *odorant-binding protein*, a dimer of two identical 19 kDa subunits found in the mucus around the olfactory cilia. The major role of odorant-binding protein is to bind and to concentrate airborne odorants and then to ferry them to the tips of the cilia (Fig. 14–17b).

One particularly interesting aspect of olfactory neurons is that, unlike most other neurons, they are not permanent. In the retina, we saw that photoreceptors are continually renewing their outer segments. As we shall see in the next chapter, renewal in the adult olfactory system is accomplished by destroying *entire* olfactory neurons and replacing them by new neurons. The new neurons arise from precursor cells in a manner similar to the formation of neurons during embryonic development. The axons of the newly formed olfactory neurons must then navigate their way to their postsynaptic targets in the adult olfactory bulb.

Olfactory receptor proteins may tell the axons of olfactory neurons where to go. The axons of olfactory receptor neurons project from the nasal epithelium into the *olfactory bulb*, within the central nervous system (Fig. 14–19). Here they make connections with two types of neurons, *mitral cells* and *tufted cells*, both of which send their output further into the brain. These synaptic connections are made within large spherical structures that have a diameter of 100–200 μm and that are termed *glomeruli*. Knowing the identity of the ORs has allowed the construction of "wiring diagrams" showing the pathways by which a single receptor connects to the brain. For example, genetic strains of mice have been developed in which all of the axons of neurons that make one specific olfactory receptor can be

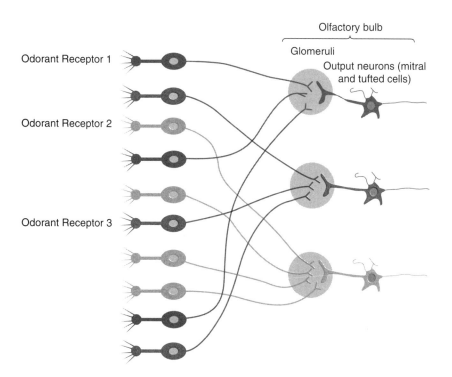

Figure 14–19. Connections of olfactory receptor neurons to the olfactory bulb. The outputs of neurons that are in different parts of the olfactory epithelium but that have the same odorant receptor, converge onto the same glomerulus.

stained and their connections traced. Thus it has been found that the receptor neurons that bear the same receptor are not clustered together, but rather are found in a mosaic-like pattern over the surface of the epithelium. The axons from these neurons, however, converge in glomeruli in the olfactory bulb (Fig. 14–19). There are about 2000 glomeruli in the olfactory bulb of a rodent, and there are about 1000 different ORs. Thus axons from neurons containing a specific OR may terminate in only one or two glomeruli that are dedicated to that receptor.

How does the axon of a specific olfactory neuron find its appropriate glomerulus? The general molecules involved in axon guidance and synapse formation will be covered in Chapters 17 and 18. The olfactory system may, however, have an additional twist. Genetic studies have shown that changing the particular OR that a receptor neuron makes alters the target that the axon finally chooses. Thus, by some means that is not yet understood, the ORs may not only function in sensory transduction but may play a role in the selection of synaptic connections.

Pheromones use a separate olfactory pathway. The olfactory system appears to be able to detect and distinguish among an enormous number of volatile substances. Some of these substances, however, have very specific significance for the behavior of an animal. For example, airborne or waterborne *pheromones* are used by many species to influence the behavior of sexual partners. The structure of these pheromones is fixed, and specific receptors that are quite distinct from the ORs have evolved for these molecules. In many mammals, the sensing of pheromones is carried out by another olfactory sense organ, termed the *vomeronasal organ*. Although the organization of this organ is similar to that of the olfactory system described above, the olfactory receptor proteins in this organ belong to two additional families of G protein–coupled receptors, the *V1R* family that contains about 35 members and the *V2R* family with about 150 members. Stimulation of these receptors can activate direct lines from neurons in the vomeronasal organ to neurons in the central nervous system that control reproductive behaviors.

Other chemoreceptors. Another important class of chemoreceptive cells is found in the lingual epithelium of the tongue. These do not need to distinguish among as varied a selection of chemical stimuli as the olfactory neurons. Taste receptors are responsible for sour, sweet, salty, and bitter sensations in food applied to the tongue. Figure 14–20a shows a picture of a taste bud, with its receptor cells. In contrast to the olfactory cells, the taste receptors do not have axons but are innervated by afferent fibers that relay gustatory information to the brain. The sensing of stimuli occurs in

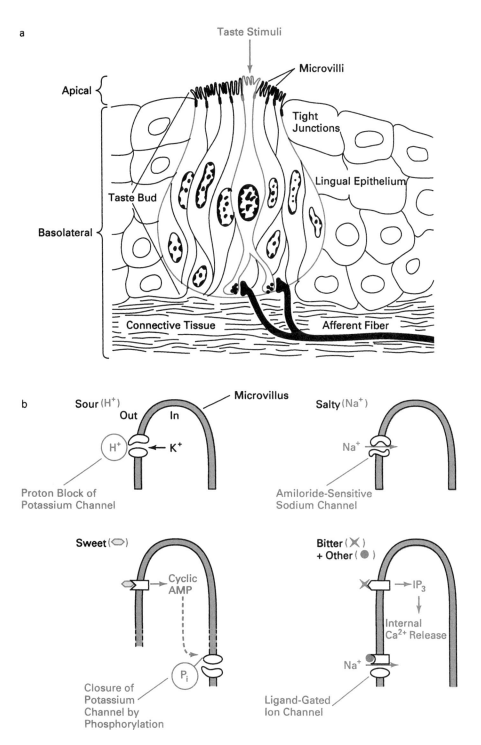

Figure 14–20. Taste transduction. *a*: Taste receptor cells within a taste bud. *b*: Some mechanisms that may transduce different taste stimuli (adapted from Kinnamon, 1988).

finger-like projections, or *microvilli*, at the surface of the taste buds. Shown in Figure 14–20b are some of the mechanisms that have been proposed to account for transduction of taste stimuli. Sourness depends primarily on the acidity of a chemical stimulus, and salty sensations are evoked by solutions with a high sodium concentration. Interestingly, responses to such substances may not occur through specific membrane receptors. Instead, transduction of acidic sourness may occur through the direct action of protons on potassium channels in the apical region of the cell. Similarly, salt may be sensed by the direct entry of sodium ions through a class of sodium channels that are blocked by the drug amiloride. Sweetness and bitterness, on the other hand, are probably transduced by specific membrane receptors for sugars, amino acids, and other chemicals. Some proposed transduction mechanisms are illustrated in Figure 14–20b; yet others may exist for particular taste stimuli.

We must not forget that chemoreceptors are used for more than just the senses of smell and taste; they also transmit information about the chemical composition of various internal fluids. The majority of these are not normally considered to be sensory systems. However, one special case that deserves mention here is the role of chemical sensitivity in what is usually ascribed to the sense of touch. Painful insect bites, or agents that cause painful local inflammation of tissue, act by stimulating nerve endings in the skin. However, much of their effect is indirect. The immediate stimulus causes the release of active substances from non-neuronal cells in the skin. These substances include peptides such as bradykinin and lipid molecules such as the arachidonic acid metabolic products called prostaglandins (Fig. 14–21a). These then act directly on the sensory neurons (Fig. 14–21b). Like the skin mechanoreceptors we considered earlier, these neurons have their cell bodies in the dorsal root ganglia. Figure 14–21c illustrates the effects of bradykinin on a type of tumor cell that, although it is not a true neuron, seems to retain many features of the neurons that respond to these locally released agents in the skin. In these cells, bradykinin evokes a transient hyperpolarization followed by a brisk neuronal discharge, which can be attributed to the activation of the phospholipase C (PLC) second messenger pathway. This is accompanied by modulation of a potassium channel by tyrosine phosphorylation.

Summary

Sensory cells have evolved pathways that allow ion channels to be regulated by external stimuli such as movement, light, or chemicals. In some cases, such as in photoreceptors and olfactory receptors, the means by

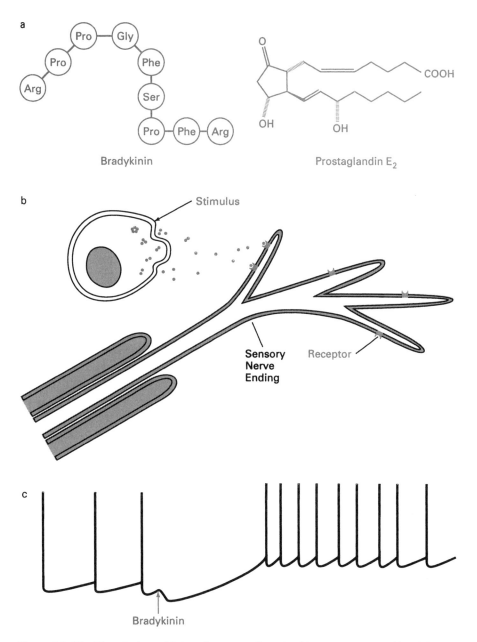

a

Pro — Gly

Pro   Phe

Arg   Ser

Pro — Phe — Arg

Bradykinin

Prostaglandin E$_2$

b

Stimulus

Sensory
Nerve
Ending

Receptor

c

Bradykinin

Figure 14–21. Chemical sensitivity of nerve endings in skin. *a*: Structure of bradykinin and one of the prostaglandins. *b*: Such substances may be released by nonneuronal cells to act locally on nerve endings. *c*: Actions of bradykinin on a hybrid neuroblastoma-glioma cell (termed an *NG-108* cell). These actions have been studied by M. Nirenberg, H. Higashida, and their colleagues.

which the external stimulus is transduced is reasonably well understood. Such cells appear to handle information in ways similar to those used by neurons that deal with information coming from a presynaptic pathway, by altering the levels of second messengers such as cyclic nucleotides, which then open or close ion channels in the plasma membrane. In contrast, in mechanoreceptors, movement may be directly linked to the gating of ion channels.

The study of sensory receptors has also uncovered some unexpected twists in signaling pathways. Ion channels that are opened directly by cyclic GMP and cyclic AMP have been found in photoreceptors and olfactory receptors. Some auditory receptors have been found to be exquisitely tuned to specific frequencies of stimulation, rather than solely to the amplitude of a sound wave. It seems possible that such mechanisms were discovered first in sensory cells because of the intense interest neurobiologists have in these cells that tell us about the outside world. On further search some of these mechanisms may also be found in nonsensory neurons.

IV

BEHAVIOR AND PLASTICITY

The previous two parts of this book dealt with the mechanisms that neurons use for intracellular and intercellular information transfer. In this final part we will discuss *behavior*, the output of the nervous system. We will also cover *plasticity*, changes in properties of individual neurons and the patterns of connections among them that lead to changes in behavior. Our discussion of plasticity will focus first on *development*, a time of rapid and dramatic changes in neuronal properties. Although our emphasis throughout this book has been on adult neurons, we begin with development because many of the cellular and molecular mechanisms that contribute to developmental plasticity are also relevant to plasticity in the adult.

Chapter 15 deals with the early events that determine whether an immature cell develops into a neuron or into some other cell type. It also covers the factors that govern *neuronal survival*, both during the formation of the nervous system and in response to damage to the brain later in life. This is followed in Chapter 16 by an account of the many molecules that regulate the growth of neuronal precursors and their *differentiation* into adult nerve cells. Once an immature neuron begins to extend an axon, this axon must find its way, often over very long distances, to its synaptic target. The role of various protein molecules in this process of *pathfinding* is summarized in Chapter 17. Such molecules play an important role in guiding neuronal processes through the extracellular matrix and over the surfaces of other cells. Specific cell surface molecules also tell neurons when they have reached an appropriate synaptic target and can stop migrating. In Chapter 18 we discuss *synaptogenesis*, the formation of the complex chemical synapse that occurs when an axon reaches a suitable target. During development and also in the adult, synapses can be continually formed and eliminated. The mechanisms that contribute to the *selective maintenance* of some synapses therefore are also presented in this chapter.

The ways in which *networks of interconnected neurons* can generate behavior is the subject of Chapter 19. Certain small groups of neurons that can mediate surprisingly complex behavioral outputs have been analyzed in detail. These analyses have provided insights into the way individual neurons are uniquely tailored to their role in a network and the way changes in their cellular properties alter the output of the network. *Computational models* based on biological data can be used to investigate this organization and to make quantitative predictions that can be tested by further biological experiments. Finally, in Chapter 20 we end the book with a discussion of *learning and memory*. These fundamental features of animal behavior, the ability to modify behavior as a result of experience (learning) and to maintain the new behavior, often for as long as the animal lives (memory), have fascinated scientists for many years. Recent advances in our understanding of neuronal properties and their modulation (see Chapters 11 through 13), and of the selective stabilization of synaptic pathways (see Chapter 18), are providing new insights into the cellular and molecular mechanisms of learning and memory.

15

The Birth and Death of a Neuron

R adical changes in the structure and connections of neurons occur during the development of the nervous system. Immature neurons are subject to chemical and mechanical influences that cause them to migrate to various locations in the nervous system, to extend axonal and dendritic processes toward other cells, and then to make and break synaptic connections with these cells before a final pattern of branching and connections is established. A full account of the different stages of neuronal development is beyond the scope of this book, which focuses on the properties of adult nerve cells. Nevertheless, neuronal plasticity in the adult animal may utilize mechanisms that are active during development, a period of profound plastic changes in neuronal structure and function. Furthermore, many of these mechanisms may also contribute to the maintenance of neuronal form and connections in the adult. In this chapter, we shall therefore first give a brief and general account of the normal course of neuronal development, and discuss some of the molecules involved in the earliest steps of the formation of the nervous system. We shall cover how new neurons come into being, both during development and in the adult. Finally, we shall discuss the mechanisms that lead to the death of a neuron. The following three chapters will cover molecules that determine the existence and properties of select groups of neurons, the growth of axons, and the formation of synaptic contacts.

Cell Determination

Early in the development of a vertebrate embryo, there exist three layers of cells. The cells that are destined to become neurons are found in the most external layer termed the *ectoderm*. Immediately under the ectoderm

375

lies a layer of cells termed the *mesoderm*. The first step in neuronal development is the determination of cells in the ectoderm to become neuronal precursors. This process is often called *neural induction* (Fig. 15–1).
In the nervous system of vertebrates, this appears to result from the action of *neural inducers*—diffusible molecules—released from nearby cells
in the mesoderm. After this stage the cells in the ectoderm can develop
only into neurons, glial cells, or a limited number of other cell types.

Some of the most critical experiments for our understanding of neural
induction have come from studies of the African frog *Xenopus laevis*. In
normal development, only a small part of the external ectoderm layer, that
situated at the most dorsal (top) side of the embryo, develops into neural
tissue. The remainder of the ectoderm develops into *epidermis*, the external skin of the animal. This occurs both in an intact embryo and in a culture dish. The *animal cap* is a layer of ectoderm that stretches from the
dorsal to the ventral side of the embryo. When any part of the animal cap

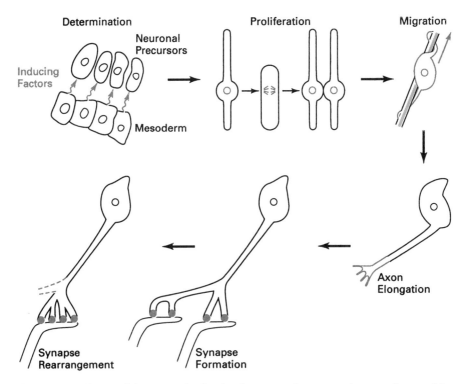

Figure 15–1. Some of the stages in the development of neurons that are discussed in
this and the next three chapters.

is dissected out from the embryo and is maintained in a culture dish, its cells develop into epidermis (Fig. 15–2).

In the 1920s, the biologist Hans Spemann found that when a small, specific part of the developing embryo, which has now come to be termed the *Spemann organizer*, is grafted onto the ventral part of a recipient embryo, it causes the ectodermal cells at that position to develop a secondary nervous system. Again, this experiment can be recreated in a culture dish. If the animal cap of ectodermal cells is cultured together with the Spemann organizer, its cells take on the appearance and molecular properties of neural tissue (Fig. 15–2). The Spemann organizer is an important source of neural inducers. A variety of these molecules have been found, and they have been given names such as Noggin, Chordin, Follistatin, and Cerberus. Application of any one of these to the ectodermal cells induces the formation of neural tissue.

How do these neural inducers work? An important clue came from the finding that if ectodermal cells are completely dissociated from each other before culturing, they eventually take on many of the characteristics of neurons or glia (Fig. 15–2). In such solitary confinement, they send out long processes from their cell bodies and synthesize proteins that are normally restricted to the nervous system. This discovery led to the sugges-

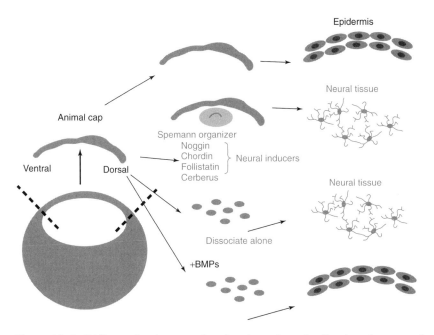

Figure 15–2. Different developmental paths of ectodermal cells when they are cultured alone, with the Spemann organizer, or with bone morphogenetic proteins (BMPs).

tion that, when left to their own devices, ectodermal cells prefer to develop into neural tissue. In a tightly packed aggregate of cells such as the
animal cap, however, the cells are exposed to factors that inhibit the formation of the nervous system and, instead, urge them to form epidermis.
Such neural inhibitors have indeed been identified. They belong to a class
of signaling molecules termed *bone morphogenetic proteins* (BMPs).

Bone Morphogenetic Proteins Are Neural Inhibitors

Bone morphogenetic proteins belong to a large family of factors termed
the *transforming growth factor-β* (TGF-β) family. Like the neuropeptides
that we considered in Chapter 8, the BMPs are first synthesized as large
precursor proteins, from which the active BMP molecule is cleaved. They
assemble into dimers and are then secreted from cells by a constitutive
pathway (see Fig. 8–5). More than 20 BMPs are known. As we shall see
in the next chapter, in addition to their ability to divert ectodermal cells
from a neural fate (which we shall discuss now), they play important roles
in the development of the nervous system at later stages.

On contacting an ectodermal cell, a BMP binds to a receptor that consists of two different subunits: the type I and type II BMP receptor subunits (Fig. 15–3a). The BMP receptor is a protein kinase that phosphorylates proteins at serine residues. When a BMP is bound, the receptor
triggers a series of signaling events, starting with the phosphorylation of
itself and of a cytoplasmic protein termed *Smad 1*. This protein is one of
a number of Smads, proteins that are involved in ferrying messages from
receptors of the TGF-β family at the plasma membrane to the nucleus of
the cell. (The term *Smad* is a hybrid word derived from the names for
these signaling molecules in flies and worms, where they were first discovered). The phosphorylated Smad 1 protein then binds another cytoplasmic protein, termed *Smad 4*, allowing the Smad1–Smad4 complex to
enter the nucleus of the cell and influence transcription. The end result of
activation of the Smad pathway in ectodermal cells is to make them into
epidermis.

The pathway from a cell that secretes BMPs to its receptors on nearby
cells is not a straightforward one. Once BMPs have been released, they
diffuse through the extracellular space, where they to bind to proteins that
are normally resident in this space. It is here, in the external environment
of the cells, that the neural inducers do their work. Inducers such as Noggin bind BMPs directly in the extracellular space, preventing the access of
the BMPs to their normal target cells (Fig. 15–3b). In the absence of the

activated Smad signaling pathway, the nucleus of the ectodermal cells carries out a program of activity designed to make a neural cell.

What Does It Mean to Be a Neuron?

How does inhibition of the Smad pathway lead to the production of neurons or other cells of the nervous system? We have already seen that neurons differ from other cells in the mix of ion channels and neurotransmitter receptors that they synthesize. Moreover, as we shall see in subsequent chapters, there are a variety of molecules that mediate physical interactions between neurons and other cells, and these must be present for a cell to function as a neuron. At the heart of the difference between a cell that is going to become a neuron and one that will eventually be an epidermal cell is their pattern of *gene expression*. Inhibition of the BMP–Smad pathway must lead to the activation of the genes that encode proteins required for the construction of a nervous system, and to the inhibition of those specific to the epidermis.

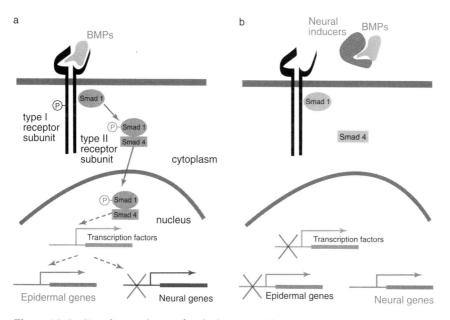

Figure 15–3. Signaling pathways for the bone morphogenetic proteins (BMPs). *a*: BMPs act though Smad proteins to activate epidermal genes and to suppress neural genes. *b*: In the presence of neural inducers, the BMP signaling pathway is inhibited, leading to the activation of neural genes (Chang and Hemmati-Brivanlou, 1998).

The regulation of neural-specific genes is a multistep process. Once the Smad1–Smad4 complex reaches the nucleus, as occurs in ectodermal cells exposed to BMPs, it binds other proteins that reside in the nucleus and then binds to specific sequences of DNA, altering the transcription of genes (Fig. 15–3a). Most of the genes that are initially influenced by the Smad pathway, however, are not those that encode proteins with day-to-day functions for epidermal or neural cells. Rather it is the synthesis of transcription factors that is first modified. *Transcription factors* are proteins that, once they are synthesized in the cytoplasm, quickly return to the nucleus, where they bind other regions of DNA that regulate the formation of epidermal or neural proteins. The BMP–Smad pathway leads to the synthesis of a particular set of transcription factors that stimulate epidermal genes and inhibit the transcription of neural genes. When the BMP–Smad pathway is inhibited by neural inducers such as Noggin, the epidermal proteins are no longer made, and other transcription factors, resident in the nucleus, allow the synthesis of neural proteins to take over. By controlling the synthesis of transcription factors, BMPs and neural inducers are able to exert orderly control over the decision to become an epidermal cell or a neural cell.

The genes for the transcription factors that turn on genes required for formation of the nervous system are termed *proneural* genes. There are many classes of transcription factors, which ultimately determine the synthesis of all cellular proteins. One class of transcription factors that are particularly important for the formation of the nervous system is the *basic helix-loop-helix*, or *bHLH*, transcription factors, so called because of a conserved pair of helices in the structure of these DNA-binding proteins. Another class of very important transcription factors contains conserved regions termed *homeodomains*. The particular mix of bHLH and homeodomain transcription factors that become activated in a cell may be the key determinant of what type of neuron that cell will eventually become.

Location, Location, Location

The type of cells that a given immature cell can eventually give rise to also depends on its position in the developing nervous system. In the early development of the vertebrate nervous system, cells are specified to form the types of cells appropriate to structures such as the forebrain or the spinal cord. If a region of cells specified to form forebrain structures is, for example, rotated by 180° during development, then it may eventually form inappropriate forebrain structures at more posterior locations. As we shall see in the next chapter, much of this specification is also brought about by factors released from mesodermal cells. Gradients of BMPs and other factors exist in the developing nervous system. The amount of a given factor to which a cell is exposed will depend on its position in the gradient. This in turn determines the particular blend of transcription factors that are synthesized, and, in this way, position controls the course of development. In addition, direct interactions with neighboring cells can induce neurons to follow different developmental paths.

Cell Proliferation

During and following the actions of factors that determine the developmental fate of a particular group of neuronal precursors, the cells begin to divide (proliferation in Fig. 15–1). During development of the vertebrate central nervous system, the embryo invaginates such that the location in which the neuronal precursor cells proliferate is adjacent to internal fluid-filled ventricles. This location is the *germinal* zone. As the cells divide, they undergo a series of changes in shape that are characteristic of dividing cells in most epithelia (Fig. 15–4a). These are, in sequence:

1. The cells send out processes that span the thickness of the germinal zone (G_1 phase).
2. As the cells synthesize DNA, the nuclei of the cells move along the processes away from the ventricles (S phase).
3. The nuclei return along the processes toward the ventricular surface.
4. The processes of the cells retract.
5. The cells divide.
6. The two daughter cells reextend processes to span the germinal zone, and the cycle begins again.

After several such cycles the cells either lose the ability to divide further and become *postmitotic*, or they migrate to another region of the developing nervous system where they undergo several more divisions before ceasing to proliferate. In the vertebrate nervous system, an immature cell that has undergone its final division and is destined to become a neuron is termed a *neuroblast*. There is some semantic confusion here in that, in invertebrates, the same term is used to describe cells that can proliferate but whose progeny are destined to become neurons.

Cell Migration

After their final division, a few cells may already be situated close to their eventual location in the nervous system. The majority, however, migrate (Fig. 15–1) considerable distances to arrive at their final destination. Dur-

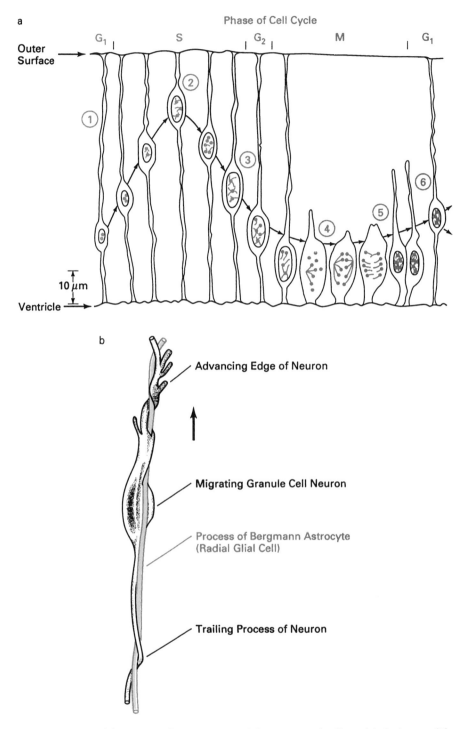

Figure 15–4. Proliferation and migration. *a*: Movements of cell nuclei during proliferation (Jacobson, 1978). *b*: The anatomical work of Pasco Rakic (1971) demonstrated the migration of neurons in the cerebellum along radial glial fibers.

ing such migration, a cell is exposed to factors released from other cells, including non-neuronal cells. It appears that such factors, in addition to direct physical interactions with other cells, play a central role in determining whether the cell will differentiate into a neuron, a glial cell, or some other cell type. Moreover, if a cell develops into a neuron, factors released by other cells influence the type of neurotransmitter it synthesizes and the specific mixture of receptors, ion channels, and other proteins that determines the characteristics of the fully differentiated neuron.

Another class of cell-to-cell interactions that occur during the migration of immature neurons determines the direction of cell migration. A clear example of this can be observed in the interaction of glial cells with developing granule cell neurons in the immature cerebellum of vertebrates (Fig. 15–4b). A class of glial cells known as *Bergmann astrocytes* is generated in the germinal zone of the developing cerebellar cortex. They differentiate into cells that extend cytoplasmic processes across the full thickness of the cortex. These radial glial fibers provide a pathway for the subsequent migration of neurons from the external surface (the external granule layer) down into the developing cortex. The cells that travel along these glial fibers eventually form a layer of granule cell interneurons in the mature cerebellar cortex.

Stem Cells

The picture we have painted of the developing brain is one in which immature cells continually assess their environment for the presence of factors such as BMPs, neural inducers, and other cells. As a result of each of these interactions, the developing cell makes a new set of proteins that determines the ultimate function of that cell in the adult brain. Like Peter Pan, however, some cells refuse to grow up. They persist from the embryo to the adult as cells that have not followed the pathways that make epidermis, neurons, glia, or other mature cell types. Such cells are termed *stem cells*.

Stem cells have the capacity for unlimited self-renewal. Each time a stem cell divides it produces two cells, one of which is identical to the original stem cell (Fig. 15–5). Depending on the environment, the other daughter cell may die, become another stem cell, or become a *progenitor* cell. The progenitor cells follow environmental cues such as those described above to produce highly differentiated descendants such as neurons or other mature cells. In fact, the progeny can usually produce many different types of differentiated cells. There is, however, no looking back. Once the progenitor cells have embarked on a course of development, they can never produce another stem cell.

The central function of stem cells may be to provide a never-ending source of progenitor cells for the replenishment of adult tissues. Stem cells may have different properties in different tissues. Very early in the development of the embryo, there are stem cells that have the capability of producing progeny that end up in every tissue of the mature organism. Such *embryonic stem cells (ES cells)* are termed *pluripotent*. In contrast, stem cells in the brain are thought to be able to generate only a more limited number of cell types that include both neurons and glia. As a result, such stem cells are often referred to as *multipotent*.

In the adult brain, *neurogenesis*, the process of making new neurons, occurs only in a few select areas. As is the case in the developing embryo, stem cells for this process are located adjacent to the fluid-filled ventricles, in the *subventricular zone*. Some of the new neurons that are born in this area then migrate along a pathway known as the *rostral migratory stream* and eventually settle in the olfactory bulb (Fig. 15–6 and Plate 9). These new neurons establish full functional connections with other cells, and become fully integrated into the neural circuits that are responsible for the sense of smell. In primates, other new neurons move into associa-

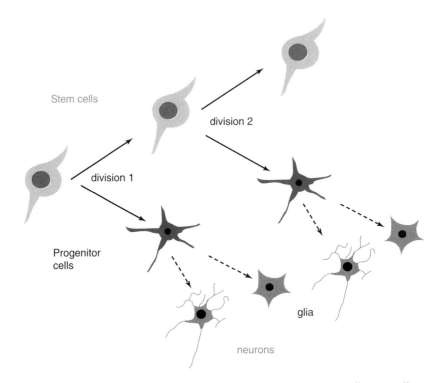

Figure 15–5. Stem cells. Division of stem cells produces more stem cells, as well as cells that eventually differentiate into mature cells of the nervous system.

tion areas of the cerebral cortex, which are likely to be important for higher cerebral functions, such as reading this book. Another site of stem cells that provide an ongoing source of neurons is the *subgranular* zone, a layer of the hippocampus. These cells provide for the replenishment of neurons in the *dentate gyrus* of the hippocampus. As we shall see in Chap-

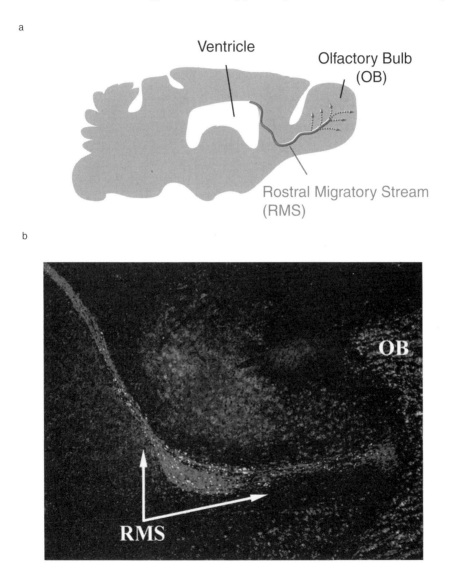

Figure 15–6. The rostral migratory stream. *a*: Path of migration of newborn neurons in the adult brain from ventricles to the olfactory bulb (Gage, 2000). *b*: A section of adult mouse brain labeled to show newly formed neurons migrating toward the olfactory bulb (OB) (van der Kooy and Weiss, 2000; see also Plate 9).

ter 20, this region is though to be important for the acquisition of new memories.

The ongoing production of new neurons in key areas of the brain suggests that new neurons may perhaps be required for some forms of learning and memory. It has been estimated that, in the mammalian brain, one new neuron is added each day for every 2000 existing neurons. The fact that the mammalian brain can make new neurons, and that these neurons can be integrated into the normal circuitry of the brain, also offers hope for the treatment of diseases such as Parkinsonism, which are caused by the death of entire populations of neurons. The implantation of stem cells or precursor cells may eventually provide a mechanism for restoring the normal complement of neurons in these areas.

The Formation of Neurons Requires Growth Factors

The formation of neurons and glia from stem cells, and their subsequent migration, both during early development and in the adult, has been investigated using many different techniques. One approach is to expose cells to radioactive thymidine or bromodeoxyridine (Fig. 15–6b). These molecules are then incorporated into DNA only in the nuclei of the newly born cells. The radioactive nuclei of these cells can be detected on a sheet of film through a technique called *autoradiography*. In some cases, dividing cells have been infected with a retrovirus, which also provides a label for all of the subsequent progeny of the dividing cells. Yet another approach has been to use stem cells that have been genetically modified to make a protein that is not found in normal stem cells. When these modified stem cells are grafted into a normal brain, their divisions and migration can be followed by the presence of the tracer protein.

The division of stem cells and precursors can also be studied in a dish. This has demonstrated that external factors are required for proliferation. Under the microscope, it is possible to watch the fate of single isolated cells taken from the forebrain. Such cells divide only in the presence of *growth factors*. When the stem cells are exposed to either epidermal growth factor (EGF) or β-fibroblast growth factor (β-FGF) they undergo cell divisions that result in the appearance of spheres made up of multiple cells. The cells in these spheres can in turn be dissociated into single cells that then produce more spheres of cells, or they can be induced to develop into glia and neurons.

The receptors for EGF and β-FGF belong to the receptor tyrosine kinases, which we covered in Chapter 12. As their names suggest, these factors were first discovered as proteins that stimulate cell division in non-neuronal cells, but they have turned out to act on neurons as well. In addition to these two proteins, many other factors have been found to influence the rate of proliferation of the stem cells and precursor cells and to determine the specific cell types that eventually differentiate from the precursors. Another important factor that may regulate the production of the olfactory neurons is *brain–derived neurotrophic factor* (BDNF). Because such factors influence the cellular properties of neurons at all stages of development, a fuller description of the actions of these factors is provided in the next chapter.

Cell Death During Development

Entire populations of neurons may arise during development only to die before a stable mature nervous system is formed. Very elegant examples of how cell death is used to build a simple nervous system have been described in invertebrates such as leeches, nematodes, and grasshoppers. For example, the nervous system of the grasshopper comprises a series of segmental ganglia along the length of the body. These ganglia are not identical and contain different numbers of neurons. Initially the pattern of cell division is similar in all of the segments. Later, the "unwanted" cells in a given segment simply die, leaving the remaining cells to establish the appropriate pattern of connections. This phenomenon has been termed *programmed cell death*. Neurons also die during development of vertebrate nervous systems. As many as three-quarters of the neurons destined for a specific neuronal pathway may die during early embryonic development. In some cases, survival of a neuron may require exposure to some diffusible *trophic factor* released by its postsynaptic or presynaptic target. Thus removal of a target, for example, of a limb bud in a chick embryo, causes the atrophy of sensory neurons that normally would innervate the limb. Conversely, implanting an extra limb partially prevents the loss of cells in the sensory ganglia. In other cases, the survival of a group of neurons may depend on exposure to a specific factor at a critical time in development.

The events that occur in a cell to bring about programmed cell death are still being unraveled. This process of dying, which has been termed *apoptosis*, is associated with a specific set of biochemical reactions that differ from those that occur during death from injury. In particular, the nucleus and the cytoplasm of the affected cells shrink, and the DNA of the cell is cleaved at specific sites (Fig. 15–7). Fragments of the dying cells are rapidly removed by *phagocytosis*, a process in which these fragments are taken up into neighboring cells or into *macrophages*, blood cells whose function it is to remove debris.

Insights into apoptosis have come from the identification of numerous proteins encoded by "death genes" in the nematode *Caenorhabditis elegans*, whose development proceeds through a very stereotyped pattern of selective cell death. The first of these genes identified, termed *ced-3*, encodes a protease that becomes activated in the cytoplasm of cell that is destined to die, resulting in the destruction of cellular proteins and the breakup of the nuclei. Mammals have a number of proteases that are counterparts of the ced-3 enzyme, and these are termed *caspases*.

Life and Death Decisions Are Made by Mitochondria

Clearly, caspases are dangerous enzymes. Yet they exist even within mature neurons, and must normally be maintained in an inactive state. The activation of these proteases occurs only when an irrevocable decision has been made that it is appropriate for a cell to die. This decision is gener-

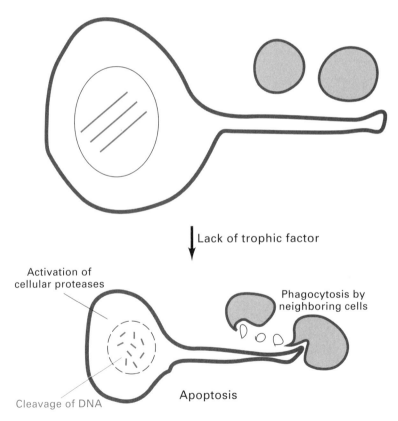

Figure 15–7. Programmed cell death. Lack of trophic factors leads to proteolysis of cellular proteins, cleavage of DNA, and removal of cell fragments by adjacent cells.

ally made by a second class of death genes, those that encode the Bcl-2 family of proteins. The Bcl-2 family proteins can function as ion channels, and they carry out their work in the outer membrane of mitochondria (Fig. 15–8). In neurons, the greatest density of mitochondria is found at synaptic endings.

To understand how the Bcl-2 proteins regulate apoptosis, we must review some basic properties of mitochondria. These organelles have two membranes, a highly invaginated inner membrane and a smooth outer membrane. Between the two membranes is the *intermembrane space*. The best-known function of mitochondria is to make the ATP that powers all cellular functions. An important component in the pathway that uses oxygen to drive ATP synthesis is the enzyme *cytochrome c*, which normally resides in this intermembrane space. In response to external signals that induce apoptosis, cytochrome c is released from the intermembrane space into the cytoplasm, where it binds and activates caspases, triggering apoptosis. The first enzyme that is directly activated by binding to cytochrome c is *caspase 9*. This enzyme, in turn, activates another caspase, *caspase 3*, leading to a chain of biochemical reactions that destroy cellular DNA and other cellular constituents (Fig. 15–8). In neurons, the external signal that triggers this sequence of events is typically the withdrawal or loss of trophic factors. We shall cover the biological actions of several of these neuronal factors in the next chapter.

The Bcl-2 family of proteins appears to be a key regulator of the per-

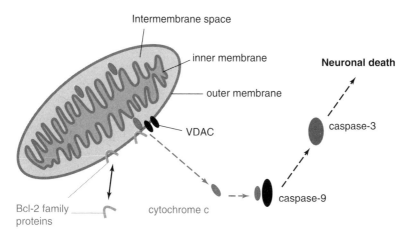

Figure 15–8. Regulation of the permeability of the outer mitochondrial membrane by Bcl-2 family proteins and by VDAC. Release of cytochrome c from the mitochondria into the cytoplasm activates caspases, leading to apoptosis.

meability of the outer mitochondrial membrane. Bcl-2 proteins come in two flavors, those that promote apoptosis (*pro-apoptotic*) and those whose function is to prevent programmed cell death, termed *anti-apoptotic* proteins. The Bcl-2 protein itself is anti-apoptotic, as is its relative Bcl-x$_L$. Pro-apoptotic members have names such as Bid, Bad, and Bax. Some of these proteins have been shown to be ion channels. In contrast to the plasma membrane channels that we covered in the first few chapters of this book, however, the Bcl-2 channels are not integral membrane proteins, and they are not inserted into membranes by a secretory pathway (see Fig. 8–5). Instead, they bind to cellular membranes directly and insert their ion channel pore region across the membrane. In fact, while some of the Bcl-2 family proteins are bound to the outer mitochondrial membrane at all times, others are usually bound to proteins in the cytoplasm, but can shuttle between the cytoplasm and the mitochondrial membrane. This occurs in response to changes in the external factors that induce apoptosis.

The Bcl-2 channels are not the only proteins that control the permeability of the outer mitochondrial membrane. A major protein component of this membrane is VDAC, the Voltage-Dependent Anion Channel (Fig. 15–8). In contrast to Bcl-2 proteins, VDAC is a bone fide integral membrane protein. Nevertheless, it again differs from the familiar plasma membrane channels in a very important respect. When VDAC is open, its conductance is 10 to 100 times greater than that of the plasma membrane channels. Thus, in addition to ions such as chloride and potassium, the open channel can conduct metabolites such as ATP and even small proteins. The opening and closing of VDAC can be regulated by many metabolites and proteins in the intermembrane space, and there is evidence that, in addition to being ion channels in their own right, the Bcl-2 family proteins control the opening of VDAC.

When activated by external signals, the pro-apoptotic Bcl-2 family members, perhaps acting in concert with VDAC, allow the passage of cytochrome c across the outer mitochondrial membrane, leading to the activation of caspases. In mice in which the genes for either caspase 9 or caspase 3 have been deleted, there is an excessive overall production of neurons, because of the lack of neuronal apoptosis. Paradoxically, this excessive production leads to the death of the animals before birth. Of course it is essential that cell death occur only in "unwanted" neurons. In some way that is not yet fully understood, signaling pathways that activate anti-apoptotic Bcl-2 proteins render the mitochondria resistant to the action of the pro-apoptotic proteins and prevent death of the cells. Thus the development of the nervous system represents a battlefield in which different external factors vie for control of the permeability of the mitochondrial membranes of the neurons.

Excitotoxic Cell Death

Programmed cell death is a normal aspect of development and also occurs to a limited extent in the adult brain, so as to compensate for the continual formation of new neurons and glia from stem cells. However, neurons can also die by other, more pathological, mechanisms. Neurons become damaged and may die when deprived of oxygen, a process termed *hypoxia*. This occurs during *ischemia*, when blood supply to part of the brain becomes impaired, causing a lack of both oxygen and glucose. Loss of neurons as result of hypoxia and ischemia causes the disabilities that follow a stroke and is a major cause of death in many countries. In contrast to the orderly slow biochemical changes that precede apoptosis, neuronal death in response to lack of oxygen and glucose can be very rapid. Such cell death has been termed *necrosis*, and it is usually accompanied by swelling of the cells, rather than the physical shrinkage that is characteristic of programmed death.

A multitude of undesirable cellular events occurs within neurons following deprivation of oxygen (Fig. 15–9). A fall in ATP levels results in

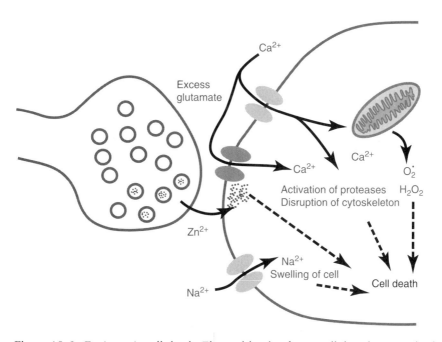

Figure 15–9. Excitotoxic cell death. Elevated levels of extracellular glutamate lead to the influx of calcium and sodium. Cell swelling and the destruction of cellular components can lead to rapid necrosis. Apoptotic mechanisms may also be triggered, leading to delayed cell death if neurons survive the early excessive stimulation.

an inability of cells to maintain their normal resting potentials and ionic gradients. The depolarization that follows causes the release of the excitatory neurotransmitter glutamate. The loss of ATP also compromises the activity of the uptake mechanisms that normally pump extracellular glutamate back into the cytoplasm. This leads to *excitotoxicity*, a major cause of neuronal death. The actions of glutamate during excitotoxicity produce abnormally high levels of intracellular sodium and calcium ions, both as a result of depolarization and by direct influx of calcium ions through the NMDA subclass of glutamate receptors. Several biochemical processes have been implicated in this rapid form of neuronal death, including the activation of calcium-dependent proteases and the destruction of the cytoskeleton.

Even if a neuron manages to survive these early events, it may still be doomed. Some of the events occuring during excitotoxicity can produce more delayed reactions and can even trigger the biochemical reactions of apoptosis, resulting in delayed cell death. Calcium entry into the mitochondria may also trigger the formation of reactive oxygen species such as superoxide ions and hydrogen peroxide, which contribute to cell death. Another agent that has been suggested to be a participant in the execution of neurons is the zinc ion. At many excitatory synapses, a proportion of presynaptic vesicles are filled with high levels of zinc (Fig. 15–9). It has been suggested that when zinc ions are released during normal neurotransmission, they may play a role in shaping postsynaptic responses. During the excessive amounts of secretion and depolarization that occur during ischemic brain damage, however, large amounts of released zinc are taken up by the postsynaptic neurons, where they accumulate in the cell bodies. By mechanisms that have not been fully established, such accumulation of zinc may lead to the delayed death of the postsynaptic neurons.

Summary

The development of the nervous system requires the participation of a variety of factors that influence neuronal determination, proliferation, migration, and differentiation. The earliest steps in the formation of a neuron involve the actions of factors such as the bone morphogenetic proteins and neural inducers. Acting on cells that still have the potential to develop into many different types of cells, these factors control the synthesis of transcription factors and determine whether the complement of genes that becomes activated corresponds to those required for building a neuron. The birth of new neurons occurs at a high rate early in development but, in some brain regions, persists in adults. The normal formation of the nervous system also requires the death of many neurons. Decisions as to whether a specific neuron survives or perishes during development are made by factors that control the permeability of the outer mitochondrial membrane. In the adult nervous system, death of neurons can be brought about by excessive excitatory stimulation. The interplay between neuronal birth and death is fundamental for the formation and function of the nervous system.

Neuronal Growth and
Trophic Factors

*I*t is safe to say that we are only beginning to understand the multiplicity of signals that determine whether a cell will differentiate into a neuron, and whether it survives or dies before development is complete. The previous chapter briefly covered some of the major events that occur during development of a neuron. We saw that the neural inducers, together with the bone morphogenetic proteins (BMPs) play a key role in the early steps of making a nervous system. The growth factors epidermal growth factor (EGF) and β-fibroblast growth factor (β-FGF) are required for the proliferation of some of the cells that will eventually become components of the brain. Clearly, the real picture is much more complex. In any part of the brain, there are many different types of neurons, with different morphologies, diverse patterns of synaptic connections, and different electrical properties. These cells coexist with other cell types such as glia or sensory cells. The resultant properties of any specific mature neuron result from its exposure during development to the action of many different external factors, including those secreted by cells far away and those on the surface of neighboring cells. This chapter will cover some more of the molecules that act on developing neurons and their precursors.

General Actions of Growth Factors and Trophic Factors

Table 16–1 lists some of the factors that influence the fate and specific properties of cells in the nervous system. The names these factors have been given are rather varied. Some terms, such as fibroblast growth factors or bone morphogenetic proteins, are purely descriptive (although, as we have seen, the description may not indicate the real function of a factor). Other more colorful names, such as *Sonic Hedgehog* or *frizzled*, exist because they were first used to describe mutant animals in which some aspect of normal development had been perturbed. A favored animal for such genetic experiments is the fruit fly *Drosophila*. We have already seen in Chapter 5 how a study of mutant flies termed *Shaker* led to the characterization of a family of potassium channels. The names of the mutants are now used to refer to the normal genes and to the protein factors or receptors they encode. Other names are hybrids. For example, the term

Table 16–1 Molecular Factors that Shape Neuronal Development

Signaling Pathway	Ligands	Receptors	Transduction
TGF-β family	Bone morphogenetic proteins (BMPs), Nodal	Type I and II BMP receptors	Serine kinase receptors, Smads
Cytokines	Ciliary neurotrophic factor (CNTF), Leukemia inhibitory factor (LIF)	Cytokine receptors	JAK–STAT pathway
Fibroblast growth factor (FGF)	β-FGF	FGF receptor	Receptor tyrosine kinase
Epidermal growth factor (EGF) family	EGF	EGF receptor	Receptor tyrosine kinase
Neurotrophins	NGF, BDNF	Trks	Receptor tyrosine kinase
Notch pathway	Delta	Notch	hairy, enhancer of Split
Wnt	Wnts, soluble secreted glycoproteins	Frizzled, Dally	G protein–coupled transduction
Hedgehog	Sonic hedgehog	Patched, Smoothened	Cubitus interruptus (Gli) transcription factors
Retinoic acid	Retinoic acid (RA)	RA nuclear receptors	Binding of receptor–RA complex to DNA
Steroid hormones	Estrogen, glucocorticoids	Estrogen receptor, glucocorticoid receptor	Binding of receptor–steroid complex to DNA

Wnt is a cross between the *Drosophila* mutant *Wingless* and a homologous mouse gene *int-1*.

Before we discuss the properties of some of these molecules and their receptors, it is necessary to make some general comments about the way these factors can influence the properties of a cell.

A growth factor can act either instructively or selectively. Exposure of a precursor cell to a growth factor may specifically activate genes that are required for the development of a mature neuron or glial cell. Some of the TGF-*β* family proteins have been shown clearly to function in this manner. Such an action is termed *instructive*. In contrast, many factors act by promoting the survival of cells that already express the specific properties. Such factors regulate the apoptotic and anti-apoptotic pathways that we covered in the previous chapter, and are said to act by a *selective* mechanism. As we shall see later in this chapter, many of the actions of the neurotrophins such as NGF and BDNF can be explained by this mode of action. Instructive and selective actions are, however, not exclusive, and the same growth factor can use both mechanisms at different times during development.

Timing is everything. The effects of growth factors and their signaling pathways depend on the developmental stage of the target cell. In the previous chapter, we saw that the competition between neural inducers and BMPs determines which cells of the ectoderm will develop into the nervous system. Once this important decision has been made, however, the BMPs (and the inducers) can instruct the developing cells to become particular types of neurons or other cell types. We shall encounter these actions again very shortly when we discuss how the forebrain comes to differ from the spinal cord and why motorneurons form in the ventral but not the dorsal regions of the spinal cord. Later in this chapter, when we cover the *Notch/Delta* pathway, we shall cover the role that timing is thought to play in the formation of the different types of cells that exist in the retina.

The relative amount of different factors is critical. Development is shaped by the coordinated action of many factors that originate in different locations. As we shall see in the case of the *Notch/Delta* pathway, some factors that induce a cell to make a developmental decision are located on the plasma membrane of adjacent cells. Other factors that act on immature neurons and their precursor are secreted by non-neuronal cells located outside the developing nervous system. In the previous chapter, we have already emphasized that the position of an immature cell in the developing nervous system determines how much it is exposed to different factors. Spatial gradients are known to exist for many of the factors listed in Table 16–1. As a result of these gradients, cells in different locations are exposed to very different ratios of developmental factors.

Anterior–Posterior and Dorsal–Ventral Patterning

Gradients play a key role in anterior–posterior patterning. This process ensures that the forebrain develops at the anterior end of the nervous system and that the spinal cord is formed at the caudal or posterior end. As we have seen, BMPs and neural inducers are essential for the formation of neural tissue. Slightly later in development, inducers such as Noggin and Chordin, which antagonize the actions of BMPs, are essential for the normal formation of the anterior parts of the nervous system, and mutant animals in which these inducers are lacking fail to develop a normal forebrain. In the more posterior regions of the developing nervous system, additional factors are at play. For example, there exists a gradient of several members of the FGF family (termed *FGF-3* and *FGF-8*), with their concentration being greatest at the posterior end of the immature nervous system (Fig. 16–1a). Inhibition of the action of FGF during development results in embryos that have defects in trunk and tail regions. Application of FGF to forebrain cells that have been dissected away from the rest of the nervous system induces them to activate genes that are normally characteristic of hindbrain.

The actions of FGF alone cannot explain all anterior–posterior patterning. Two other factors, Wnt3A and retinoic acid (Fig. 16–1a), may also be important for producing the more posterior regions of the nervous system. *Wnts* are large secreted glycoproteins of over 300 amino acids. Their signaling pathways not fully understood, but their actions on cells may require the Frizzled receptors, which, like many of the neurotransmitter receptors described in Chapter 12, have seven transmembrane-spanning segments. Other cell surface proteins, including one termed Dally, may also be required for normal signaling by Wnts. In frog embryos, application of the Wnt family member Wnt3A can transform anterior neural tissue into posterior tissue. Moreover, the Frizzled receptor is expressed in a graded fashion with highest levels at the posterior end of the embryo (Fig. 16–1a).

Retinoic acid is a small molecule closely related in structure to retinal, the light-sensitive molecule used in phototransduction (see Chapter 14). While the precursor of retinoic acid retinol (also termed *vitamin A*) is widespread, retinoic acid is synthesized from retinol only by certain tissues and diffuses from these tissues to act on nearby targets. Its molecular action is very similar to that of steroid hormones, which we shall discuss later in this chapter. Retinoic acid readily crosses cell membranes and binds a receptor that directly binds to specific sites on DNA (termed *RABEs* for

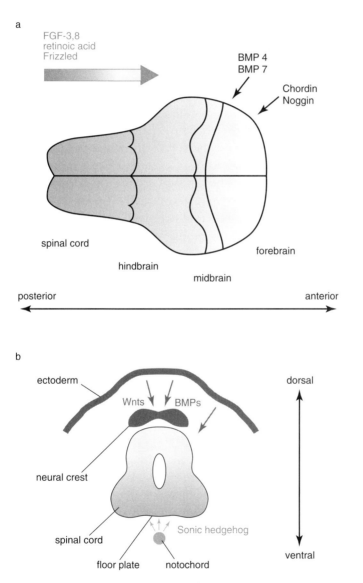

Figure 16–1. Gradients of secreted factors play a key role patterning the nervous system. *a*: Anterior–posterior gradients shape the formation of forebrain, midbrain, hindbrain, and spinal cord. *b*: Dorsal–ventral gradients determine the formation of the neural crest and different regions of the spinal cord.

Retinoic Acid Binding Elements) in the nucleus of the target cells. When applied to intact embryos, retinoic acid inhibits the formation of the proteins that mark the anterior parts of the nervous system and promotes the activation of genes characteristic of posterior regions. Thus this small molecule acid, in combination with Wnts and FGFs, may contribute to anterior–posterior patterning of the nervous system.

Gradients also contribute to dorsal–ventral patterning. Within the spinal cord, motor neurons are located ventrally, as is the *floor plate*, a structure composed of epithelial cells that extends the entire length of the spinal cord and into the brain (Fig. 16–1b). As we shall see in the next chapter, cells in the floor plate play an important role in guiding axons to their targets. Other types of neurons are located in the dorsal parts of the spinal cord. Located even more dorsally, between the developing spinal cord (also termed the *neural tube*) and the ectoderm, is the *neural crest*, which, as we shall see later, is a collection of cells that eventually make neurons whose cell bodies lie outside the central nervous system (the sympathetic and parasympathetic nervous systems), as well as other cell types.

A gradient for the factor *Sonic Hedgehog* is instrumental in determining the different properties of cells along the dorsal–ventral axis (Fig. 16–1b). This factor is first synthesized in the notochord, a non-neural tissue that lies beneath the spinal cord. If the notochord is transplanted to the dorsal side of the developing spinal cord, motor neurons as well as the floor plate develop on the dorsal, rather than the ventral, side. Conversely, if the notochord is eliminated, the ventral part of the cord fails to develop and cells from the dorsal regions take over the ventral area. This occurs because the developmental fate of the ventral cells is normally ensured by the diffusion of Sonic Hedgehog from the notochord. At later stages of development, Sonic Hedgehog is also synthesized in cells of the floor plate, further reinforcing the gradient of this factor from the ventral to the dorsal nervous system.

Sonic Hedgehog is a member of the Hedgehog family of secreted proteins. The way that Hedgehog proteins influence the properties of cells is still being established, in large part by studies in the fruit fly *Drosophila*. Hedgehog proteins are first secreted in an inactive form and must become activated by removal of their C-terminal domain (Fig. 16–2). This is accomplished by the N-terminal region of the Hedgehog protein itself, which contains a protease domain. Activation can occur, however, only after the protein binds the membrane lipid cholesterol on the surface of a cell. The activated cholesterol-bound Hedgehog protein then binds a membrane receptor termed *Patched*. This 12-transmembrane segment protein exists in a complex with *Smoothened*, a member of the 7-transmembrane G–coupled receptor family. Through steps that are not yet fully understood, stimulation of the Patched/Smoothened receptor results in the translocation of a protein termed *cubitus interruptus* from the cytoplasm to the nucleus. Before stimulation, cubitus interruptus is bound to the cytoskeleton, through its association with proteins that tether it to microtubules. After stimulation, cubitus interruptus enters the nucleus to stimulate the transcription of specific genes. Mammalian homologs of the cubitus interruptus gene are termed *Gli* genes.

While a gradient of Sonic Hedgehog from the notochord shapes the destiny of the ventral spinal cord, a similar scenario is being played out on the dorsal side of the developing spinal cord. A variety of factors, including BMPs, are released form the overlying epidermis and from the *roof plate*, a dorsal group of cells analogous to the floor plate. Some of these,

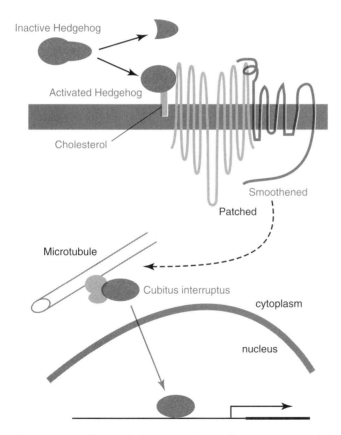

Figure 16–2. The Hedgehog signaling pathway. In *Drosophila*, the activated Hedgehog ligand, bound to cholesterol, activates the Patched–Smoothened receptor complex, ultimately resulting in translocation of the cubitus interruptus transcription factor from microtubules to the nucleus.

termed *BMP2*, *BMP4*, and *BMP7*, are required for normal development of neurons in the dorsal spinal cord and of neural crest cells. For example, BMP2 directly instructs cells of the neural crest to develop into neurons. Some Wnts, including Wnt3, which plays a role in anterior–posterior patterning, also promote the formation of neural crest cells and cells of the dorsal spinal cord.

During the development of the spinal cord, each cell along the dorsal–ventral axis is exposed to opposing signals from Sonic Hedgehog and the BMPs/Wnts. Depending on their position in the gradient, the cells encounter different ratios of these factors and activate a different set of transcription factors in their nuclei, which in turn direct the synthesis of slightly different set of proteins. As a result, the cells "know their place" and become neurons or other cells appropriate for their location.

Local Cell–Cell Interactions Shape the Development of Neurons

Within each small part of the nervous system many different types of cells may coexist. For example, the adult cerebral cortex consists of a complex meshwork of astrocytes, excitatory neurons, and inhibitory interneurons. The retina of vertebrates is a complex layered structure in which different types of neurons are situated alongside glial cells and photoreceptors. While gradients of growth factors are clearly important in the development of large regions of nervous system, it is difficult to imagine that gradients of diffusible substances alone could account for the development of different cells at such a local level. We shall now give a brief account of two *Drosophila* mutations, termed *Notch* and *sevenless*, to illustrate how these mutations provided major insights into neuronal differentiation. Unlike the soluble factors discussed above, the factors encoded by these genes are components of membranes and require direct cell-to-cell contact to exert their effects on neuronal differentiation.

The Notch *locus.* During normal development of *Drosophila*, a strip of cells along the ventral midline of the embryo comes to form the *neurogenic region* (Fig. 16–3a).The cells in this region develop either into neuroblasts, which give rise to neurons along the ventral cord of the fly, or into dermoblasts, which eventually form the epidermis over the ventral cord. (Remember that *Drosophila* is an invertebrate, and that neuroblasts therefore divide to give rise to neurons.) Under normal conditions, about one-quarter of the cells in the neurogenic region form neuroblasts. However, in a class of mutant flies first noted early in this century, the cells that normally become dermoblasts turn into neuroblasts, resulting in hypertrophy of the nervous system and loss of the ventral epidermis.

The defect in these animals was localized to a stretch of DNA termed the *Notch* locus. A complete deletion of the DNA in this region produces the change in the fate of the precursor cells for the epidermis described above. This in turn causes the death of the embryo. Other mutations of the DNA in this region are not always lethal but result in a variety of abnormalities of development affecting particularly the eyes and wings. The *Notch* locus encodes a large protein of 2703 amino acids (Fig. 16–3b). The predicted structure of this protein has some features of both a growth factor and a receptor within the same molecule. It has one stretch of hydrophobic amino acids that spans the plasma membrane. Near the amino terminal of the protein there is a sequence of 38 amino acids that contains six cysteine residues. Variants of this 38 amino acid sequence, each con-

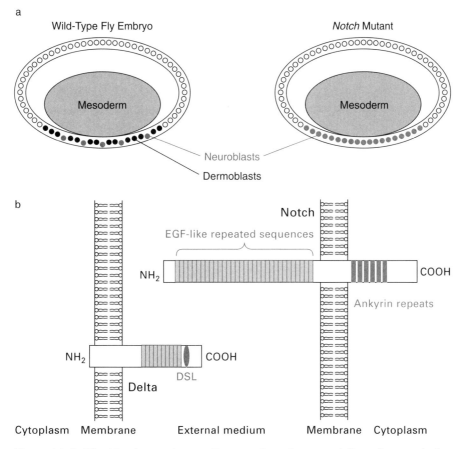

Figure 16–3. The *Notch* mutation. *a*: Cross section of a normal fly embryo and of a Notch mutant, with its overabundance of neuroblasts. *b*: The sequence of the Notch protein was deduced by Spyros Artavanis-Tsakonas (1995) and colleagues. Notch binds the Delta ligand on adjacent cells.

taining six cysteines, are repeated in tandem throughout most of the 1700 amino acids that lie on the extracellular side of the membrane. Each of these repeated sequences is very similar to a region that exists in EGF and related growth factors that we have already encountered. It has therefore been suggested that the EGF-like repeats in the Notch protein act as a form of membrane-immobilized growth factor. The intracellular domain of Notch does not resemble any of the receptors that we have considered thus far, but also contains a set of repeated domains that are essential for its normal function. These six intracellular repeats resemble the protein *ankyrin*, a protein of red blood cells that anchors the cytoskeleton to a transporter in the plasma membrane, and are therefore termed *ankyrin repeats*.

Notch does indeed function as a receptor. The ligand for this receptor is a protein termed *Delta*. In flies, deletion of the gene encoding Delta produces the same alterations in development as the loss of Notch. Unlike most of the ligands that we have considered thus far, however, Delta is also a membrane-bound protein (Fig. 16–3b). Like Notch, the Delta protein has several EGF-like repeats in its extracellular domain. It also contains a region rich in cysteines termed the *DSL* motif (named for Delta-Serrate-Lag-2; the names of three other proteins that contain this motif), which is essential for binding of Delta to Notch. Unlike Notch, however, Delta is simply a membrane-bound ligand, and does not appear to be a receptor. Thus its short intracellular domain is not required for normal signaling.

Initially all precursor cells in the epidermis are equivalent and have both Notch and Delta in their plasma membranes. The Notch receptors in each cell bind Delta ligands on neighboring cells (Fig. 16–4a). When Notch receptors and Delta ligands are balanced in this way there is a stalemate in which each cell prevents its neighbor from differentiating. With time, however, it appears that biochemical feedback mechanisms amplify small natural fluctuations in the activity of these signaling proteins. Thus cells with high levels of Delta *lower* the activity of their own Notch receptors, but become surrounded by cells with *raised* Notch activity. The cells with low Notch activity then develop into neuroblasts, while their neighbors with high Notch activity become dermoblasts. This process of interaction between adjoining cells has been termed *lateral inhibition* or *lateral specification*.

Further genetic experiments have shed light on the signaling pathway that has been adopted by the Notch receptor. At least one component is a protein colorfully termed *Suppressor of Hairless* [Su(H)]. This protein of 594 amino acids is present in the cytoplasm, where it associates with the ankyrin repeats on the intracellular domain of Notch. When Notch binds its ligand Delta, Su(H) is released and translocated into the nucleus of the cell, where it acts as a transcription factor and contributes to changes in the activity of genes required to form dermoblasts.

Homologs of Notch and its partner Delta are found in all species. They are found in the membranes of many dividing cells and their role is not

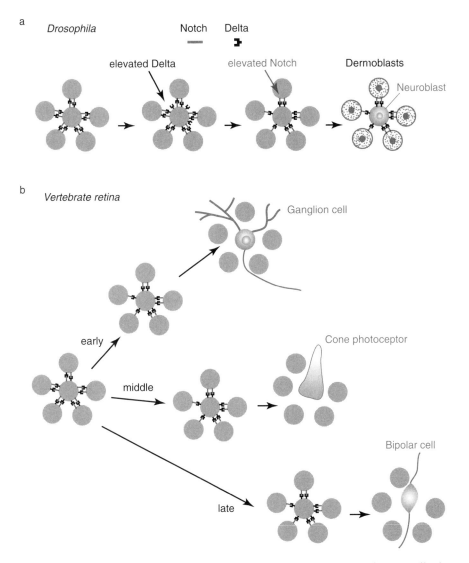

Figure 16–4. Lateral specification by Notch–Delta interactions. *a*: Adjacent cells that are initially equivalent differentiate into dermoblasts or neuroblasts through changes in the relative levels of Notch and Delta in their plasma membranes. *b*: The time during development when Notch levels become elevated in cells of the developing vertebrate retina may determine the cell types that are eventually formed.

specific to the formation of the nervous system. Rather, they seem to be required for many situations in which interactions between adjacent cells result in a switch in the direction of their development. One example of where Notch/Delta signaling has been implicated in the formation of different cells in the nervous system is in the vertebrate retina. In addition to the photoreceptors that respond directly to visual stimuli, the retina contains glia and several types of neurons that process these stimuli before sending them to the brain. These neurons include the ganglion cells, whose axons send the visual information into the central nervous system, and bipolar cells, which are interposed between the photoreceptors and the ganglion cells. The different cell types differentiate from precursor cells at various stages during the formation of the retina (Fig. 16–4b). It has been possible to manipulate the levels of Notch or to block the activity of Delta at these stages. The results of such experiments indicate that cell–cell interactions mediated by this pathway lead to the formation of each of these cell types. Interestingly, it appears that the time at which Notch becomes elevated in a cell is a key factor in deciding what that cell will become. Early in the formation of the retina, an elevation of Notch leads to ganglion cells, whereas elevation at later times produces cone photoreceptors and, even later still, bipolar cells.

Sevenless. Another *Drosophila* mutation that has provided the insight that direct cell–cell interactions determine the formation of specific types of neurons is the *sevenless* mutation. This mutation alters the fate of a photoreceptor named R7 in the compound eye of the fly. The eye of a fruit fly comprises several hundred units termed *ommatidia*, each of which contains a precise arrangement of eight photoreceptor neurons, R1–R8 (Fig. 16–5). As is typical of photoreceptors, these cells have elongated processes, termed *rhabdomeres*, that contain the photosensitive pigments. The elongated rhabdomeres are aligned around a central axis. One of these cells, R7, is specialized to respond to ultraviolet light. Six of the cells, R1–R6, span the length of the ommatidium. The rhabdomeres of the other two cells, R7 and R8, span only half the length of the ommatidium each, with cell R7 sitting on top of R8. Situated directly above these sensory neurons is a group of four cone cells whose function is to synthesize non-neuronal components of the overlying eye structure including the cornea. (These cone cells are themselves non-neuronal and are not to be confused with cone photoreceptors of the vertebrate retina.)

During normal development, the cells that make up an ommatidium arise from an amorphous collection of precursor cells. Cells that can be recognized as R1–R8 and the cone cells come into being in a fixed sequence, with R7 being the last sensory neuron to form. In the *sevenless* mutant, however, the R7 cell does not develop. Instead, the cell that would normally have become R7 differentiates into one of the overlying cone cells (Fig. 16–5).

As in the process of cell differentiation mediated by Notch/Delta that we discussed above, the normal formation of cell R7 requires the interaction of a membrane-bound ligand with a membrane receptor on an adjacent cell. In this case, however, this interaction does not occur by lateral specification in a field of equivalent cells, as occurs in the neurogenic region. Rather, it takes place between two different types of cells, neuron R8 and the cell destined to become R7, a process termed *inductive signaling*. The *sevenless* gene locus encodes a large transmembrane receptor protein. Like many other receptors involved in cellular development, the cytoplasmic side of this receptor is a protein kinase that phosphorylates proteins on tyrosine residues. It has been shown that development is abnormal when this receptor tyrosine kinase is defective in cell R7 itself, but not when it is defective in other cells in the eye. Moreover, there exists a second gene, termed *Son of sevenless*, or *Sos*, that is required for signal transduction by the sevenless receptor. As we shall see in the next section, when we cover the actions of the neurotrophins, the Sos protein is a key

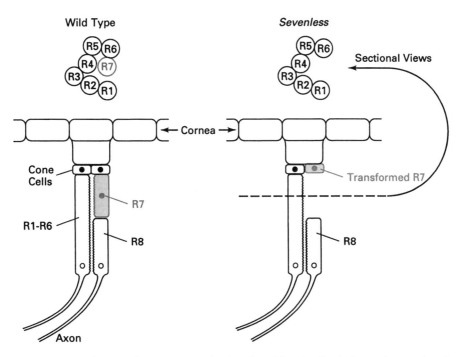

Figure 16–5. The *sevenless* mutation. Sectional and longitudinal views of normal and *sevenless* ommatidia (Palka and Schubiger, 1988).

intermediary in the transduction of signals that are activated by many different receptor tyrosine kinases (see Fig. 16–9).

The ligand that is required to transform a precursor cell into sensory neuron R7 is found in cell R8, the cell that lies immediately below R7. This ligand is encoded by the *bride of sevenless* gene, also termed the *boss* gene. The boss ligand is a membrane protein with seven transmembrane-spanning regions and a large extracellular domain. As in the case of *sevenless*, mutants with defective *boss* genes fail to make an R7 neuron. According to this scheme, the precursor cell above R8 develops into a cone cell in the absence of the signal arising from the boss ligand in R8. The binding of boss in the R8 neuron to sevenless in the precursor cells is followed by the uptake of the receptor–ligand complex into the cytoplasm of the R7 precursor by endocytosis. There the sevenless–boss complex can be detected in membranous structures termed *multivesicular bodies*. When the sevenless receptor is successfully activated by the boss ligand, the appropriate proteins to build the ultraviolet-sensitive R7 sensory neuron begin to be synthesized.

While the Sevenless receptor is unique to *Drosophila*, the internal signaling pathway that is triggered upon activation of this tyrosine kinase receptor is highly conserved in both vertebrates and invertebrates. As we shall see in the next section, this pathway is used not only by receptors that can be activated by immobilized ligands such as the boss protein but also by soluble factors that shape the properties of neurons.

The Neurotrophins

By engendering the activation or inhibition of specific transcription factors in the nucleus of their target cells, the cell–cell interactions that we discussed above instruct the nucleus of a cell to follow a particular developmental path. We have seen that gradients of soluble factors also promote the synthesis of proteins that determine the eventual phenotype of a neuron. A major role for certain soluble factors, however, is to prevent the apoptotic death of subtypes of cells. In particular, a family of proteins termed the *neurotrophins* is important for neuronal survival during development and for the maintenance of neurons in adult life. The first example and the most thoroughly characterized of these factors is nerve growth factor (NGF).

Nerve growth factor. The first clues to the existence of NGF came from experiments by E. Bueker in 1948 that demonstrated that if a muscle tumor is implanted into the body wall of an embryo, the tumor becomes innervated by neurons from the sensory and sympathetic ganglia along the spinal cord. This innervation is accompanied by a great increase in the size of the ganglia that project to the tumor. These experiments were followed up by Rita Levi-Montalcini and Victor Hamburger, who provided evidence for the existence of a soluble substance that promotes the growth of neurons in these ganglia. To characterize this substance, Levi-Montalcini developed a simple bioassay. She placed small pieces of tissue containing sensory neurons or neurons from the sympathetic nervous system into a culture dish. The addition of cells from the muscle tumor was then found to produce a very dramatic stimulation of the growth of neurites out of the explant (Fig. 16–6a). (The term *neurite*, or *neuritic branch*, is used to describe either an axon or a dendrite, and is a particularly useful term when it has not been established whether the growing process is in fact an axon or a dendrite.)

Subsequent experiments by Levi-Montalcini and Stanley Cohen found that certain tissues other than muscle tumors could also provide the neurite-inducing factor. In an attempt to characterize the molecular properties of NGF, Cohen treated a crude preparation of the factor with snake venom, which contains a phosphodiesterase that should degrade nucleic acids but leave proteins intact. Surprisingly, the snake venom alone was found to be active in inducing neurite outgrowth, and was shown subsequently to contain high amounts of NGF. In mice, the submaxillary salivary gland, an anatomical homolog of the snake gland that secretes venom, was also found to be very rich in NGF. The salivary gland was the source from which the protein was eventually purified.

Structure of nerve growth factor. As we shall describe below, NGF is a complex of three different types of protein. However, its biological activity on sympathetic and sensory neurons resides entirely in a complex of two identical peptide chains that have a molecular weight of 13,259 each (Fig. 16–6b). This homodimer has been termed the β *subunit* of NGF. Although there is only one gene for the β subunit, the RNA that is transcribed from this gene may be spliced in four alternative ways to yield four different messenger RNA species. The proteins produced by these messenger RNAs differ by up to 20 amino acids. Different tissues use different splicing alternatives, and thus the precise structure of the β subunit can vary from tissue to tissue.

In the submaxillary gland of mice, NGF consists of a complex of three different proteins, in which the β subunit is combined with two α subunits and two γ subunits (Fig. 16–6b). (This large complex has a sedimentation coefficient of 7 Svedberg [S] units and is therefore sometimes termed *7 S NGF*, in contrast to the β subunit alone which has been called

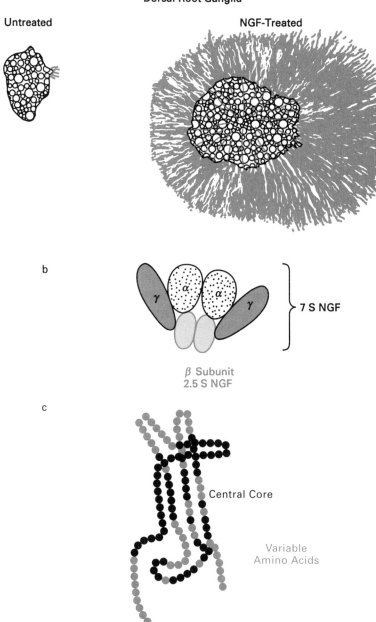

Figure 16–6. Nerve growth factor (NGF) *a*: Growth of neurites from sensory ganglia is induced by NGF. *b*: The structure of 7 S NGF. *c*: Structural studies have established that the β subunit of NGF has a central core with external loops. The organization of the peptide chain of β-NGF is shown, with the amino acids that are most different in the other neurotrophins shown in blue.

2.5 S NGF.) The γ subunits are peptidases that appear to play a role in the formation of mature β subunits, which are cleaved from a slightly larger precursor protein. The role of the α subunits is unknown. It is also not known whether NGF exists as this three-protein complex in all of the tissues in which the biologically active β subunit has been detected.

Direct measurements of the levels of NGF in various tissues, as well as the use of DNA probes to detect messenger RNA coding for the β subunit, have shown that NGF is synthesized at a low rate by a variety of tissues that are innervated by sympathetic neurons. The reason for the atypically high levels in salivary glands and in the saliva of mice is not known. Levels of NGF may also become elevated on injury to a nerve, when it appears to be synthesized by Schwann cells.

Actions of nerve growth factor during development. Despite its name, NGF is not a true growth factor. It does not appear to cause the mitosis of neurons or their precursor cells. NGF and the other neurotrophins that will be described below do, however, have a profound influence on the existence, shape, and activity of neurons. Some of the different actions of the neurotrophins are listed in Table 16–2. Thus it is clear that NGF plays a role in the normal development of sympathetic neurons and in their maintenance in adult animals. For example, injection of antibodies to NGF into embryonic or newborn mice results in the complete abolition of the sympathetic nervous system. Injection of antisera to other growth factors does not have as specific an effect. Destruction of the sympathetic nervous system also occurs in older animals that are deprived of biologically active NGF by repeated injections of anti-NGF antisera, although a more prolonged period of application is required than in the embryo or newborn.

Table 16–2 Actions of the Neurotrophins

Neuronal survival	Prevention of the death of neurons
Nerve growth	Stimulation of the elongation of both axons and dendrites
Nerve sprouting	Stimulation of the sprouting of both axons and dendrites of adult neurons (see Chapter 17)
Anabolic actions	Increasing the size of neuronal somata
Differentiation	Inducing the synthesis of proteins required for a neuronal phenotype
Modulation of transmission	Increasing the synthesis of neurotransmitters, neuropeptides, and their synthesizing enzymes
Electrical properties	Altering the activity and levels of ion channels

Conversely, injection of NGF itself into immature animals causes an enlargement of the sympathetic ganglia. Generally similar results are obtained with sensory neurons, although it appears that antisera to NGF are able to induce a depletion of sensory neurons only when applied early in embryonic development.

On the basis of these sorts of experiments, the hypothesis has emerged that target cells destined to be innervated by sympathetic or sensory neurons provide NGF to ensure the survival of their synaptic inputs. It may be that NGF acts to inhibit the mechanisms that would normally lead to cell death in this population of cells. A localized source of NGF may also provide a chemical signal for the directional growth of axons during development of the sympathetic nervous system (see Chapter 17). Indeed, experiments with isolated cells in culture, as well as with the intact nervous system, have demonstrated that neurites will grow in the direction of an increasing gradient of NGF. However, studies using cDNA probes to measure the amounts of messenger RNA for NGF during development have shown that major synthesis of NGF begins only after sympathetic neurons have reached their targets. Dependence on NGF for survival also begins at this time.

Only a limited set of cells respond to nerve growth factor. Although sympathetic and sensory neurons are the major neuronal types that are sensitive to NGF, a small number of other types of neurons also respond to this factor. For example, there exists a population of cholinergic neurons in the septum that projects to the hippocampus. If the axons of these neurons are cut, the cells normally die. Application of NGF prevents the death of these cholinergic neurons but does not affect the survival of other types of neurons in the septum. NGF also acts on certain non-neuronal cells such as chromaffin cells in the adrenal medulla, which can be induced to synthesize catecholamines and to extend neurites on treatment with NGF.

Brain-derived neurotrophic factor and the other neurotrophins. As mentioned above, NGF promotes the survival of sensory neurons at an early stage in development but becomes ineffective as the cells mature. A more prolonged survival of sensory neurons can be achieved by treating them with extracts from the brain. When the component responsible for this more prolonged trophic action was purified, it was found to have a structure very similar to that of NGF, and was termed *BDNF* for **Brain-Derived Neurotrophic Factor**. Molecular cloning revealed that there are several other closely related members of this neurotrophin family, termed *NT-3*, *NT-4/5*, and *NT-6*. The rather odd name NT-4/5 resulted from the finding that the fourth and fifth neurotrophins to be discovered were in fact the same factors isolated from different species. Each of these molecules has a central core region that is very similar to that of β-NGF, but they differ from each other in the structure of the loop regions (Fig. 16–6c) and at their amino and carboxyl terminals. In contrast to NGF, which acts only on a limited number of types of neurons, the other neurotrophins are widely distributed in the brain, both in neurons and in glial cells, as well as in peripheral tissues such as muscle. Correspondingly, they are able to promote the survival of a wide range of neurons, including many motor neurons and other central neurons such as dopamine-containing neurons from the substantia nigra (see Fig. 10–6). Recall from Chapter 13 that BDNF can also influence the excitability of mature neurons (see Fig. 13–9).

The Trk Receptors for the Neurotrophins

Nerve growth factor and the other neurotrophins produce their effects on neurons by binding to two types of receptors that span the plasma membrane, the *Trk* receptors and a glycoprotein termed *p75* (Fig. 16–7). The specificity of action of the different neurotrophins is conferred by the actions of the Trk proteins, which form homodimers whose extracellular domains comprise a tight binding site for a neurotrophin. The intracellular

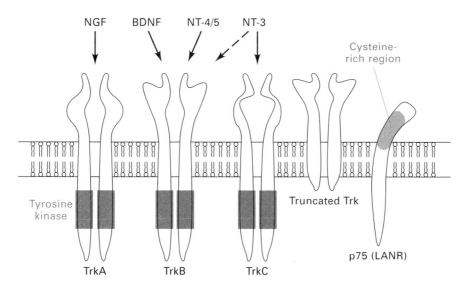

Figure 16–7. Neurotrophin receptors. Neurotrophins such as NGF bind full-length and truncated Trk receptors, as well as the low-affinity neurotrophin receptor p75. There is some cross-talk between different neurotrophins and their Trk receptors.

part of these receptors contains an enzyme activity that is a *tyrosine ki-nase*. One of the events that occurs when NGF or one of the other neu-rotrophins binds to a Trk receptor is that the tyrosine kinase activity is stimulated, resulting in the autophosphorylation of the receptor molecule. Each activated kinase domain causes phosphate groups to be transferred from ATP to tyrosine residues on the other chain of the Trk receptor. This sets in motion the chain of events described below.

There are three known Trk proteins, TrkA, TrkB, and TrkC (Fig. 16–7). The actions of NGF are mediated specifically by TrkA. As expected, there-fore, the TrkA receptor is found only on a few types of neurons, prima-rily sympathetic and sensory neurons and a small number of other neu-rons in the brain. In contrast, both TrkB and TrkC are found on most neurons. TrkB binds both BDNF and NT-4/5, while NT-3 acts primarily through TrkC. It appears, however, that a limited amount of cross-talk may occur between one neurotrophin and the preferred receptor for an-other neurotrophin.

Both the TrkB and TrkC receptors exist in a full-length and a trun-cated form. By alternative splicing of mRNA, the genes for TrkB and TrkC produce a truncated form of these receptors that is missing the intracel-lular kinase domain (Fig. 16–7). In contrast to the full-length form of these tyrosine kinase receptors, which are found only in neurons, the truncated forms exist predominantly on non-neuronal cells such as astrocytes and oligodendrocytes. The roles of these truncated receptors are not known, but it is possible that they comprise part of a mechanism that leads to the uptake of neurotrophins from the extracellular space and thereby controls the local concentrations of these factors.

A second membrane protein to which all of the neurotrophins bind is p75, sometimes termed *LANR* (**L**ow-**A**ffinity **N**eurotrophin **R**eceptor) (Fig. 16–7). This protein is unrelated in structure to the Trk proteins, but is a member of another family of receptors, the *tumor necrosis factor* (TNF) receptors. By itself, p75 is unable to mediate any of the actions of NGF or the other neurotrophins. Indeed, somewhat surprisingly, stimulation of LANR by NGF in the absence of the Trk receptors actually triggers, rather than inhibits, apoptosis. Nevertheless, the presence of this low-affinity re-ceptor in neurons appears to potentiate the TrkA signaling pathway and is important for some of the actions of NGF. For example, in animals in which the *p75* gene has been deleted, much higher than normal concen-trations of NGF are required to ensure survival of sympathetic neurons. Moreover, such animals have fewer sensory neurons than normal, and the axons of many of their sympathetic neurons fail to reach their normal targets.

Signaling pathways for the neurotrophins. The effects of the neurotrophins are so diverse that they must certainly engage a variety of different signaling pathways. Some of their actions are rapid and very local. For example, application of NGF to a restricted part of a sensory neuron produces effects on the morphology of its neurites that occur within 30 sec and are confined to the local area of application (see Chapter 17). From Table 16–2 we can see, however, that many neurotrophin actions result in changes in the rate at which specific proteins are synthesized by the neuron. This requires that a signal be sent from the axon terminals, where the neuron encounters the neurotrophin, back to the cell body, where gene transcription and protein synthesis occur. This appears to be accomplished through internalization of the neurotrophin by endocytosis, after which it is carried back to the soma by retrograde transport (Fig. 16–8).

Following binding of a neurotrophin such as NGF to its receptor, many of the subsequent effects on neurite outgrowth and gene transcription involve a protein known as *ras*. The ras protein is a 21 kDa phosphoprotein that binds GTP and is homologous to other GTP-binding proteins such as the rab protein (Chapter 8) and the G protein α subunits that couple neurotransmitter receptors to the formation of second messengers (Chapter 12). It is found in most eukaryotic cells, and was first discovered as a protein encoded by a proto-oncogene (for a discussion of proto-oncogenes see Chapter 18). When the ras protein is activated, it sets in

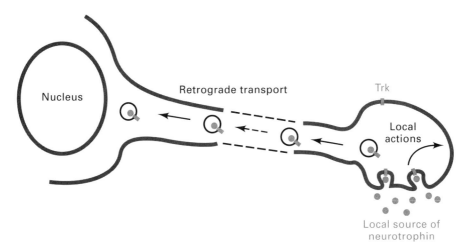

Figure 16–8. Sites of neurotrophin action. After binding to Trk receptors in the plasma membrane, neurotrophins can act locally, or they can be ferried back to the nucleus by retrograde transport.

motion a cascade of events involving the sequential activation of a chain of protein kinases.

The pathway for the activation of ras by the TrkA receptor is shown in Figure 16–9a. On binding NGF, the receptor dimerizes, so that each intracellular kinase in each peptide chain is able to phosphorylate specific

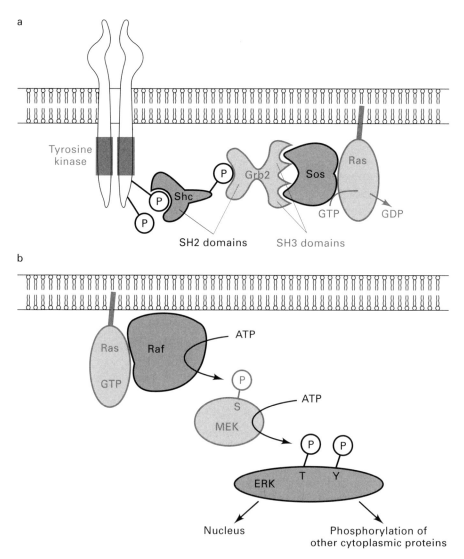

Figure 16–9. The ras/raf/MEK/ERK pathway. *a*: Pathway linking activation of a Trk receptor to the exchange of GTP for GDP on the ras protein. *b*: In its GTP-bound form, ras recruits the raf kinase to the plasma membrane and triggers a cascade of phosphorylation events, including the phosphorylation of MEK and ERK.

tyrosine residues on the other chain. Once phosphorylated, these tyrosines serve as points of attachment for proteins that contain structures termed *SH2 domains* (for Src Homology 2, because the Src protein kinase was the first protein in which these domains were found). Such domains are found in many signaling proteins and their function is simply to bind phosphotyrosine. One SH2 domain–containing protein that binds to phosphotyrosines on the TrkA receptor is the Shc protein, which, after binding, becomes phosphorylated by the receptor (Fig. 16–9a).

The Shc protein acts as the first part of a bridge that links the receptor to the ras protein. The second part of the bridge is an "adaptor" protein termed *Grb2*. This adaptor contains an SH2 domain, which allows it to bind to the tyrosine phosphorylated Shc protein. Grb2 also contains two *SH3 domains*. Like SH2 domains, SH3 domains allow signaling molecules to link to each other. Instead of binding to phosphotyrosines, however, SH3 domains recognize specific amino acid sequences that contain a proline and several hydrophobic amino acid residues. The SH3 domains on Grb2 join this adaptor to the third part of the bridge, the Sos protein (the signaling protein first found in ommatidial development, as described above).

The binding of Sos to Grb2 at the inner surface of the plasma membrane forms the final link, bringing Sos in contact with ras. Sos proteins promote the exchange of GDP on ras for GTP, thereby putting ras into an active state. The ras molecule then sets off a sequence of protein kinase reactions beginning with the activation of the raf kinase.

From ras *to* raf *to* MEK *to* ERK. Like some other GTP-binding proteins, ras is linked to the membrane by a lipid tail (see Chapter 12). In its GTP-bound state, ras recruits a protein kinase termed the *raf kinase* from the cytoplasm to the plasma membrane. On moving to the plasma membrane, the raf kinase becomes activated and phosphorylates another protein kinase, termed *MEK*, at serine residues, thereby activating this second kinase (Fig 16–9b). MEK is unusual among protein kinases in that it has the ability to add phosphates to both serine/threonine and to tyrosine residues. In turn, the activated MEK enzyme phosphorylates yet another protein kinase, *ERK* (for Extracellular Response Kinase, sometimes also called a *MAP kinase*, for Mitogen-Activated Kinase). This phosphorylation occurs on a threonine and a tyrosine residue. It is after this point in the kinase cascade that the multiplicity of effects of the neurotrophins can be understood. In addition to phosphorylating numerous cellular proteins, the activated ERK enzymes also enter into the nucleus where they act on transcription factors that alter the rate at which the messenger RNA for specific proteins is synthesized.

PC12 cells and the mechanism of NGF action. Although NGF acts on only a limited set of neurons in the nervous system, there exists a cell line that has been particularly useful in studies of the signaling pathways activated by this neurotrophin. These PC12 cells were derived from a tumor of adrenal chromaffin cells, termed a *pheochromocytoma*. Like sympathetic and sensory neurons, chromaffin cells are derived from the neural crest, and the TrkA and p75 receptors are present in the plasma membranes of PC12 cells. Treatment of the cells with NGF stimulates neurite outgrowth. Evidence that this effect of NGF involves the ras/raf/MEK/ERK pathway has come from experiments using a mutant form of ras that is diminished in its ability to hydrolyze GTP. By analogy with other G protein subunits, such a mutant ras protein would be expected to be chronically activated. In fact, injection of such a mutant ras protein directly into the cytoplasm of PC12 cells induces morphological differentiation similar to that induced by NGF (Fig. 16–10). Injection of the unmutated, and therefore unactivated, normal ras protein does not produce this effect. The injection of antibodies to the normal ras protein has been found to block the effect of NGF on PC12 cells.

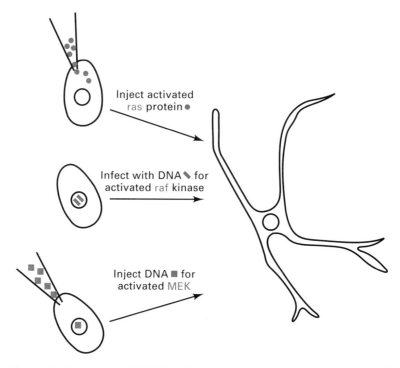

Figure 16–10. A role for the ras/raf/MEK pathway in neurite outgrowth. Injection of activated ras protein, or introduction of DNA for activated raf or MEK enzymes, which leads to the synthesis of the activated proteins within PC12 cells, causes the extension of neurites.

The kinases that act downstream of ras can also induce neurite out-growth in PC12 cells. For example, an activated form of the raf kinase can be introduced into these cells by inserting the DNA encoding the en-zyme into the genome of a retrovirus. On infection with the retrovirus, the cells begin to synthesize the activated enzyme and to extend neurites, mimicking the effect of NGF. Similar results are obtained on injection of DNA encoding a mutated MEK enzyme that is active even when not phos-phorylated (Fig. 16–10). Moreover, it is possible to make another form of mutated MEK, which is inactive but which blocks signaling by competing for the normal cellular raf kinase. Injection of DNA encoding this inhib-itor MEK prevents the action of NGF on neurite outgrowth.

Other signaling pathways are also used by the neurotrophins. Experiments such as those described above indicate that the ras/raf/MEK/ERK pathway is a key element in the actions of the neurotrophins. It is, however, not the only signaling pathway activated by the Trk receptors. The phosphoty-rosines on Trk receptors may engage a variety of other signaling mole-cules. For example, a form of the enzyme phospholipase C, termed *PLCγ*, is recruited to activated Trk receptors through its SH2 domains (Fig 16–11). This enzyme is then activated by tyrosine phosphorylation, and results in the formation of diacylglycerol and inositol trisphosphate, sec-ond messengers that were discussed in Chapter 12.

While the ras/raf/MEK/ERK pathway is required for full differentia-tion of many neurons, it is not required for the very important action of neurotrophins in protecting neurons from apoptosis. The effects of NGF on the survival of PC12 cells can proceed in the absence of an activated ras protein. The pathway that appears to be required for cell survival is the activation of the enzyme *PI3 kinase* (phosphatidylinositol-3-kinase). This enzyme causes the phosphorylation of phosphatidylinositol, which, as we saw in Chapter 12, is part of the DAG/IP$_3$ signaling pathway. The actions of PI3 kinase, however, constitute a signaling pathway that is com-pletely distinct from the DAG/IP$_3$ system (Fig. 16–11). The lipid second messengers produced by PI3 kinase activate a cytoplasmic serine/threonine kinase termed *Akt*. It is thought that this kinase, in turn, may influence the activity of Bcl-2 family proteins in neuronal mitochondria, which, as we saw in the last chapter, results in protection of cells from apoptosis.

Cytokines and the JAK–STAT pathway

Another class of molecules, structurally unrelated to the neurotrophin fam-ily, has also been found to be required for the survival of many types of neurons and to influence their cellular properties. These molecules were first found to influence the differentiation of cells in the blood and the immune system and are termed *cytokines*. In contrast to the neurotrophins, the cytokines act on membrane receptors that are not themselves tyrosine kinases. Instead, the cytokine receptors stimulate the activity of soluble cytoplasmic tyrosine kinases termed *JAKs* (Janus kinases). There are four known JAK kinases, each of which has seven conserved regions termed *JH domains* (Fig. 16–12a), and can themselves undergo phosphorylation in the JH1 domain that contains the active site of the enzyme.

One molecule that acts through the cytokine pathway is ciliary neurotrophic factor (CNTF), which was first described as a factor required for the survival of neurons of the ciliary ganglion of chicks, and is a potent survival factor for many types of neurons. CNTF can also induce the differentiation of astroglia from precursor cells. On the surface of cells,

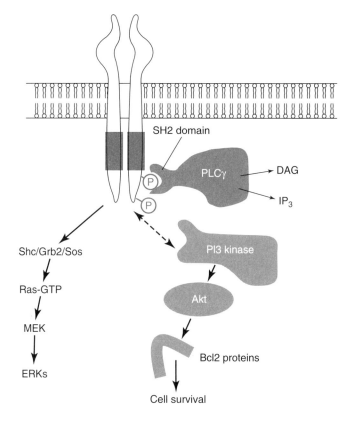

Figure 16–11. Multiple intracellular signaling pathways are activated by the neurotrophins. These include the PI3 kinase pathway, which promotes cell survival, as well as the ras/raf/MEK/ERK and PLCγ pathways. DAG, diacylglycerol; IP$_3$, inositol trisphosphate.

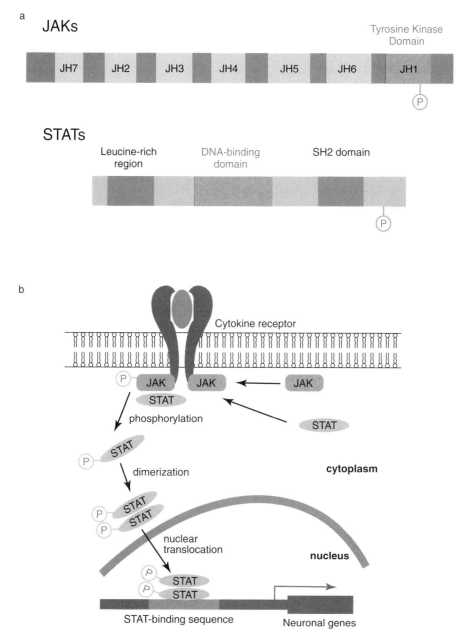

Figure 16–12. The JAK–STAT signaling pathway. *a*: Structures of the JAK kinases and their STAT substrates. *b*: Following binding of cytokine to its receptor, STATs are phosphorylated, leading to activation of specific genes.

421

CNTF binds to a protein termed *CNTFRα* (CNTF-receptor *α*), which forms a complex with two other proteins, LIFR*β* (leukemia inhibitory factor receptor *β*) and gp130 (Fig. 16–13). On activation by CNTF, the receptor complex is able to bind a JAK kinase, which becomes activated and phosphorylates substrate proteins knows as STATs (Signal Transducers and Activators of Transcription) (Fig. 16–12a). Seven such STAT proteins are currently known. These proteins contain SH2 domains that allow them to bind other proteins that are phosphorylated on tyrosine residues, as well as a region rich in leucines. Once a STAT is phosphorylated, these regions allow it to form a dimer with another STAT and then enter the nucleus. There they bind to DNA at regions termed *STAT-binding sequences*, which are situated upstream of genes that become activated on exposure of the cell to CNTF (Fig. 16–12b).

Factors that make a cholinergic neuron. One of the best-studied examples of how cytokine signaling influences the properties of neurons has come from work with cells that form the sympathetic and parasympathetic nervous

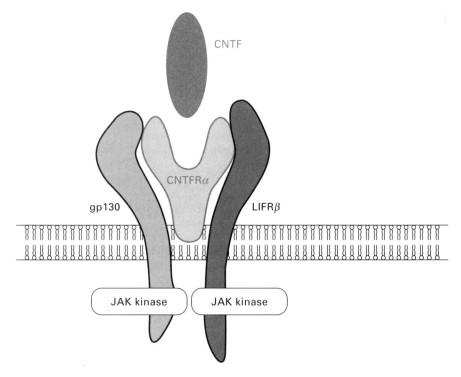

Figure 16–13. The ciliary neurotrophic factor (CNTF) receptor. This receptor is a complex of three proteins that, when bound to CNTF, activates JAKs, cytoplasmic tyrosine kinases.

systems. These cells migrate from the neural crest (Fig. 16–14), a column of undifferentiated cells at the dorsal margin of the neural tube that we first encountered when discussing the development of the spinal cord (Fig. 16–1). Neurons of the sympathetic nervous system, which arise from the central portion of the developing spinal cord, synthesize the enzymes required for the production of norepinephrine, which they use as a neurotransmitter. In contrast, neurons of the parasympathetic nervous system, which develop largely from the anterior developing spinal cord, synthesize and secrete acetylcholine as their major transmitter.

The development of the biochemical machinery to produce either the adrenergic or the cholinergic transmitter system is not determined by the position in the neural crest from which the cells migrate, but rather by a factor that the cells encounter during their migration away from the neural crest. When immature adrenergic neurons are isolated in culture they maintain the ability to make norepinephrine. However, if these neurons are cultured in the presence of non-neuronal cells such as heart cells or other cell types that normally receive a cholinergic input, the cells stop synthesizing tyrosine hydroxylase, the rate-limiting enzyme in the pathway

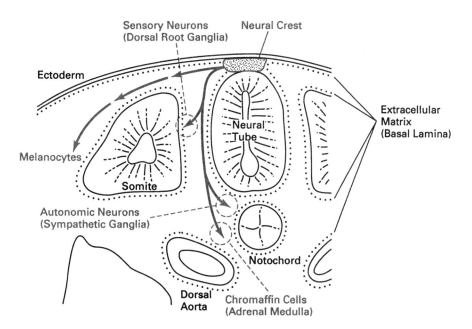

Figure 16–14. The neural crest. A cross section through the trunk region of a chick embryo. Cells that migrate from the neural crest region develop into sensory, sympathetic, and parasympathetic neurons, as well as other cell types. Also shown is the extracellular matrix of the basal lamina (see Chapter 17). (Modified from Sanes, 1983.)

for synthesis of norepinephrine (see Chapter 10). Instead, the neurons now synthesize choline acetyltransferase and make acetylcholine their transmitter. There are several different factors, secreted into the medium from different tissues, that can produce this result. One of these, which can be purified from the medium secreted by heart cells, is *leukemia inhibitory factor* (LIF), which has also been termed *cholinergic differentiation factor* (CDF). A second factor is CNTF itself. Both of these factors signal to the nucleus through the JAK–STAT pathway. Some other factors that produce the same results may also be associated with the membranes of cells with which the migrating neurons come into contact.

Although the type of transmitter can be modified by CDF/LIF in immature cells taken from young animals, adrenergic neurons from older animals are insensitive to its actions. Thus, there exists a critical period in development during which such factors are able to exert their effects. A particularly interesting aspect of the action of CDF/LIF is that its activity is strongly dependent on the amount of electrical activity in the neurons. Direct electrical stimulation of the cultures of neurons or depolarization with solutions containing a high concentration of potassium ions prevents the action of the cholinergic factor and maintains the adrenergic phenotype. This inhibition of the action of cholinergic factor by electrical activity is due to calcium entry through voltage-dependent calcium channels. Thus it is possible that the activity of calcium channels during development serves to fix the choice of transmitter in neurons of the autonomic nervous system.

Other Trophic Molecules

Another factor that promotes the survival of motor neurons and of other neurons, such as dopaminergic neurons in the central nervous system, is *glial cell line–derived neurotrophic factor* (GDNF), which comprises a ~40 kDa dimer of two glycoproteins linked by disulfide bridges and is related to the BMPs and the TGF-β family of growth factors.

In addition to these neurotrophic molecules, which were discovered because of their ability to prevent different types of neurons from dying, there are other trophic factors, first discovered as true growth factors, that stimulate cell division in non-neuronal cells. Many of these molecules and their receptors are present within neurons and glial cells or in the peripheral targets of neurons. When applied to neurons they have been found to have many of the trophic actions listed in Table 16–2. Among such factors are some we have already encountered, such as *acidic fibroblast growth factor* (aFGF), which is present within motor neurons, and *basic fibroblast growth factor* (bFGF), which is present within astrocytes that surround the somata of motor neurons (Fig. 16–15). Receptors for both of these molecules are found on the surface of motor neurons and both substances aid in the survival of motor neurons that have been isolated in culture. Another trophic factor *insulin-like growth factor-1* (IGF-1) is able to stimulate the sprouting of axons (see Chapter 17).

Two trophic factors are better than one. A simple concept arising from the discovery of NGF is that the normal target of a neuron provides the factor that is required for its survival. This concept must be modified for some of the other factors that have trophic effects on neurons. For example, both BDNF and CNTF improve the survival of embryonic motor neurons. BDNF is found in target muscles and may be a true target-derived factor. CNTF, on the other hand, is present in the myelinating Schwann cells that envelop the axon of the motor neurons (Fig. 16–15). Both of these factors may be required for the normal maintenance of motor neurons. For example, in a mutant strain of mice termed *wobbler* that normally suffers progressive loss of motor neurons, application of both factors produces

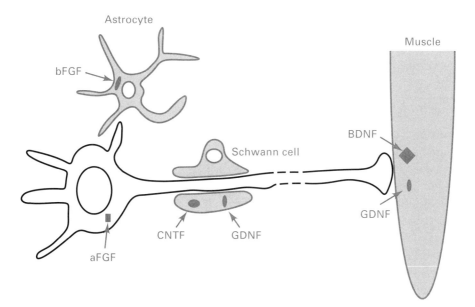

Figure 16–15. Trophic factors for motor neurons. Important sources of trophic molecules are glial cells and the innervated muscle (modified from Nishi, 1994). aFGF, acidic fibroblast growth factor; bFGF, basic fibroblast growth factor; BDNF, brain-derived neurotrophic factor; CNTF, ciliary neurotrophic factor; GDNF, glial cell–derived neurotrophic factor.

full survival of motor neurons, whereas treatment with either one alone produces only partial benefits.

As expected for target-derived trophic factors, BDNF and the other neurotrophins begin to be made in neuronal targets before the time in development when cell death occurs. Thus the motor neurons that are exposed to BDNF and other trophic factors at this time are allowed to survive. In contrast, CNTF begins to be synthesized in the Schwann cells at the time of myelination, well after the time of naturally occurring cell death. It is only after this time that the neurons come to depend on CNTF. This fact can readily be observed in mutant mice in which the gene for CNTF has been deleted. The motor neurons of such animals develop normally up to the time of myelination. Thereafter, as the animals mature, there is a progressive decrease in the size of the somata of these cells. This is followed in turn by the death of a proportion of the motor neurons.

In addition to CNTF, yet other trophic agents are present in cells that are not the natural targets of these neurons. As we mentioned above, both aFGF and bFGF act on motor neurons, and their effects may synergize with those of the other factors. For example, bFGF is present in astrocytes adjacent to the somata of the motor neurons and may have a *paracrine* mode of action (that is, it may act on an adjacent cell). By contrast, aFGF is present within the motor neurons themselves and may therefore be an *autocrine* factor (it may act on the same cell that releases the factor) (Fig. 16–15).

One of the questions that still has to be resolved is how and when motor neurons come to be exposed to these factors. The neurotrophins appear to be typical secretory proteins that are released by muscle cells and other neuronal targets. In contrast, CNTF in the Schwann cells, bFGF in astrocytes, and aFGF in the neurons are cytoplasmic proteins without a signal sequence that would be expected for normal secretion (see Chapter 8). The action of these factors on motor neurons must therefore occur by a less conventional mechanism.

Because of the importance of trophic factors, it would be expected that the genetic knockout of a trophic factor or its receptor would seriously impair development. In some cases this is true. Elimination of a factor or its receptor produces characteristic deficits in the numbers of specific types of neurons and, at later stages of development, may be lethal. For example, elimination of the *TrkA* gene in mice results in the destruction of the sympathetic nervous system, as expected for a mutation that blocks the effects of NGF. Nevertheless, in many other cases the effects of eliminating a trophic factor are not as profound as might be expected. For example, loss of the TrkA receptor does not alter the cholinergic neurons in the septum that are sensitive to NGF. In addition, elimination of BDNF does not impair the development of motor neurons (although it does produce a partial loss of sensory neurons, where it acts as an autocrine trophic factor). Such surprising results may be explained by the fact that survival of many neurons can be regulated by multiple factors acting together and by the fact that there is cross-talk between some of the receptors (see Fig. 16–7), so that one factor may be able to substitute in part for the loss of another.

Steroid Hormones

For many cells in the nervous system, appropriate development depends on the action of hormones secreted by other organs in the body. Some of these are listed in Table 16–3. In contrast to peptide hormones, steroid hormones are lipid soluble and readily enter the brain from the blood. They also cross cell membranes without the need for specific carriers or receptors in the plasma membrane. There is evidence, based primarily on the finding of receptor proteins for steroid hormones in the cytoplasm of neurons or glial cells, that each of these hormones influences the nervous system. In most cases, the different receptor proteins are localized to specific groups of neurons rather than being uniformly distributed throughout the nervous system.

How do steroid hormones work? The best-understood mode of action of these hormones is through a class of receptor proteins that, in the presence of the hormone, directly bind DNA in the nucleus, allowing the transcription of specific genes. The general structure of these receptor proteins is shown in Figure 16–16a. There is a high degree of homology in the regions of DNA binding and of hormone binding in the different receptors for this class of hormones. Figure 16–16b shows part of the sequence of the DNA-binding region of the receptors, which is rich in the amino acid

Table 16–3 Steroid Hormones Important for Neuronal Development

Class	Example	Source
Androgens	Testosterone	Gonads
Estrogens	β-Estradiol (estrogen)	Gonads
Progestins	Progesterone	Gonads
Glucocorticoids	Corticosterone	Adrenal gland
Mineralocorticoids	Aldosterone	Adrenal gland

cysteine. These are believed to form a coordination complex with zinc ions, producing two *zinc fingers*, structural features that allow proteins to bind DNA.

When a cell is exposed to hormone, the receptors bind the hormone and undergo a structural change that allows the DNA-binding regions to interact with specific short sequences in the DNA of the cell. These DNA sequences have been termed *hormone response elements* (HREs). They are found in the proximity of genes coding for proteins whose expression is regulated by the steroid/thyroid family of hormones. Although the exact position of the HRE relative to the structural gene encoding the protein itself may vary in different genes, the sequence of the HRE is very similar for each of the genes that is regulated by a specific hormone. The sequence of the HRE in the gene for prolactin, a peptide whose synthesis is regulated by the steroid hormone estrogen, is shown in Figure 16–16c.

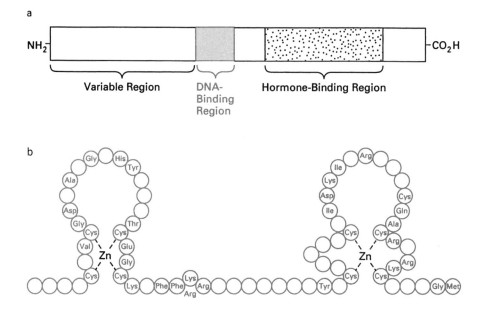

c   **Hormone Response Elements**

G C A T T T T [T G T C A] C T A [T G T C C] T A G A G T

DNA Sequences Recognized by Receptor

Figure 16–16. Steroid receptors. *a*: Outline of the three distinct regions found in these receptors. *b*: Amino acid sequence of a DNA-binding region. The named amino acids are found in nearly all receptors of this family. *c*: DNA sequence within the prolactin gene required for binding the estrogen receptor (Evans, 1988).

Organizational effects of steroid hormones. Examples of the neuronal action of such hormones have come from studies of the role of the gonadal steroids in the control of reproductive behaviors. Differences exist between the brains of males and females in the size and synaptic connections of several well-defined groups of neurons. One such group in rat brain is the *sexually dimorphic nucleus of the preoptic area* (SDN-POA), which is five times larger in males than in females. The increased number of neurons in males results from the action of testosterone during development. Thus, if a female rat is treated with testosterone during late embryonic development and over the first 10 days after birth, the SDN-POA develops as in a male (Fig. 16–17). Interestingly, this action of testosterone is not mediated by a receptor specific for testosterone. Enzymes exist within the neurons that convert testosterone into estrogen. This process is termed *aromatization* (Fig. 16–17). Thus estrogen is actually the active hormone within the cells, and treatment of immature females with compounds such as diethylstilbestrol, a highly active analog of estrogen, also causes the male pattern of development of the SDN-POA.

    The action of a steroid hormone to alter this developmental pathway is an example of what have been termed *organizational* effects of steroid

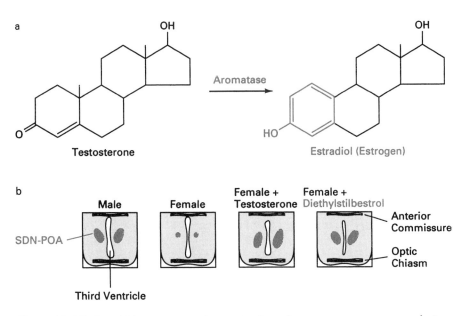

Figure 16–17. Steroid hormones. *a*: Aromatization of testosterone to estrogen. *b*: Sections through the sexually dimorphic nucleus of the preoptic area (SDN–POA) were prepared by Roger Gorski (1989) and colleagues, using normal male and female rats and steroid-treated female rats.

hormones. In particular, the action of the hormone is permanent and is restricted to a critical period during development. For example, treatment of female rats with testosterone later than 6 days after birth cannot alter the size of the SDN-POA. It is not yet known which specific steps in neuronal development (Fig. 15–1) are sensitive to testosterone and estrogen.

Activational effects of steroid hormones. The role of steroid hormones is not confined to the organization of specific neuronal pathways during development. The hormones also regulate the properties of many mature neurons and thereby influence the onset of specific animal behaviors. Again, such effects are particularly obvious in reproductive behaviors and have been termed *activational* effects. For example, the morphology and extent of dendritic branching in neurons that innervate muscles involved in copulation remain sensitive to changes in testosterone in adult male rats. Another well-studied effect is the action of estrogen and progesterone in the onset of lordosis behavior in female rats. During this behavior, the female rat assumes a characteristic body posture that indicates sexual receptivity. Groups of neurons that control lordosis behavior are found in the ventromedial nuclei within the hypothalamus. An elevation of the levels of estrogen produces morphological changes in these neurons, increasing the size of their somata and increasing the synthesis of a variety of proteins, including the receptors for progesterone. Subsequent elevation of progesterone levels, as would normally occur during the estrus cycle, induces the synthesis of further proteins that are essential for lordosis behavior to occur.

The nature of the changes in neuronal properties and possible synaptic remodeling that are induced by the consecutive actions of estrogen and progesterone is not yet understood. However, it is known that estrogen increases synthesis of the neuropeptide Met-enkephalin and of receptors for the peptide oxytocin in the ventromedial nuclei, and that receptors for other transmitters, such as GABA and acetylcholine, may decrease in number. The steroid hormones may be considered to be agents that prime neuronal pathways for the occurrence of stereotyped reproductive behaviors.

Regulation of neurons by testosterone in songbirds. One of the clearest examples of the influence of steroid hormones on the properties of a neuron is found in songbirds, such as canaries. In this case, the hormones produce profound plastic changes in the properties of adult neurons. This emphasizes the fact that there are commonalities in mechanisms of developmental and adult plasticity. During the breeding season, adult male canaries generate a song made up of a fixed pattern of individual sounds, termed *syllables*. This stereotyped pattern of syllables is termed a *stable song*. Although in any one bird the song pattern remains relatively fixed during the spring reproductive season, the specific pattern of syllables that comprises the stable song is lost in the months that follow. At this time the animals vocalize variable patterns of syllables, termed *plastic song*, and may generate new syllables that were not used in prior years. In the next breeding season, the bird acquires a brand new pattern of syllables in its stable song.

One group of neurons that controls singing in canaries is found in the forebrain, and is termed the *nucleus robustus archistriatalis* (RA, Fig. 16–18a). These neurons receive inputs from another nucleus in the forebrain, the *higher vocal center* (HVA). A number of RA neurons project in

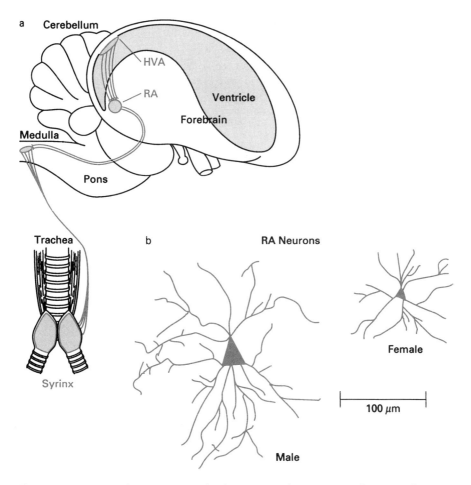

Figure 16–18. Steroid actions in songbirds. *a*: Canary brain circuits that control singing were identified by Nottebohm (1989) and colleagues. HVA, higher vocal center; RA, nucleus robustus archistriatalis. *b*: Morphology of neurons in the nucleus robustus archistriatalis of male and female zebra finches (Gurney, 1981).

turn to motor neurons in the medulla. These send connections directly to muscles of the syrinx that produces the sounds comprising a song. The RA and HVA nuclei are several times larger in adult male canaries than in females, whose songs are much less elaborate than those of the males. In the RA nucleus, it has been shown that this difference arises from an increase in the number of neurons as well as in the extent of dendritic branching and synaptic connectivity in the male (Fig. 16–18b). Treatment of a female canary with testosterone increases the size of the RA and HVA nuclei, inducing the growth of dendrites and new synaptic connections. Restructuring of these neurons by testosterone also evokes a stereotyped pattern of singing comparable to that of the male.

Further evidence that testosterone plays an ongoing role in maintenance of the form and connections of these neurons comes from measurements of testosterone in male canaries throughout the year. During summer and early fall, levels of testosterone in the blood are low. At this time, variable plastic song predominates. Thereafter testosterone levels rise and the RA and HVA nuclei double in size. As this occurs the pattern of song changes to the stereotyped stable song, which is dominant in the spring.

Steroids regulate neurogenesis. In the previous chapter, we saw that, even in the adult, neurons continue to be generated and undergo migration to specific areas of the brain. One interesting aspect of the remodeling of neural form and connections in song birds is that not only can preexisting connections be modified by hormones, but also the addition of new neurons is a key feature of the remodeling. When radiolabeled thymidine, which incorporates into the DNA of dividing cells, is injected into the brain of an adult songbird, a variety of neurons become labeled, including those of the HVA nucleus, although not those of the RA nucleus. As in a normal developing brain, neurogenesis in adult birds occurs in a zone of precursor cells adjacent to the ventricle, after which the cells migrate along radial glial cells to their final destination and establish the form and connections of mature neurons (see Fig. 15–1). Over 1.4% of the neurons in the HVA are newly generated each day. It appears that this neurogenesis represents a turnover of neurons, rather than a continual increase in cell number throughout the life of the animal. The formation of the neurons and their migration into the HVA is stimulated by estrogen. Because neurogenesis occurs at about the same rate in both males and females, and at times when new patterns of song are not being elaborated, the significance of new neurons in the HVA for singing behaviors is not yet known.

What is the mechanism of steroid action in the nervous system? Studies such as those described above suggest that in many neurons, proteins that influence development and the eventual pattern of dendritic branching and synaptic connections may be encoded by genes coupled to HREs for steroid and related hormones. Nevertheless, some neurons that are highly sensitive to the steroid estrogen appear not to possess the estrogen receptor, indicating that the effects of the steroid must be indirect. For example, the newly generated neurons whose formation is stimulated by estrogen do not have the estrogen receptor. Moreover, the pharmacology of steroid responses does not always match that of the classic steroid receptors. In addition, it has been found that some steroids can act directly at the plasma membrane of a neuron, enhancing responses to the neurotransmitter GABA. Such findings demonstrate that there is much we do not yet understand about the mode of action of these hormones in the nervous system.

Summary

The development of the nervous system requires the participation of a variety of factors that influence neuronal determination, proliferation, migration, and differentiation. Molecular genetic approaches using *Drosophila*, as well as other creatures whose genetics is well understood, have provided insights into the mechanisms of action of some of these developmental factors. The fate of a developing neuron may be directed by its interaction with ligands that are bound to the surface of adjacent cells. Soluble molecules, such as the neurotrophins, which are released from neuronal targets or nearby cells, also determine the fate of a neuron. Some of these factors recruit intracellular signaling pathways that are coupled to the activation of receptor tyrosine kinases, while others use cytokine signaling pathways. Hormones released from remote organs, including steroid hormones, can also profoundly influence neuronal form and function in the developing as well as in the adult nervous system.

17

Adhesion Molecules and Axon Pathfinding

We know that the electrical activity of neurons can be transformed and modulated in ways that allow a neuron to control specific behaviors. Electrical behavior, however, is not the only aspect of neuronal activity that is subject to regulation by other cells or external stimuli. Structural features, such as the number, size, and type of synapses that a neuron makes, can also be modified. Furthermore, the entire shape of a mature neuron's dendritic branches may alter over time. This is illustrated in Figure 17–1, which shows tracings of the dendrites of a neuron of the superior cervical ganglion in the intact nervous system of a mouse. This cell was injected with a fluorescent dye and drawings were made immediately of the shape of its dendrites. After a period of several weeks in the intact animal, the ganglion was again exposed and drawings were made of the fluorescent cell. Clear changes in dendritic branching pattern, and by inference in the synaptic connections on the dendrites, occur during this time. Although the factors that control such changes in cell form are largely unknown, these experiments lend support to the idea that long-term regulation of neuronal activity in the mature nervous system may be accompanied by rearrangements of neuronal structure and connections. To examine such rearrangements, we must first understand the factors that lead to specific patterns of branching during formation of the nervous system.

Axon Outgrowth During Development

Once an immature neuron has reached its final location in the nervous system, it must establish contacts with its appropriate synaptic partners by extending axonal and dendritic branches toward these partner neurons

435

(see Fig. 15–1). In some cases, a neurite may have been established even during cell migration. For example, in the case of the developing granule cells of the cerebellum that we discussed in Chapter 15, some neurite extension occurs before the cells migrate along the Bergmann glial cell. A trailing neurite is then left along the length of the glial fiber and eventually becomes the axon of the granule cell. In general, however, neurite extension occurs after cell migration.

The growth cone. The outgrowth of neurites is guided by a specialized region of the cell known as the *growth cone*, which is found at the leading tip of a neurite. Growth cones can be investigated in cell culture, where neurite extension can be examined readily under the microscope. Figure 17–2 illustrates the major features of the growth cone region (see also the cover illustration). The *central core* is an extension of the neurite process itself and is rich in microtubules that provide the structural support for axoplasmic transport (see Chapter 2). Using video-enhanced microscopy, bidirectional transport of granules can be observed up to the central core. In addition, the core of the growth cone is rich in mitochondria, endoplasmic reticulum, and vesicular structures.

Surrounding the central core is a region that is generally devoid of organelles but very enriched in the contractile protein *actin*. Time-lapse pictures of these regions, which are known as *lamellipodia*, reveal the existence of undulating waves of movement that have been termed *ruffling*. Finally, very thin straight processes known as *microspikes* or *filopodia* are found at the extremities of the lamellipodia. These, like the lamellipodia, are rich in actin. The microspikes are in constant motion, extending from and retracting back into the lamellipodia. Growth of the neurite occurs

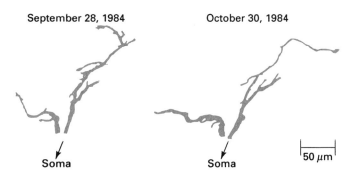

Figure 17–1. Remodeling of dendrites. A neuron in the superior cervical ganglion of a mature mouse was injected with a fluorescent dye by Purves and Hadley (1985). The two drawings show the change in shape of its dendrites over a period of 1 month.

when a microspike extends and then, instead of retracting, remains in place while the lamellipodium advances toward the end of the microspike (Fig. 17–3). New microspikes then extend from the newly advanced border of the lamellipodium.

What makes the growth cone move? The movement of the growth cone is associated with a continual cycle of polymerization and depolymerization of actin. At the very leading edge of the growth cone, actin proteins are continually assembled into the structural long filaments termed *F-actin*. This assembly of actin filaments is balanced by the ongoing depolymerization or cleavage of these filaments at the other end of the lamellipodium, at its junction with the central core of the growth cone (Fig. 17–4a). To link these cycles of synthesis and destruction, there is a continual *retrograde flow* of the actin cytoskeleton back from the leading edge toward the central core. The retrograde flow of F-actin accounts for the undulating waves of movement that can be observed with video-enhanced microscopy and is believed to be generated by molecular motors, comparable to those we encountered in Chapter 2. Such motors must therefore be anchored to the plasma membrane or to some component of the central core.

The rate at which a growth cone extends along a surface or *substrate* depends on how strongly the growth cone adheres to the substrate. A simple model that has been proposed for the elongation of a neurite is shown in Figure 17–4b. According to this model, the rate of growth depends on the strength of physical coupling between the F-actin cytoskeleton and the substrate. As we shall see later, in the membranes of neurons there are many molecules known to serve as such physical links from the cy-

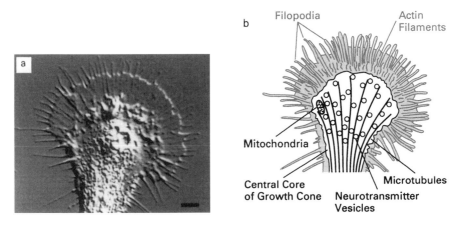

Figure 17–2. The growth cone. *a*: Photograph of the growth cone of an *Aplysia* neuron in cell culture (Forscher and Smith, 1988). *b*: Components of a growth cone.

toskeleton to the outside world. If such coupling is weak or absent, the retrograde flow of actin proceeds normally and is not coupled to the substrate. In this condition, the substrate is said to be *nonpermissive* for growth, and the growth cone remains stationary (Fig. 17–4a). In contrast, if the F-actin cytoskeleton is tightly coupled to the substrate, this coupling prevents or slows the flow of actin filaments back toward the central core. Instead, the formation of new actin filaments at the leading edge now leads to the forward extension of the growth cone. Such stronger coupling is said to occur on *permissive* substrates (Fig. 17–4b).

A neurite does not elongate simply by extending its cytoskeleton. The increase in overall size of the cell requires that new plasma membrane must continually be added as the growth cone makes its way toward its target. Experiments using fluorescent lipids have revealed that there is a continual flow of membrane lipids toward the growth cone. Incorporation of new lipids into the plasma membrane appears to occur at the soma and along the entire length of the growing axon.

Axonal pathfinding. The growth of an axon in the nervous system does not proceed randomly but follows a relatively precise pathway toward its target. Moreover, the pathway that an axon follows is specific to the cell itself, and may be very different from that of neighboring cells. An example of this is shown in Figure 17–5, which illustrates the growth of the axons of motor neurons in the embryonic spinal cord of a zebrafish. Three such motor neurons, termed *RoP*, *MiP*, and *CaP* (for rostral-, middle-, and caudal-primary motor neurons), are found in each segment of the body of a zebrafish. Initially, the growth cones of all three cells extend ventrally in the same direction away from the cell bodies. After a short period of

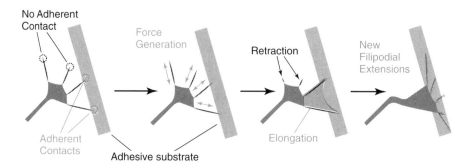

Figure 17–3. Scheme showing how continual extension and retraction of microspikes, coupled with the adhesion of microspikes to the selected substrate, may guide the direction of a growth cone.

growth, however, the axon of the MiP cell turns sharply and continues to extend dorsally between the dorsal muscle and the spinal cord. The other two axons continue ventrally until the junction of the dorsal and ventral muscles is encountered. At this point the axon of the RoP cell turns laterally while the CaP cell continues to grow ventrally. The three neurons come to innervate different muscles in each body segment of the zebrafish.

Another clear example of stereotyped branching patterns is in the grasshopper embryo, whose relatively simple nervous system has allowed the mapping of the precise pattern of navigation of the axons of several different identified neurons. On encountering a specific feature of the environment, such as another neuron or a glial cell, the growth cone of an axon may be forced to follow one pathway while that of a neighboring neuron may continue in another direction toward its appropriate target. It has been observed that when a growth cone reaches such a *landmark cell*, it may actually extend its filopodia deep into that cell. It is possible that such interactions produce biochemical changes that alter the adhesivity of membranes and thereby change the subsequent migration of axons.

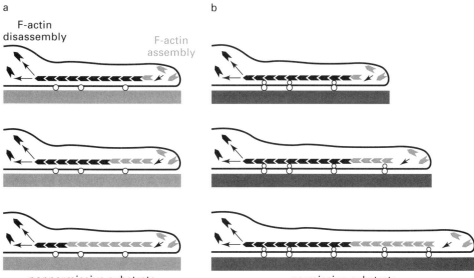

Figure 17–4. Actin assembly in the lamellipodium. *a*: Experiments by Paul Forscher and colleagues suggest that on a surface that is nonpermissive for axon elongation, F-actin filaments are not closely linked to the surface, leading to persistent retrograde flow of newly assembled F-actin. *b*: When the F-actin cytoskeleton is coupled to the substrate, polymerization of F-actin at the leading edge leads to forward extension of the growth cone.

In some cases, as in the growth of nerve tracts, a large number of axons initially may all grow in the same direction. A bundle of closely associated axons is called a *fascicle* and the formation of such bundles is known as *fasciculation*. In the growth of a fascicle of axons, the first neuron to enter the pathway follows cues from the environment. This neuron is frequently called the *pioneer cell*. The growth cones of the subsequent axons may extend along the axon of the pioneer neuron to form the fascicle. It appears, however, that these follower neurons sometimes have the ability to make the appropriate navigational decisions in the absence of the fibers of pioneer cells.

Both adhesion and guidance are required for directed growth. Such stereotyped patterns of branching and directed growth of axons have been described in a variety of systems in both vertebrates and invertebrates. What mechanisms might give rise to such stereotyped behavior? We have already seen that adhesion of the growth cones and microspikes to their substrate are important for elongation. Thus, one of the factors that control the direction a growth cone follows is the *differential adhesion* of different growth cones to other cells and surfaces that are encountered along the way. The general problem of how a cell adheres to, and interacts mechanically with, its environment is not specific to the nervous system. Neurons, however, are remarkable in the degree of specificity that is required to control both

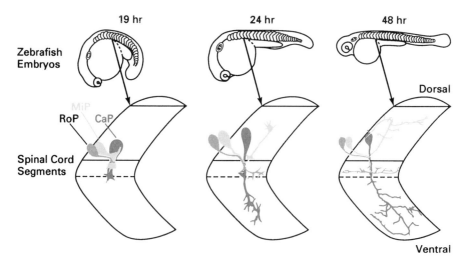

Figure 17–5. Axonal pathfinding. The embryonic development of the spinal cord of a zebrafish was studied by Westerfield and Eisen (1988) by following the paths of motor neurons that were filled with fluorescent dyes. The branching of each of these three neurons follows a stereotyped pattern to innervate a different set of muscles.

the differential navigation of growing axons and dendrites and the eventual establishment of synaptic contacts. Molecules involved in cell-to-cell adhesion are known as *cell adhesion molecules* (CAMs) (Table 17–1). The CAMs and a related class of adhesion molecules termed *cadherins* physically glue the membrane of a cell to that of an adjoining cell or to noncellular components of the extracellular space (Fig. 17–6). The way these molecules shape the growth of axons will be covered later in this chapter.

Physical adhesion, however, is only part of the story. There exist molecules whose sole function is to provide directions to the growing axon. In contrast to cell adhesion molecules, these *guidance molecules* do not need to be present in sufficient abundance to provide mechanical adherence. Rather, they simply relay messages from the external environment to the growth cone. Some of these molecules and their known receptors are listed in Table 17–1. Guidance molecules can either be soluble molecules that are secreted from a distant target or can be present on the surfaces along which the growth cone makes its journey (Fig. 17–7). Diffusion of an attractant molecule from a distant source causes a growth cone to turn and extend toward the source, a phenomenon known as *chemoattraction* (Fig. 17–7a). Conversely, in a gradient of a repulsive molecule, the growth cone experiences *chemorepulsion*, and turns away from the source (Fig 17–7b). For the case of attractant or repulsive guidance molecules on cell surfaces, a growth cone will turn onto or away from such surfaces, but only after the growing neurite has touched the surface (*contact-dependent* attraction or repulsion; Fig. 17–7c,d).

Because these guidance molecules do not directly affect the strength of physical adhesion between the growth cone and its substrate, there must be other cellular mechanisms that are regulated by these factors. The most likely end result of the interaction of a growth cone with a guidance fac-

Table 17–1 Cell Adhesion and Guidance Factors and Their Receptors

Adhesion Factor	Receptor	Guidance Molecule	Receptor
Substrate molecules fibronectin, laminin	Integrins	Semaphorins	Neuropilins, plexins
Cell adhesion molecules (CAMs)	CAMS	Netrins	UNC-40, *C. elegans* DCC, vertebrates Frazzled (*Drososophila*) UNC-5 (Repulsive)
Cadherins	Cadherins	Nogo	Unknown
		Ephrins	EphA and EphB receptors

tor is a change in the rate of polymerization of actin at the site of the interaction. The formation of the actin cytoskeleton within lamellipodia and filopodia is regulated by a family of small GTP-binding proteins termed *Rho* proteins. These proteins are related to the ras protein that is involved in the signaling action of receptor tyrosine kinases (see Chapter 16). At least three proteins in this family, Cdc42, Rac, and Rho itself, are thought to regulate the actin cytoskeleton in the growth cones of neurons. Experiments in which these activated proteins have been introduced into neurons suggest that Cdc42 and Rac promote an attractive response, whereas activated Rho triggers repulsion by causing the local disassembly of actin.

Second messengers and neurotransmitters modulate axonal growth. The signaling pathways by which the neuronal guidance molecules act on the Rho family of proteins are not yet known. It should be pointed out, however, that a single guidance molecule can be an attractant for one cell and a repulsant for another. Moreover, as we shall see later, the same molecule can be both attractive and repulsive to different parts of the same cell or to the same cell at different times. Such versatility exists, in part, because the state of second messenger signaling within a neuron at the time it encounters the guidance factor can influence the response. For this reason, agents such as neurotransmitters or growth factors that alter second messenger pathways may participate in forging the amount and direction of axonal growth. Examples of the action of such nonconventional guidance molecules will be given later in this chapter. We shall turn first to a discussion of the properties of the various molecules that guide the extension of neurites.

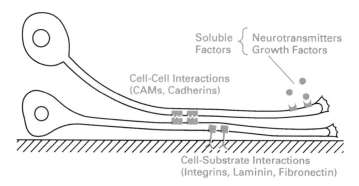

Figure 17–6. Factors that determine the amount and direction of neuritic growth. These include the interaction of a neuron with other cells, with the substrate, and with soluble molecules released by other cells.

Cell–Substrate Adhesion

What is extracellular matrix? We have stated that the ability of a neuron to adhere to specific surfaces that it encounters plays a major role in its migration to the appropriate site in the nervous system and in its extension of neurites toward the appropriate targets. For some types of neurons, much of their migration and axon elongation occurs not over the surface of other cells but through an extracellular matrix that is relatively devoid of cells. This matrix is required as a physical substrate for migration and can have a profound influence on the properties of cells in contact with it. For example, the normal division and differentiation of many cells, such as Schwann cells, require interaction with this matrix. Because the fixed components of this extracellular space are relatively simple compared to the chemical composition of cell membranes, much of what has been learned about neuronal adhesion and neurite outgrowth has come from the study of cell–substrate interactions.

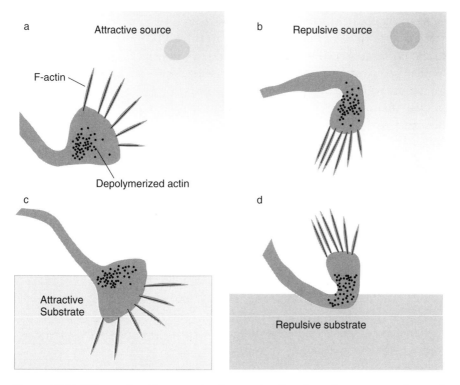

Figure 17–7. Effects of guidance molecules on the direction of movement of growth cones. *a*: chemoattraction; *b*: chemorepulsion; *c*: contact-dependent attraction; *d*: contact-dependent repulsion.

Substrate adhesion molecules. The space surrounding many non-neuronal cells is filled with a loose latticework of glycoproteins and sugars. Close to the membrane of cells that are not migrating through the space, this latticework becomes denser and forms a *basement membrane* (Fig. 17–8a). The major components of this latticework are listed in Table 17–2. Of particular interest are the proteins *fibronectin* and *laminin*. These can be obtained in purified form, and their effects on cell adhesion and neurite outgrowth can be assessed by culturing isolated neurons in tissue culture dishes whose surface has been coated with these proteins. Both substances readily promote the adhesion and extension of neurites by several types of neurons. Figure 17–8b illustrates the structures of fibronectin and laminin. Both are very large glycoprotein complexes that contain several distinct domains, each of which appears to have a specific role in binding other components of the extracellular matrix or in binding to cell membranes and promoting neurite outgrowth. Thus they may be considered a major part of the "glue" that attaches cells to the matrix.

The attachment of fibronectin and laminin to cells is mediated by receptor proteins termed *integrins*, which are located in the plasma membrane of many neurons and other cells (Fig. 17–8b). For example, the extracellular domain of the integrin fibronectin receptor binds to the sequence of amino acids Arg-Gly-Asp-Ser that is found in the fibronectin molecule. Similar sequences are found in many molecules that bind to other integrins in a wide variety of nonneuronal cells. The integrins are composed of two subunits. The α subunit regulates the specificity of interactions with different ligands; the short cytoplasmic domain of the β subunit of the integrins binds directly to components of the actin cytoskeleton. This provides a direct link between the intracellular scaffold of the cells and the external latticework (Fig. 17–8a).

The integrins do more than provide a mechanical link for the extracellular matrix. As in the case of some other receptor molecules, the binding of a ligand induces the clustering of these receptors in the plasma membrane. As this occurs, a number of tyrosine protein kinases associate with the integrin–cytoskeleton complex, and thereby become activated. For example, the ras/raf/MEK/ERK pathway, covered in the last chapter, as well as the protein kinase C pathway, is activated upon stimulation of integrins. It is not yet known, however, if all of the effects of extracellular matrix molecules on parameters such as neurite outgrowth are mediated through the integrin family of receptors.

Role of extracellular matrix in migration of neural crest cells. As we have already seen in Chapter 16, one of the preparations most favored by developmental neurobiologists is the *neural crest*, a collection of cells on the dora

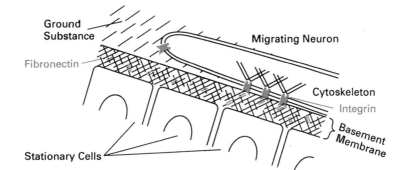

Ground Substance

Migrating Neuron

Fibronectin

Cytoskeleton

Integrin

Basement Membrane

Stationary Cells

b

Fibronectin
Dimer, $M_r \sim 450,000$

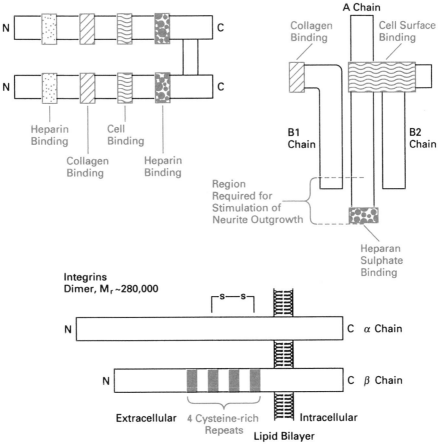

N

C

N

C

Heparin Binding

Cell Binding

Collagen Binding

Heparin Binding

Laminin
Trimer, $M_r \sim 800,000$

A Chain

Collagen Binding

Cell Surface Binding

B1 Chain

B2 Chain

Region Required for Stimulation of Neurite Outgrowth

Heparan Sulphate Binding

Integrins
Dimer, $M_r \sim 280,000$

S—S

N

C α Chain

N

C β Chain

Extracellular   4 Cysteine-rich Repeats

Intracellular

Lipid Bilayer

Figure 17–8. Neuron–substrate interactions. *a*: The extracellular matrix. *b*: The structure of some molecules involved in cell–substrate interactions.

445

sal edge of the developing neural tube. Cells that are destined to become neurons of the sympathetic or sensory ganglia arise from the neural crest. In addition to sympathetic and sensory neurons, neural crest cells may develop into melanocytes, Schwann cells, and cells of the adrenal medulla. The analysis of this system of cells has been central to the identification of many of the molecules involved in neural differentiation. Figure 16–14 shows the directions in which cells from the neural crest migrate to their final destination. The pathways through which these cells travel are relatively devoid of cells but are filled with extracellular matrix containing fibronectin. Levels of fibronectin in this matrix are high during the period of migration but drop after migration has ceased. Moreover, the ability of neural crest cells to adhere to a collagen matrix has been shown to depend directly on fibonectin.

Cell–Cell Adhesion

Although the extracellular matrix plays an important role in the migration of cells and the extension of neurites in the periphery, the central nervous system does not possess a well-defined extracellular matrix. Basement membranes are found only along the cerebral blood vessels and lining the fluid-filled cerebral ventricles, and thus the movement of neurons and their axons in the central nervous system occurs largely over other cells. Moreover, even in the peripheral nervous system, much of the growth of axons occurs over the surface of epithelial cells and other axons. In contrast to the molecules described above, which have been termed *substrate adhesion molecules* (SAMs), the physical association of the membranes of two cells occurs through cell adhesion molecules (CAMs).

Cell adhesion molecules. Cell adhesion molecules were initially discovered by Gerald Edelman and colleagues using suspensions of cells from chick retina. When such cells are dissociated in culture, they reaggregate read-

Table 17–2 Some Components of the Extracellular Matrix

Collagens	A family of glycoproteins rich in proline

Fibronectin
Laminin
Chondronectin
	Elongated glycoproteins that bind to receptors
	    on cell membranes and also to other components
	    of extracellular matrix such as the collagens

Hyaluronic acid Chondroitin sulfate Heparan sulfate	Glycosaminoglycans—unbranched disaccharide polymers

ily into clumps of cells. Antibodies that can specifically prevent this reag-gregation were made and then used to isolate a membrane glycoprotein that binds to these antibodies. The first protein to be isolated in this way, termed *N-CAM* for neuronal-CAM, is one of a family of cell adhesion molecules that has now been found to be expressed on neurons and on a wide variety of other cells. Figure 17–9 shows the similarity of N-CAM to three other CAMs, which represent only some of the known CAMs. Ng-CAM is an adhesion molecule found on specific axonal tracts. Myelin-associated glycoprotein (MAG) is a glial cell adhesion molecule. Fasciclin II, as will be described below, is a glycoprotein expressed on a subset of grasshopper neurons. The extracellular part of these molecules has a se-ries of domains that each contains about 50 amino acids between two cys-teine residues. By forming -S;-S- bridges, these can form the domains into

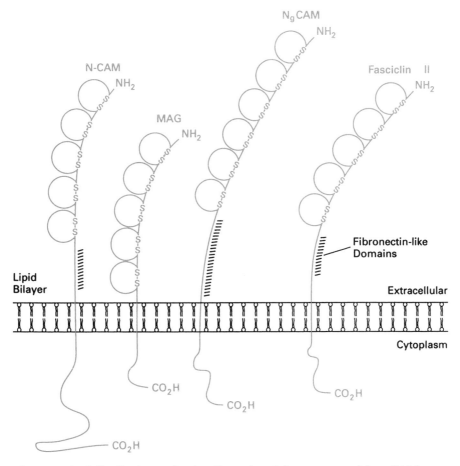

Figure 17–9. Cell adhesion molecules. Examples of the structure of four CAMs.

loops. Very similar structures (termed *immunoglobulin C2 type domains*) are found in *immunoglobulins*, molecules involved in the mounting of immune responses by lymphocytes. The CAMs are therefore considered to belong to the immunoglobulin superfamily.

Most of the CAMs are believed to cause cell–cell adhesion by binding to the same CAM on an adjacent cell. Thus N-CAM molecules on one cell bind directly to N-CAM molecules on its neighbor, providing *homophilic* interactions between the cells. However, as shown in Figure 17–9, some of these molecules also contain regions of homology to fibronectin. These latter regions (termed *type III domains*) include the sequence Arg-Gly-Asp-, which is used in binding to the integrins. This suggests that these molecules may interact with cell surface proteins in more than one way. Another important family of related cell adhesion molecules is the cadherins. N (for neuronal)-cadherin is the best-studied example in the nervous system, although it is also found in non-neuronal cells. Like the CAMs, an N-cadherin molecule binds to another N-cadherin on an adjacent cell. In contrast to the CAMs, however, this binding requires the presence of external calcium ions.

A central test for the involvement of the CAMs and cadherins in normal development has been to expose developing cells to antibodies raised against specific adhesion molecules. For example, antibodies that block the homophilic binding of N-CAM or N-cadherin have been shown to disrupt the normal development of the retina into sharply defined cell layers (Fig. 17–10). Another test for the role of N-cadherin in the extension of

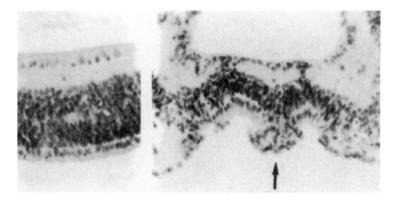

Figure 17–10. Disruption of retinal fragments by antibodies to N-cadherin. The effects of antibodies on the structural integrity of embryonic chick retina were tested by M. Takeichi and colleagues. *Left*: Photograph of a stained section of a normal fragment incubated with a control antibody for 4 days. *Right*: Fragment incubated with the antibody to N-cadherin. The arrow points to the broken photoreceptor layer (Matsunaga et al., 1988b).

axons from the retina has been to place fragments of retina onto a single layer of cells that do not normally express N-cadherin on their surface. In this condition, although retinal cells in the explant possess N-cadherin, no neurites extend out from the retinal fragments onto the monolayer of cells. When, however, the cells constituting the monolayer are induced to make N-cadherin by introduction of an active gene for this adhesion protein into the cells, vigorous neurite outgrowth is observed (Fig. 17–11).

Do CAMs *and cadherins account for specificity of axon guidance?* Earlier in this chapter we illustrated that growing axons make specific decisions about the direction in which they extend, and that these decisions may differ from those of neighboring axons (Fig. 17–5). The differential adhesion of the growing neurite to specific molecules on the surface of nearby cells appears to be central in the choice of the pathway that an axon will follow, and there is evidence that cell adhesion molecules may be involved in these choices. Because the prototype molecules N-CAM and N-cadherin are widely distributed throughout the nervous system, they are generally viewed as acting as a relatively nonspecific glue that may aid cells in migrating and extending processes through surrounding tissue. In contrast,

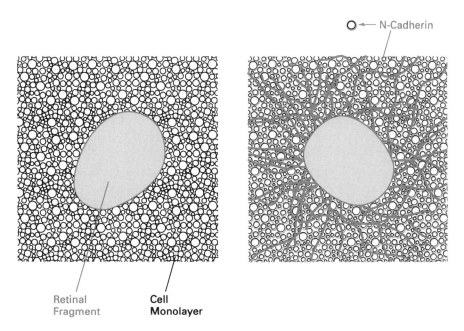

Figure 17–11. N-cadherin guides optic nerve fibers over the surface of other cells. Shown here is another experiment by M. Takeichi and colleagues (see Fig. 17–10). Fragments of retina, placed over a layer of cells that lack N-cadherin, do not extend neurites from the explant. When the cells forming the layer are modified to express N-cadherin, outgrowth occurs (Matsunaga et al., 1988a).

some of the other CAMs, such as Ng-CAM and fasciclin II, are found only in specific neurons and in specific tracts of axons. Moreover, such CAMs may appear on the surface of neurons transiently, at specific times during development, and their appearance may be localized to areas of membrane in contact with certain other cells.

An instructive example of the possible role of a CAM, fasciclin II, in the selective guidance of axons is provided by work on grasshopper embryos. In very early embryos, fasciclin II is found on the surface of all ectodermal cells. At a later stage, however, it can be detected only on a subset of cells and neurons within each segment of the developing nervous system. Figure 17–12 illustrates the disposition of fasciclin II in three neurons, termed MP1, dMP2, and vMP2, which adhere to the mesectodermal cells at the midline. Axon outgrowth from these three cells occurs initially over the surface of glial cells and along a basement membrane. At this stage the axons and growth cones do not contain fasciclin II, although the cell bodies do (Fig. 17–12a). In time, the axons of two of these neurons, MP1 and dMP2, which grow in a posterior direction, begin to approach the axons of other MP1 and dMP2 neurons that are located in adjacent segments. At this time, these two neurons begin to express fasciclin II over their entire membrane, including that of the growth cones (Fig. 17–12b). When the axons reach the next segment, they cease to navigate along the basement membrane, and now adhere to the axons of MP1 and dMP2 neurons in this segment, forming a fascicle of axons (Fig. 17–12c). When the developing embryo is incubated with antibodies to fasciclin II, the ability of these axons to recognize each other and to form this MP1/dMP2 fascicle is selectively impaired.

In contrast to the MP1 and dMP2 neurons, the vMP2 neuron extends its axon in an anterior direction. This axon eventually joins the axons of other vMP2 neurons to form an independent fascicle of vMP2 neurons (Fig. 17–12c). Although the soma of vMP2 expresses fasciclin II, at no stage does the axon or growth cone appear to bear this adhesion molecule. Still later in development, the fasciclin II at the soma of all three neurons is lost, while that in the MP1/dMP2 axons remains (Fig. 17–12d).

The picture that emerges from these and similar results is that adhesion molecules arise on the surface of growing neurons, at specific times and places, to provide an adhesive "road surface" that routes the axonal traffic in appropriate directions. Thus, for the vMP2 neuron described above, fasciclin II at the soma provides transient adhesion to the mesectodermal cells, while another CAM, as yet unidentified, may provide adhesion to the axons of other vMP2 neurons. For the MP1 and dMP2 neurons, the same CAM, fasciclin II, contributes to adhesion both to the mesectodermal cells and to the other homologous axons.

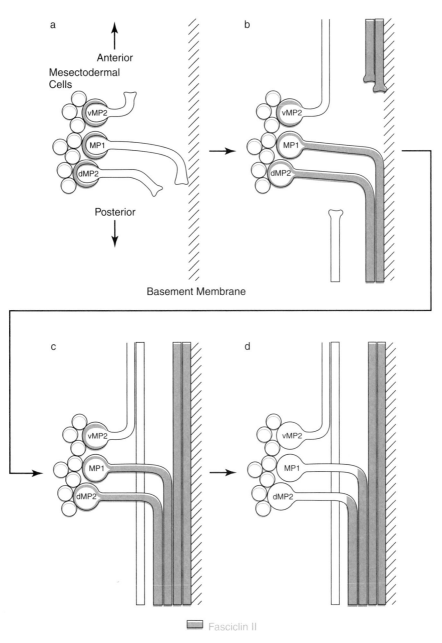

a

Anterior

Mesectodermal
Cells

vMP2

MP1

dMP2

Posterior

Basement Membrane

b

vMP2

MP1

dMP2

c

vMP2

MP1

dMP2

d

vMP2

MP1

dMP2

Fasciclin II

Figure 17–12. Changes in cell adhesion molecule (CAM) distribution during axonal growth. Corey Goodman and colleagues used immunocytochemistry to study progressive changes (*a–d*) in the localization of the cell adhesion molecule fasciclin II during axonal outgrowth from three grasshopper neurons (Harrelson and Goodman, 1988).

Diversity of cell adhesion molecules. A relatively large number of specific cell adhesion molecules must exist if they are to account for the many different paths that growth cones of different axons take as they move toward their final destination. Some that have been described to date have been given such poetic names as amalgam, neurofascin, and contactin. Many more, perhaps some with structures unrelated to the immunoglobulin superfamily, are certain to be discovered. In addition, considerable diversity could in principle be generated by expressing different forms of the same basic molecule. For example, the N-CAM protein exists in three closely related forms of different length. These all share the same extracellular domain but differ in the length of the C-terminus region. Two of these cross the plasma membrane, as shown in Figure 17–9, whereas the third lacks the membrane-spanning and cytoplasmic domains and is anchored to the cell membrane through an inositol-containing lipid.

It is likely that, in addition to changes in the expression of different CAMs, modifications of a CAM that is already expressed may produce a progressive change in the adherent properties of a cell or a neurite. For example, much of the sugar that is bound to the N-CAM protein consists of an oligosaccharide termed *polysialic acid.* During development of the chick brain, there is conversion of an embryonic form of N-CAM to an adult form. This occurs due to a progressive loss of polysialic acid, from about 26% of the weight of the N-CAM molecule in the embryo to only 9% in the adult. This reduction in bound oligosaccharide produces a marked increase in the adhesive power of the N-CAM molecule, perhaps because the polysialic acid hinders the normal adhesive interactions.

Molecular Guidance Cues

The cell adhesion molecules that we considered in the last section bind to similar molecules on the surface of adjoining cells, providing the homophilic interactions between these cells. As we mentioned earlier, other types of cell–cell interactions, as well as gradients of soluble factors, also guide growth cones to their appropriate destinations. Four of the best-characterized classes of guidance factors are the semaphorins, the netrins, Nogo, and the ephrins (Table 17–1). We shall discuss the first three in this chapter, and cover some of the action of the ephrins in the next chapter when we deal with synapse formation.

Semaphorins. A very important class of guidance molecules are the semaphorins, which can exist either as fixed membrane glycoproteins or as soluble proteins that are secreted from cells (Fig. 17–13a). Moreover, they can provide either attactant or repulsive cues to an advancing growth cone. All semaphorins contain a large conserved extracellular sequence termed the *semaphorin domain*. In addition, semaphorins can be divided in nine classes according to other characteristic features such as immunoglobulin C2 domains. The membrane semaphorins have a single transmembrane

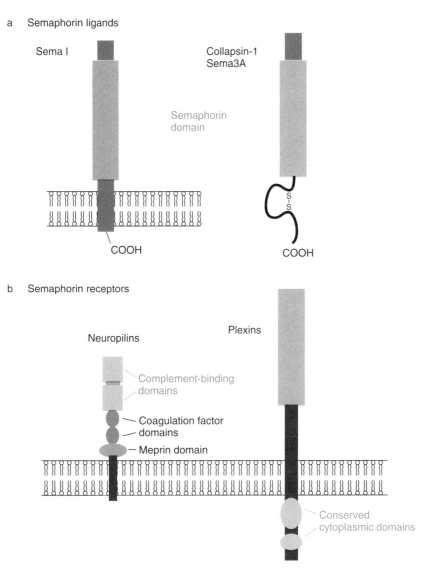

Figure 17–13. Semaphorin molecules and their receptors. *a*: G-sema I is a membrane-bound semaphorin ligand in grasshopper cells. Collapsin is a soluble semaphorin isolated from chick cells. *b*: Neuropilins and plexins are two structurally distinct receptors for semaphorins.

domain with a very short cytoplasmic tail, which is not thought to play a role in signaling beyond anchoring the protein in the cell membrane. Like cell adhesion molecules, semaphorins are present on subsets of axons and on non-neuronal cells along which growth cones travel. In contrast to the adhesion molecules, however, the presence of semaphorins in the membranes of dissociated cells does not cause the cells to aggregate into clumps. Rather, changes in direction of advancing growth cones are effected by biochemical changes produced by local activation of membrane receptors.

Two very different types of receptors on neurons are known to bind semaphorins (Fig. 17–13b). The first, termed the *neuropilins*, contain domains first identified in proteins involved in blood coagulation, the *complement-binding* and *coagulation factor* domains. They also contain a *meprin* domain, named after a conserved domain in meprin proteases, which is thought to be required for certain protein–protein interactions. The second class of receptors are the *plexins*. Technically, these are semaphorins, since they possess a large extracellular semaphorin domain. In contrast to the semaphorin ligands, however, the plexins have two large cytoplasmic domains that are conserved and that are likely to participate in signal transduction once the extracellular domain binds a semaphorin ligand.

Semaphorin signaling in grasshopper neurons. We turn again to a specific type of neuron in the embryonic nervous system of the grasshopper for an example of growth cone guidance by a semaphorin. The cell bodies of these neurons, termed Ti1 pioneer neurons, are present in the limb buds of the grasshopper, and during development their axons extend from the periphery into the central nervous system (Fig. 17–14a). As the axons first grow away from the cell bodies, they chart a course directly toward the central nervous system. At one point on their journey, however, they encounter a layer of epithelial cells that extends in the dorsal–ventral direction. These epithelial cells have on their surface a semaphorin termed *G-sema I*. The growing axons are not able to cross this barrier of epithelial cells. Instead, on contacting the surface of these cells, the growing axons stop and then reorient their growth ventrally along the distal edge of the semaphorin-containing cells. It is only after the filopodia of the axons contact another type of cell, the Cx1 neurons, that the growing axons cross the epithelial cells and proceed in the direction of the central nervous system (Fig. 17–14a).

The change in the direction of growth that occurs when the Ti1 growth cones meet the epithelial cells can be attributed to the presence of G-sema I on the epithelial cells. For example, the cells can be exposed to antibodies against G-sema I during the period of axon outgrowth, thereby pre-

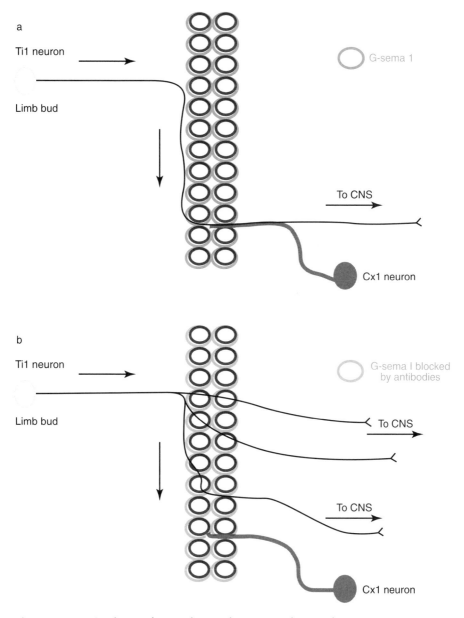

Figure 17–14. Guidance of axons by repulsion. *a*: In the grasshopper nervous system, the Ti1 neuron in the limb bud sends its axon toward the central nervous system (CNS). On encountering a layer of epithelial cells bearing G-sema I on their surfaces, the axon is diverted ventrally until it contacts the processes of the Cx1 neurons, where it crosses the G-sema I barrier. *b*: Preincubation of cells with an antibody to G-sema I neutralizes its repulsive effect, allowing axons to cross the epithelial cells.

venting these molecules from interacting with the growth cones. When this happens, the ingrowing axons are able to extend directly across the stripe of epithelial cells (Fig. 17–14b).

A single semaphorin can be both attractive and repulsive. G-sema I causes the axons of Ti1 neurons to follow a particular path because of its repulsive effect on their growth cones. Similar effects on axonal growth cones of many vertebrate neurons occur with *Sema3A*, one of the soluble semaphorins. In common with its membrane-bound relatives, Sema3A contains a large semaphorin domain (Fig. 17–13a). Instead of a transmembrane segment, however, Sema3A contains an immunoglobulin C2 type domain. This type of semaphorin was first discovered as a soluble factor that causes the collapse of the actin cytoskeleton in the growth cones of chick sensory neurons. As expected, such a collapse of the lamellipodium prevents further elongation of the axon, and because of this biological action, the chick homolog of Sema3A was given the name *collapsin-1*.

The major output of the cerebral cortex of mammals occurs from pyramidal neurons, which send their axons down into the white matter underlying the cortex. These neurons receive and integrate synaptic inputs on their apical dendrites, which extend towards the external surface of the cortex, also termed the *pial surface*. During development, Sema 3A guides the orientation of both the axons and dendrites of the pyramidal cells, but in opposite directions. This can be detected by placing the cell body of a single isolated pyramidal neuron on top of a slice of immature cerebral cortex. If the cell placed on the cortical slice is labeled with a fluorescent marker, the growth of its axon and dendrites can be followed in culture for several days. As is the case for normal pyramidal neurons, the growth cones of the dendrites of the labeled cell move toward the pial surface, whereas the growing axon extends in the opposite direction, toward the white matter and the underlying ventricle (Fig. 17–15). The identity of dendrites can be confirmed by staining the processes with the microtubule-associated protein MAP-2, a marker for dendrites.

A variety of approaches have shown that a gradient of Sema3A, which originates close to the pial surface, shapes the orientation of both axonal and dendritic growth. For example, elimination of the action of Sema3A by gene knockout or blocking of its neuropilin receptor by applying antibodies to the slices impairs the orientation of axons and dendrites. The endogenous gradient can also be altered by placing non-neuronal cells that have been engineered to express high levels of Sema3A onto the slice near the white matter. When this occurs, the pyramidal cells now orient their axons away from the new source of Sema3A, and their dendrites now extend toward the Sema3-expressing cells.

How is it that a single guidance molecule can produce attractant and repellant actions on different parts of one pyramidal neuron? Clues to this question have come from an examination of the effects of second messengers on the actions of Sema3A. As mentioned above, application of Sema3A to certain neurons in culture causes collapse of growth cones. When Sema3A is applied in a gradient from a micropipette close to the end of the growing axon, it causes repulsion, resulting in a change in the direction of growth away from the pipette. If, however, the neuron is first treated with agents that elevate levels of the second messenger cyclic GMP (see Chapter 12), the axon now orients toward the source of Sema3A (Fig. 17–16a). Although other explanations are possible, it is likely that cyclic GMP also contributes to the different orientation responses of the axons and dendrites of pyramidal neurons. The soluble enzyme guanylate cyclase (Fig. 12–10) is preferentially localized in the growing dendrites of the cells (Fig. 17–16b) and inhibition of this enzyme or of the cyclic GMP–dependent protein kinase completely disrupts the orientation of dendrites

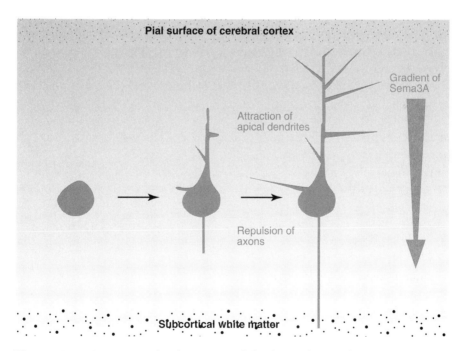

Figure 17–15. Sema3A guides the axons and dendrites of cortical pyramidal neurons in opposite directions. Work by Anirvan Ghosh and colleagues has shown that single pyramidal neurons placed on a slice of immature cerebral cortex orient their axons away from a source of Sema3A at the pial surface, while growing dendrites are oriented into the gradient (Polleux et al., 2000).

toward the apical surface. The factors that first produce the asymmetry in guanylate cyclase activity or the effect that this eventually has on actin polymerization in the growth cones are, however, not yet known.

The netrins–soluble guidance molecules related to laminin. A second class of guidance molecules, which are structurally unrelated to the semaphorins, are the netrins (*netr* is a Sanskrit word for "one who guides"). Like peptide neurotransmitters and other secreted molecules, the netrins are first synthesized with a signal sequence, which allows them to enter the secretory pathway; the signal sequence is likely to be cleaved shortly after synthesis (see Fig. 8–6). The remainder of a netrin molecule bears a strong resemblance to part of the B2 chain of the extracellular matrix protein laminin (see Fig. 17–8). Like the B2 chain of laminin, the netrins contain several EGF repeats and the sequence of amino acids Arg-Gly-Asp that is a recognition signal for many of the integrin receptors (Fig. 17–17). Like the semaphorins, netrins can exert either attractive or repulsive actions on growing axons.

Netrins were first purified as chemoattractive factors that come into play during the development of the spinal cord. Neurons termed *commissural neurons* differentiate in the dorsal part of the spinal cord and then send their axons in a stereotyped pattern toward the ventral part of the spinal cord (Fig. 17–18a). At the ventral midline of the spinal cord lies the floor plate, a structure composed of epithelial cells (Chapter 16). The

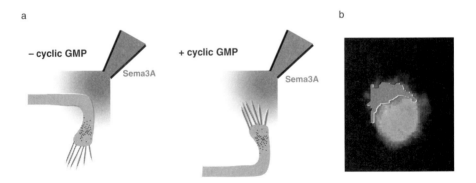

Figure 17–16. Effects of cyclic GMP on orienting of neurites. *a*: Experiments by Mu-Ming Poo and co-workers showed that the repellant action of Sema3A can be converted to attraction by treating the cells with activators of the cyclic GMP pathway (Song et al., 1998). *b*: Preferential localization of guanylate cyclase immunoreactivity (*blue*) to the apical pole of a pyramidal neuron that has not yet extended dendritic branches (Polleux et al., 2000).

floor plate extends the entire length of the spinal cord and into the brain. Chemoattractant molecules released from these floor plate cells guide the growing axons of the commissural cells around the circumference of the spinal cord on their path ventrally. This can be demonstrated by placing explants of the dorsal spinal cord in proximity to pieces of the floor plate. In such explanted tissues, the growing axons reorient themselves toward the floor plate cells.

Within the spinal cord there are two netrins: netrin-1 is present only in the floor plate cells themselves, while netrin-2 is found more diffusely in the ventral half of the spinal cord (Fig. 17–18a). When applied to explants of the dorsal spinal cord, both netrins stimulate the outgrowth of neurites. The direction of this outgrowth depends on the source of the netrin. For example, it is possible to make an artificial source of secreted netrins by transfecting a kidney cell line with the gene for netrin-1. When a clump of such transfected cells is placed next to an explant of the dorsal spinal cord, the secreted netrin-1 causes the reorientation of axon outgrowth toward the transfected cells (Fig. 17–18b). For some neurons, such as certain motor neurons, whose axons grow in a direction away from the midline, netrins exert a repulsive rather than attractive influence.

Netrins are found in both vertebrates and invertebrates. Indeed, the first described netrin, known as UNC-6, was found by genetic studies in the nematode (UNC refers to Uncoordinated, reflecting the phenotypes of mutations in such proteins). In all these species netrins are present in cells near the midline of the brain and play a role in attracting the axons of neurons that will cross from one side of the brain to the other. Tracts of such axons are termed *commissures*. Mutant mice in which netrin-1 is present only in very low amounts fail to develop several commissures, including the *corpus callosum*, the major commissure that is composed of axons joining the two cerebral hemispheres.

There are at least two known receptors for the netrins. One major class of netrin receptor is proteins of the DCC family (for Deleted in Colorectal Cancer). In vertebrates, these include the DCC protein itself and a re-

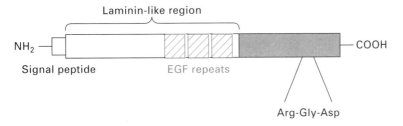

Figure 17–17. Structure of a netrin.

lated receptor termed *neogenin*. In *Drosophila*, the corresponding receptor is termed *Frazzled*, and in nematodes, *Unc-40*. (The very different styles for naming proteins in flies and worms probably reflects the personalities of the investigators.) A surprising finding that has been made using certain *Drosophila* neurons (including the dMP2 neuron of Fig. 17–12) is that guidance of their axons by netrins does not require the presence of the receptor on the neuron itself. Instead, it is found on the surface of cells along which the growing axon navigates. Thus, rather than being a receptor in the true sense, the Frazzled protein may be a binding molecule that immobilizes the soluble netrins and ensures that the growing axon detects the appropriate concentration of netrins along its path.

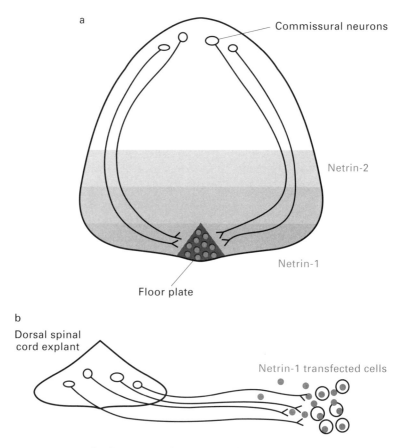

Figure 17–18. Netrins guide the axons of commissural neurons in the spinal cord. *a*: The normal course of commissural axons toward the floor plate. *b*: The axons of commissural neurons are guided from an explant of the dorsal spinal cord toward cells transfected with netrin-1.

Another class of netrin receptor is termed the *UNC-5* family of proteins. These receptors are present on neurons that are repulsed by netrins and are required for this repulsive action. As in the case of the semaphorins, however, attraction and repulsion are fickle and subject to the state of second messenger signaling in the growing neuron. In the case of neurons isolated from the frog spinal cord, however, it is cyclic AMP, not cyclic GMP, that switches the response. Spinal cord neurons that are normally attracted to a source of netrin-1 can be made to extend their axons in the opposite direction if the cells are treated with agents that inhibit the cyclic AMP–dependent protein kinase. As for the semaphorins, it is likely that these second messengers alter the dynamics of actin assembly by Rho proteins.

In addition to the netrins, semaphorins, and the cell adhesion molecules that we have covered, there are many new guidance molecules whose roles are being investigated. These include factors or receptors termed *Derailed*, *Slit*, *Robo*, *Comm*, and *HGF/SF* (Hepatocyte Growth Factor/Scatter Factor). Each of these is thought to play a role in shaping the final wiring diagram of the nervous system. Another guidance molecule, Nogo, may, however, participate in a special case of axonal guidance that occurs only after the normal wiring pattern has become established.

Nogo. A severe form of repulsion of axons occurs after damage to nerve fibers of the adult central nervous system. The devastating effects of injuries to the brain and spinal cord are due to the fact that, once they have been severed, axons of neurons within the central nervous system fail to regenerate. This is because mammalian neurons are not able to extend neurites over the surfaces of oligodendroglia, the cells that make the myelin sheath of central neurons. During development, most axonal pathfinding has already occurred by the time the myelin sheaths begin to form. The repulsive effect of oligodendroglia is due to the presence in these cells of proteins that selectively repulse growth cones. A membrane protein termed *Nogo*, which bears no relationship to the other guidance factors we have discussed, appears to be the major repulsive factor in these glial cells.

Nogo is present in oligodendroglia but is absent in Schwann cells, the glial cells that make the myelin of peripheral nerves. For this reason, axons of the peripheral nervous system are frequently capable of regenerating. It is possible, however, to induce growing axons to cross oligodendroglia by applying antibodies to Nogo. Such antibodies neutralize the inhibitory effect of Nogo and allow axons to extend actively over the glial membranes. As might be imagined, the ability to manipulate neuronal pathfinding after injuries has enormous clinical implications.

The Regulation of Growth Cones by Neurotransmitters and Neurotrophins

The recognition and binding of immobilized and soluble guidance molecules by receptors on the surface of a neuron have many analogies with the interaction of a neurotransmitter or growth factor with its receptor. Moreover, we have seen that changes in cyclic AMP and cyclic GMP levels can alter the direction of growth. Thus it is not surprising that growth factors, neurotrophins, and even neurotransmitters themselves can influence neurite outgrowth. An early example was provided by the neurotrophin nerve growth factor (NGF). As we saw in Chapter 16, neurons from the sympathetic ganglia and sensory neurons from dorsal root ganglia are sensitive to NGF, responding to the presence of this factor with profuse outgrowth of neurites. It turns out that the direction from which NGF is applied alters the way the growth cones respond. If a gradient of NGF is established by leakage of NGF from a pipette tip in a culture dish, the axons of cultured neurons extend toward the tip of the pipette. When injections of NGF are made into the brains of newborn rats, aberrant growth of neurites from sympathetic ganglia toward the injection site occurs. Because, during the course of development, the axons of sensory and sympathetic neurons come to rely on the trophic actions of NGF only after they have established their axon pathways, it is unlikely that NGF itself acts as a chemoattractant within the nervous system.

The application of neurotransmitters, and even the onset of electrical activity within an axon, may modify the growth of neurites. Figure 17–19 illustrates the actions of the neurotransmitter serotonin on an identified neuron of the mollusc *Helisoma*. This neuron, termed *B19*, may be placed in cell culture where it normally extends neuritic branches. Application of serotonin to the growing cell, however, abruptly terminates the elongation of the neurites and causes loss of lamellipodia in the growth cones. In contrast, the growth of cells that do not bear serotonin receptors is unaffected by this transmitter (Fig. 17–19a).

This regulation of neurite growth by neurotransmitters occurs locally through receptors on the growth cones themselves, and does not require signals from the cell body. By severing a neurite just before the region of the growth cone, it is possible to isolate growth cones from the remainder of the cell (Fig. 17–19b). Interestingly, such isolated growth cones continue to extend along the substrate for a considerable time after they have been severed from their cell bodies. Isolated growth cones of neuron B19 respond to serotonin in the same way as those on intact B19 cells, indicating that inhibition by serotonin is a local event occurring at the growth cone itself.

While the action of serotonin described above is inhibitory, some transmitters stimulate axon outgrowth. For example, application of the peptide substance P stimulates axon outgrowth in some cultured mammalian neurons. Experiments with the calcium indicator dye fura-2 (see Chapter 9) have shown that changes in the amount or the direction of growth are associated with changes in the levels of intracellular calcium

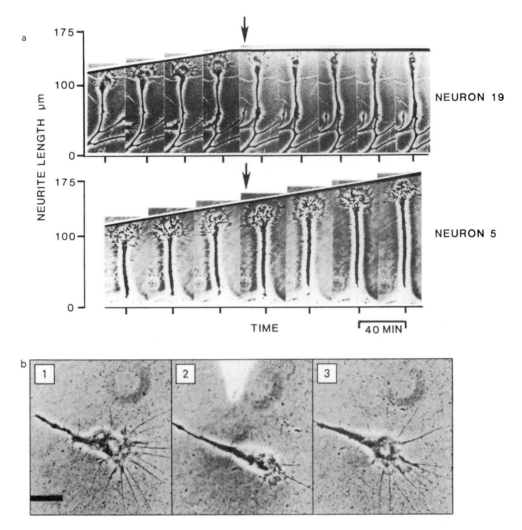

Figure 17–19. Inhibition of growth cones by neurotransmitter. *a*: Experiments by Ben Kater and colleagues showed that application of serotonin (5-HT) to *Helisoma* neuron B19 inhibits growth of its neurites. Neuron B5 is unaffected by serotonin. *b*: Serotonin also inhibits an isolated B19 growth cone (*1*), when applied from an external pipette (*2*). Growth recovers when serotonin is removed (*3*) (Haydon et al., 1984).

within the growth cone. One line of thinking is that normal extension of growth cones occurs only when the calcium concentration in the growth cone is within a range of concentrations permissive for growth. Neurotransmitters that act to change intracellular calcium levels, moving them into or out of this permissive range, stimulate or inhibit growth. In the same way, electrical activity itself can also influence neurite extension, by allowing calcium entry through voltage-dependent calcium channels. For example, direct electrical stimulation of neurons such as B19 prevents axon elongation. In some cases, neurotransmitters exert influences similar to those of bone fide guidance molecules. For example, when embryonic neurons of the spinal cord of frogs are exposed to microscopic gradients of acetylcholine applied from a nearby pipette, their growth cones consistently turn in the direction of the pipette.

Because most of these studies have been carried out using neurons in cell culture, the relevance of the effects of neurotransmitters and electrical stimulation to axonal growth in the intact nervous system is not yet established. It does seem likely, however, that these influences shape the final branching patterns at times when synaptic contacts are being established.

Biochemical Properties of Growing Axons

Secretion of proteases. To reach their targets in intact developing tissues, growing neurites must penetrate other tissues and forge their way through extracellular matrix. To aid their progress, growth cones appear to secrete *proteases*, enzymes that partially digest proteins in the extracellular matrix. One way this can be demonstrated readily is by plating neurons in cell culture on a dish covered with a layer of protein, such as fibronectin, laminin, or gelatin, that has been modified chemically so as to fluoresce. Degradation of the proteins is detected as loss of fluorescence near the cell and the growth cone. The release of proteases must, of course, be selective and controlled because, as we have seen, many extracellular proteins are important in cell adhesion. In addition to aiding the mechanical progress of a growth cone, it is possible that such extracellular proteolysis serves as a cell-to-cell signal to trigger responses that follow contact of one cell by the growth cone of another. In the next chapter we shall encounter one of the actions of *Kuzbanian*, a protease whose activity has been found to be essential for normal axonal extension.

Synthesis of GAP-43. An interesting protein that is strongly suspected of influencing the ability of axons to grow is *GAP-43*, which is short for 43 kDa growth-associated protein. What is the evidence that GAP-43 is associated with neuronal growth? During the extension of axonal branches, the pattern of proteins that is synthesized at the soma and then transported down to the tip of a developing axon differs from that in fully formed nerves. Figure 17–20 illustrates the pattern of newly synthesized proteins transported along the axons of neurons in the retina of a hamster. These proteins were labeled by injecting a radioactive amino acid into the retina. Four hours later, they were extracted from the *superior colliculus*, a brain area that receives extensive synaptic input from the retina. The pathway from the retina to the colliculus in mammals closely resembles the retino-tectal pathway in lower vertebrates that is described in the next chapter. The two-dimensional separation of proteins by gel electrophoresis shows that several proteins are either enriched or depleted in a 2-day-old animal relative to adult animals. Among these, one protein in particular, GAP-43, is present in large amount in the growing cells. However, it undergoes a decrease of 90% or more in the several weeks that follow the period of maximal growth.

GAP-43 is a highly acidic protein. Its synthesis and transport occur at a high rate during periods of axonal extension in many different neuronal pathways. When axonal outgrowth is stimulated in cultured cells, for example, by NGF, GAP-43 is one of the proteins whose synthesis is induced. Moreover, when a pathway in the mammalian nervous system is severed, the synthesis of GAP-43 may be markedly stimulated. This occurs only in those cases in which the pathway regenerates, but it is not seen in tracts

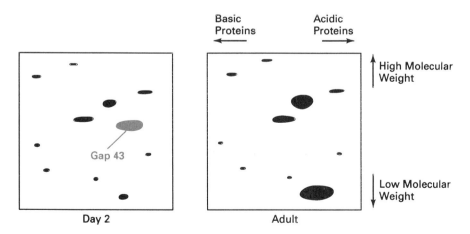

Figure 17–20. GAP-43. Representation of a two-dimensional separation of newly synthesized proteins transported along axons of retinal ganglion cells in a 2-day-old hamster and in an adult (Benowitz and Routtenberg, 1987).

in which no regeneration occurs. Such findings suggest that GAP-43 may be an important component of the neurite outgrowth process.

The growth cones of developing axons also contain GAP-43. Highly purified growth cones can be prepared by centrifugation techniques, and GAP-43 is a major component of such preparations. The primary structure of GAP-43, which is known from the cloning of the DNA encoding the protein, does not have the hydrophobic sequences characteristic of integral membrane proteins. However, GAP-43 may be closely associated with the internal surface of the plasma membrane of growth cones and may regulate the dynamics of actin at this location. Moreover, the introduction of GAP-43 into non-neuronal cells promotes the extension of filopodia and of processes resembling neurites. GAP-43 does not disappear altogether during development and can be detected readily in certain regions of adult brain. It is a phosphoprotein and can be phosphorylated by the enzyme protein kinase C. It is therefore possible that this intriguing protein plays a role in plastic changes in the adult nervous system.

Summary

Developing neurons extend neurites, which become the axons and dendrites of the adult neuron. These neurites follow specific paths and branch in characteristic ways. The leading tip of the neurite, the growth cone, appears to sample the extracellular environment and contribute to decisions about the direction of neurite extension.

Molecules of various types are essential for appropriate pathfinding by growing neurites. For example, neurites grow selectively toward or away from certain soluble factors, including the semaphorins, netrins, and neurotransmitters. In addition, a variety of adhesion molecules play a primary role. These include protein molecules in the membrane of the neurite and in the extracellular matrix that mediate specific adhesion of the neurite to the substrate over which it is growing. Other membrane proteins promote the adhesion of neurites of different cells to each other in specific patterns. Some of these molecules and mechanisms that regulate neuronal development and differentiation may also regulate neurite outgrowth in adult nervous systems, either during recovery from injury or in response to novel stimuli from the environment.

18

Formation, Maintenance, and Plasticity of Chemical Synapses

*F*ollowing cellular determination and neurite elongation, developing neurons form the specific synaptic connections that are essential for brain function (Fig. 15–1). One particularly striking aspect of the formation of synapses is its extraordinary sensitivity to patterns of electrical activity in the developing pathways. We will now describe synaptogenesis during development and its guidance by the pattern of electrical stimulation to which an immature neuron is exposed. Synaptogenesis is not, however, restricted to the developing nervous system. We have hinted that reorganization of neuronal form and function occurs in the adult nervous system, and in fact mature neurons retain most of the machinery necessary for restructuring their synaptic connections by mechanisms similar to those operating in development. We will therefore provide some examples of synaptic plasticity in adult neurons. Finally, we will describe some of the changes that occur in the properties of cells once synaptic contacts have been established.

Synaptogenesis During Development

Morphological changes during synapse formation. When growing axons approach the cell on which they will finally make synaptic contacts, changes occur in the shape of their growth cones (Fig. 18–1). The lamellipodia that are characteristic of rapid growth shrink in size and the filopodia extend from the tip of the neurite in an irregular pattern. This change in the appearance of growth cones is associated with a slower rate of elongation.

When the growth cone finally contacts a cell with which it forms a synapse, a further change takes place in its structure. The lamellipodium and filopodia disappear as neurotransmitter vesicles from the central core region advance into the tip of the neurite. The point of contact is then transformed into a full-fledged synapse with the accumulation of material in the synaptic cleft and the thickening of the postsynaptic membrane to form a *postsynaptic density*. Functional synaptic communication, however, can occur as soon as the neurite contacts the postsynaptic cell. Indeed, experiments in cell culture have demonstrated that even extending growth cones are capable of releasing neurotransmitter.

As described in Chapter 8, some neurons do not contact their targets directly but release neurotransmitter locally to influence neighboring cells without making specialized synaptic contacts. Changes in the terminals of these cells must also occur when their axons have reached their final destinations. An example of how terminal morphology can change without synapse formation is given in Figure 18–2, which shows the change in structure of a growth cone of an *Aplysia* bag cell neuron in cell culture following elevation of cyclic AMP levels. The actin-rich lamellipodium is invaded by microtubules and other organelles from the central core region to produce a club-like ending that is packed with secretory granules. Although such changes can be induced experimentally in cell culture, it is not known whether second messengers such as cyclic AMP play a role in similar transformations of growth cones in the nervous system.

What determines the choice of postsynaptic target? How specific is this interaction of a growing axon with its target? Can the axon of a motor neu-

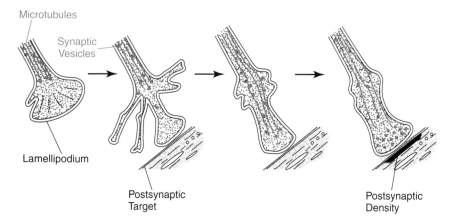

Figure 18–1. Synapse formation. Transformation of a growth cone into a presynaptic ending.

ron, for example, form a synapse on any muscle cell, or is there a strict one-to-one recognition of a specific muscle cell or a particular neuron? It appears that the very earliest stages of synapse formation are rather indiscriminate. This lack of early specificity in connections can be seen in cell culture, where neurons make synapses with other neurons or muscle cells that are not their normal targets. It is only in time that a finely tuned pattern of specific point-to-point connections emerges in the developing brain.

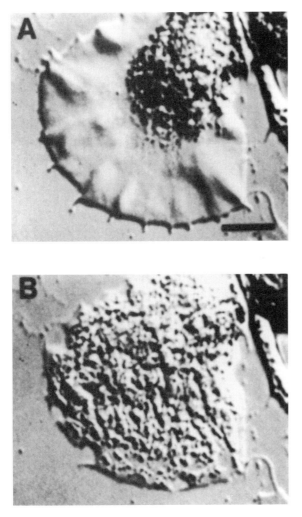

Figure 18–2. Changes in structure of a growth cone in cell culture. Photographs of the growth cone of an *Aplysia* neuron before (*A*) and after (*B*) treatment with drugs that elevate cyclic AMP levels (Forscher et al., 1987).

The progression in time to an increasingly specific pattern of synaptic connections can readily be explained by the finding that synapse formation occurs in two very distinct phases. There is an early phase of synapse formation that is relatively indiscriminate. This is followed by a second, more prolonged phase during which some synapses are stabilized while others are eliminated. It is this fine-tuning and pruning of contacts during the second phase that achieves a highly ordered final pattern of synaptic connections.

The two phases of synapse formation. The first phase of synapse formation is closely related to the process of neural pathfinding that we considered in the previous chapter. An extending axon does not make synaptic contacts with every cell that it encounters on its path. When it reaches an appropriate synaptic target, therefore, some signal must be generated that instructs the growing cell to slow its growth, contact the postsynaptic cell, and form a synaptic terminal. This initial phase of synapse formation may be termed *target selection*. As we shall see in specific examples of synapse formation in the mammalian brain, this initial phase may produce a pattern of synaptic connections that is relatively coarse-grained compared to the final pattern that is seen in the adult. Another characteristic feature of this first phase is that it generally is independent of ongoing electrical activity in the growing neurons. Thus, target selection usually occurs normally even in the presence of drugs, such as tetrodotoxin, that block neuronal action potentials (see Chapter 6).

The initial phase of synapse formation is followed by a second phase that has sometimes been termed *address selection*. During this second phase a major remodeling of the original pattern of connections occurs. The initial synaptic contacts may expand or retract and may withdraw altogether. A neuron whose process has retracted from one postsynaptic cell may subsequently form a more stable synapse on another cell. Because of this second phase, synapse formation during development is a relatively protracted process. For example, in the mammalian brain, the number of synapses formed may increase over a period of many weeks or months after birth. Thereafter the total number of synapses declines toward that of the adult. Moreover, in some cases synapses continue to be made and broken during adult life.

As will be described below, the fine-tuning of synaptic connections during the second phase appears to result in large part from the competition of different axons for the same postsynaptic cell. A second very important aspect of this fine-tuning process is that it depends on, and is entirely shaped by, the pattern of electrical activity that occurs in the synaptic pathway. One of the most thoroughly studied and clearest examples of the way that activity-independent (first phase) and activity-dependent (second phase) mechanisms contribute to final choice of synaptic target is to be found in the visual system of vertebrates.

Synapse Formation in the Visual System

The retinotectal system. In many lower vertebrates, the major neuronal projection from the *retina* extends from the optic nerve to part of the midbrain known as the *optic tectum*. This pathway controls many of the rapid visual reflexes of such animals. A feature of this pathway that has attracted much attention from developmental biologists is the particularly clear point-to-point mapping of the input from different parts of the retina to corresponding points on the surface of the tectum. Such mapping can readily be demonstrated by shining points of light on the retina and recording electrophysiological responses in the tectum. As shown in Figure 18–3a, points of light that fall on the ventral retina triggers responses in the dorsal tectum, whereas stimulation of cells in the dorsal retinal produces responses in the ventral tectum. Similarly, retinal neurons that respond to light falling on the anterior retina connect to neurons in the posterior tectum, while those activated in the posterior retina project to the anterior part of the tectum.

The chemoaffinity hypothesis for the first phase of synapse formation. Although the final connections to the tectum are arranged in an exquisitely precise array, the path that the axon of a retinal cell follows to reach its final destination may not be direct. An ingrowing axon may bypass many potential postsynaptic targets in the tectum before establishing its synaptic contacts (Fig. 18–3b). The major hypothesis to account for the specificity of these connections is the *chemoaffinity hypothesis* of Roger Sperry. The simplest form of this hypothesis states that there are specific molecules in the presynaptic and postsynaptic cells (usually thought of as being on the surface of the cells) that differ either in their chemical identities or in their relative amounts in different regions of the tectum. These differences constitute a biochemical label for each cell. The fact that cells from one region of the retina connect only to the appropriate region of the tectum is explained by the requirement of correct matching of presynaptic and postsynaptic labels for synapse formation to occur.

Many experiments support the chemoaffinity hypothesis. Some of these involve surgical manipulation of the inputs to the tectum. For example, the optic nerve of a frog can be severed and the eye rotated through 180°. The axons of the retinal cells will in time regenerate and reinnervate the tectum. Under these conditions cells in the retina form new synaptic connections with the same part of the tectum that they innervated before, even though the region of visual space projected by a given region of retina to tectal sites is now 180° different. Moreover, if half of a retina is removed, the remaining cells in the retina will reextend axons that make synaptic contacts with the appropriate half of the tectum. Initially, these axons will not innervate the remainder of the tectum, which does not bear the appropriate label. (As will be described below, however, slower remodeling

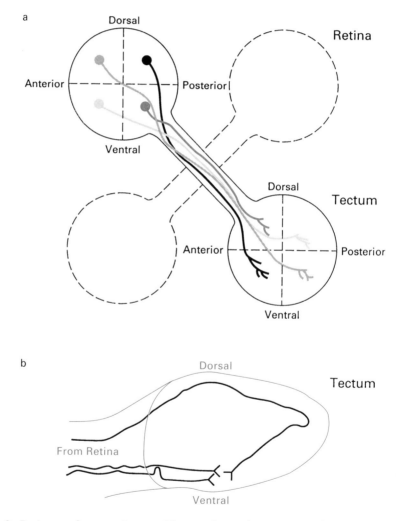

Figure 18–3. Retinotectal connections. *a*: The topology of connections. *b*: Drawings of the irregular growth of retinal axons into the ventral tectum of an adult newt (Fujisawa, 1981).

of the connections does occur, and the entire tectum is eventually innervated by the half-retina.)

Further evidence that molecules in the membrane of retinal cells may determine which region of the tectum they come to innervate has come from experiments in which the physical adhesion of retinal cells to tectal cells has been tested in a dish. Retinal cells are dissociated and then incubated with the tectum. Cells from the dorsal retina are found to bind preferentially to the ventral tectum, while cells in the ventral retina adhere more strongly to dorsal tectum. Such preferential stickiness of retinal cells matches the pattern of synaptic connections that eventually is formed by these cells.

In a variant of the above experiment, explants of retina are placed next to narrow alternating strips of cell membranes prepared from posterior and anterior tectal cells (Fig. 18–4). When a piece of the anterior retina is placed next to this striped "carpet" of membranes, the axons that grow out of the explant travel over both types of stripes. In contrast, axons from the posterior retina grow only along the stripes of membranes from the anterior tectal cells. This preference results from a repulsive factor in the membranes of the posterior tectal cells. Heating or protease treatment of the posterior tectal membranes neutralizes this repulsion and the posterior retinal cells then fail to discriminate between posterior and anterior tectal membranes. The factors that repel the axons of posterior retinal cells, causing the collapse of their growth cones, have been identified as *ephrins*. Gradients of ephrins and their receptors appear to be important components of the biochemical labels of Sperry's chemoaffinity hypothesis.

Ephrins and the Eph receptors. In many respects, ephrins and their receptors, termed the *Eph receptors*, function like the guidance molecules that we considered in the previous chapters. They are not specific to the nervous system and operate during the development of many different tissues. In the developing nervous system, like some of the other guidance molecules, they can exert either attractive or repulsive influences on axons. As we shall see later, however, there are several reasons why it may be more appropriate to consider them here in the context of synapse formation.

Ephrins come in two forms (Fig. 18–5). The ephrinA ligands (ephrins A1–A5) are extracellular proteins that are tethered to the plasma membrane by a lipid anchor (a glycosyl phosphatidylinositol, or GPI, anchor). The B class of ephrins (ephrins B1–B3) are true integral membrane proteins that posses, in their cytoplasmic domains, five highly conserved tyrosines that may undergo phosphorylation. Corresponding to these two types of ligands are two classes of receptor tyrosine kinases. EphA receptors bind clusters of ephrinA ligands, while EphB receptors bind ephrinB

ligands. The extracellular, ephrin-binding region of these receptors possesses a large globular domain, a cysteine-rich domain, and regions related
to fibronectin (type III motifs). In addition to a tyrosine kinase domain,
the intracellular region contains sites for autophosphorylation and a domain termed the *SAM domain*, through which the receptor binds other
signaling molecules. One of the interesting aspects of the ephrinB proteins
is that, following their binding to their EphB receptors, they may them-

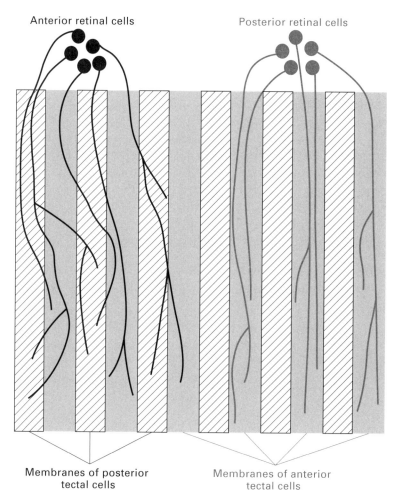

Figure 18–4. Repulsion of axons of posterior retinal axon by membranes of posterior
tectal cells. In an experiment by Boenhoeffer and his colleagues, retinal cells were allowed to extend their neurites over alternating stripes of membrane fragments from
posterior and anterior tectal cells. The posterior retinal cells avoided the stripes of posterior tectal cell membranes (Walter et al., 1987).

selves undergo phosphorylation on tyrosine residues and trigger signaling events in their cytoplasmic regions. Thus these interactions constitute a bidirectional signaling system that produces changes in two interacting cells.

Gradients of ephrins and Eph receptors in both the retina and in the tectum shape the eventual pattern of synapse formation. For example, there exist gradients of two ephrins, ephrin A2 and ephrin A5, in the tectum, with the highest levels being in the posterior tectum (Fig. 18–6). The gradient of ephrin A5 is steeper than that of ephrin A2. There is also a corresponding gradient of the EphA3 receptor, with which these ephrins may interact, in neurons of the retina, the highest levels being in posterior (or *temporal*) retina. As surmised from the experiments with alternating stripes of tectal membranes, the interaction between these receptors and ligands is a repulsive one. Thus the EphA3-bearing axons from the posterior retina fail to enter the posterior tectum and instead terminate in the anterior tectum.

The axons from neurons in the anterior (or *nasal*) retina are not sensitive to the repulsive effects of ephrins A2 and A5 and are therefore able to extend toward the posterior tectum. There may be two reasons for this. First, because of the gradient of Eph3 in the retina, these neurons lack the EphA3 receptor. This reason alone could be responsible for the pattern of

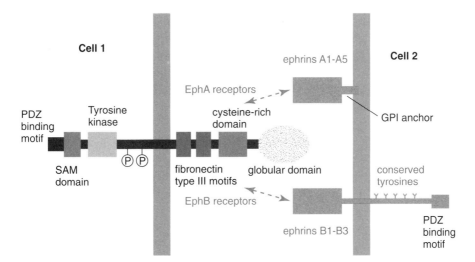

Figure 18–5. Ephrins and the Eph receptors. EphA receptors bind the lipid-anchored ephrinA ligands, while EphB receptors bind ephrinB ligands, which are integral membrane proteins. Autophosphorylation sites are shown on the receptors. GPI, glycosyl phosphatidylinositol.

anterior–posterior connections (Fig. 18–6). There appears, however, to be second set of interactions. A gradient of ephrins A2 and A5 exists in the retina, as well as in the tectum. In the retina, however, levels of these ephrins are greatest at the anterior end (Fig. 18–7a). These ephrins interact with Eph receptors in the retina itself. Although there is no EphA3 at the anterior retina, two other receptors, EphA4 and EphA5, are found uniformly throughout the retina. In some way that is not fully understood, the interaction of the Eph receptors of anterior retinal neurons with the high levels of endogenous retinal ephrins appears to make the axons of these neurons even less sensitive to the ephrins in the tectum, allowing them to make the full journey to the posterior tectum. Support for this notion is found in experiments in which cells within the posterior retina have been engineered to produce ephrin A2. When this occurs, they too are able to extend their axons to the posterior tectum (Fig. 18–7b).

Gradients of ephrins and their receptors may also regulate the dorsal–ventral synaptic connections, in addition to the anterior–posterior patterning that we have considered. Here gradients of the B class of ephrins and the EphB receptor may be implicated. For example, the ephrin B1 ligand is expressed in a high dorsal to low ventral pattern in the tectum. In

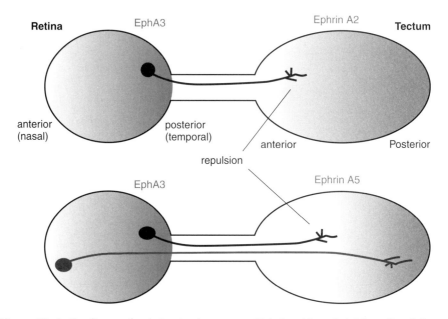

Figure 18–6. Gradients of ephrins in the tectum. Ephrins A2 and A5 in cells of the posterior tectum repel axons of neurons from posterior retina, which contain the EphA3 receptor.

chick retina, an inverse gradient of low dorsal to high ventral levels occurs for EphB2 and EphB3, receptors for the B1 ligand.

Ephrin signaling may represent the first step of synapse formation. Although we
have thus far considered the eprhins and their receptors in terms of their
ability to guide axons to their targets, there appears to be more to the
function of these proteins than simply providing a road map for growing
axons. Simply stimulating the activity of these receptors can lead to an increase in the number of synaptic sites in cultured neurons. First, the EphB
receptors have been shown to be able to bind directly to the NMDA class
of glutamate receptors. This interaction appears to result from an inter-

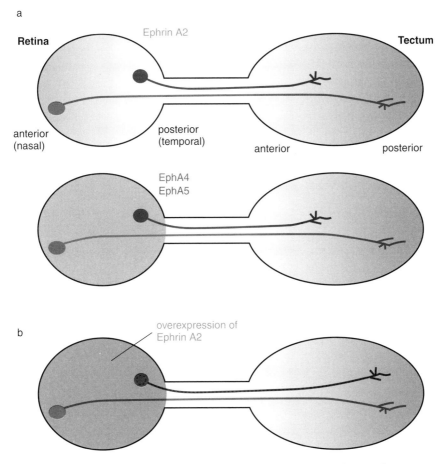

Figure 18–7. Gradients of ephrins in the retina. *a:* Normal gradients of A2 in retina
and tectum. The EphA4 and EphA5 receptors are uniformly expressed in the retina.
b: Artificial overproduction of ephrin A2 in cells in the posterior retina allows neurons to extend axons from posterior retina to posterior tectum.

action between the extracellular regions of the two proteins. As we shall see later, these receptors play a key role in the stabilization of synaptic contacts in tectal neurons. Moreover, both the EphB receptors and their Ephrin B ligands possess PDZ binding motifs at their carboxyl termini (Fig. 18–5). As we saw in Chapter 11, these motifs are present in a variety of channels, receptors, and adaptor proteins that cluster proteins containing PDZ domains at presynaptic terminals and postsynaptic densities. The picture that is emerging is that activation of these signaling molecules may, in addition to guiding an axon to its target, participate in putting together the components required to convert a cell–cell contact into a synaptic terminal (Fig 18–8).

Eph–Ephrin interactions can be reversed by proteases. The interaction between an ephrin and its Eph is a tight one. In the case of an attractive interaction between two cell membranes, as in the early steps of synapse forma-

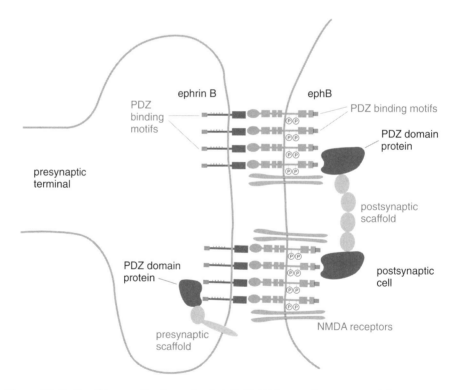

Figure 18–8. Possible contributions of ephrinB–EphB interactions to organizing synaptic contacts. EphB receptors bind NMDA receptors, and PDZ binding motifs on both ephrin Bs and their receptors may participate in the formation of presynaptic and postsynaptic scaffolds.

tion, this may not be a problem. If, however, the interaction is a repulsive one, as in the anterior–posterior labeling of axons in the tectum, the receptor and its ligand must be separated to allow the axon to find a more appropriate target. This separation involves the physical cleavage of the ephrin ligand by an extracellular protease. In the last chapter we mentioned that growing axons secrete proteases, including a metalloprotease named *Kuzbanian*. After an initial repulsive interaction between membranes, which produces biochemical changes such as changes in actin polymerization in the two sets of interacting cells, Kuzbanian in the extracellular space has been shown to cleave ephrin A that is bound to its receptor (Fig. 18–9). The cleavage leaves part of the ephrin molecule bound to the receptor, but allows the two membranes to separate. As we shall see in the next section, many of the strong attractive interactions that initially lead to synapse formation must also eventually be reversed before the process of synaptogenesis is complete.

Rearrangement of Synaptic Connections

The second phase of synapse formation in the retinotectal system. As we have already mentioned, synapse formation is a two-stage process. Once an initial set of contacts is made by the incoming axons, guided by adhesive and repulsive molecules, there follows a second prolonged period of restructuring or *sorting* of these synapses. At this time, some terminal branches and their synaptic contacts may be withdrawn from a tectal cell while the connections from other retinal neurons may be strengthened. Although

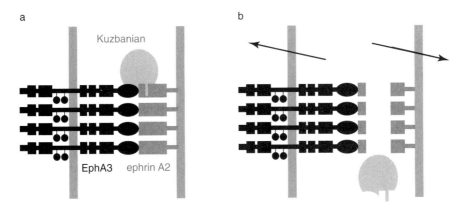

Figure 18–9. Separation of membranes by extracellular Kuzbanian. *a*: The Kuzbanian protease binds to a complex of EphA3 and its ligand ephrin A2. *b*: Cleavage allows the membranes to separate (Hattori et al., 2000).

such remodeling of connections is most obvious during the initial development of the retinotectal pathway, it is clear that in some instances this continues throughout adult life.

Particularly clear examples of the ongoing restructuring of synapses occur in frogs and goldfish. In these species, the retina and tectum continue to increase in size by the addition of new cells. In the eye, new neurons are added as a ring to the circumference of the retina. In contrast, in the tectum the new cells are added only to the posterior tectum (Fig. 18–10). Thus to maintain the correct mapping of connections from the retina to the tectum, the entire set of synapses from the retina continually retracts and reconnects to a new set of tectal neurons. In the goldfish, the retina and tectum continue to increase in size, and therefore to realign their connections, throughout adult life.

A shift in the pattern of synaptic connections also occurs in the experiment that was described above as one of the first tests of the chemoaffinity hypothesis. In this experminent, the optic nerve is cut and part of the retina is removed. Initially only the area of the tectum that corresponds to the intact retina is reinnervated by the axons from the remaining retinal cells. In time, however, branches of these axons extend to make synapses over the entire tectal area. In this way, the map of the visual field

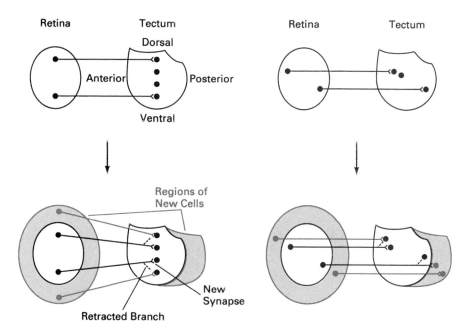

Figure 18–10. Remodeling of synaptic connections during addition of new cells. As the size of the retina and tectum increases, connections are broken and reformed to maintain the overall map of retina onto the tectum.

represented by the remaining part of the retina spreads out over the whole tectum.

Electrical activity of neurons determines the final pattern of synaptic contacts. Experiments with the tectum and with many other parts of the developing nervous system suggest strongly that the fine-tuning of synaptic connections is determined by the pattern of electrical activity in the presynaptic neurons. A given postsynaptic cell may initially be innervated by many different presynaptic cells. It appears, however, that only those inputs whose activity is correlated in time with postsynaptic activity are stabilized (Fig. 18–11). Fibers that generate weaker responses or fail to influence the postsynaptic cell altogether retract their synaptic contacts. Such fibers may, however, successfully stimulate and establish stable contacts with other postsynaptic cells.

The hypothesis that excitatory synapses are stabilized when they successfully trigger action potentials in the postsynaptic cell was proposed by the Canadian psychologist Donald Hebb in 1949. It has been used in models of both development and learning (see Chapter 20). A restatement of this hypothesis is that when a postsynaptic neuron becomes depolarized, it generates a biochemical reaction or a trophic factor that stabilizes the excitatory synapses that are firing at that time. An important aspect of this hypothesis is that a given presynaptic input to a cell need not by itself be of sufficient strength to induce a large depolarization in its target. If that input is fired at the same time as a number of other inputs and their combined action depolarizes the cell, all of these inputs will tend to be stabilized. If, in contrast, a given input fires asynchronously with most of the other inputs onto that cell, this input will tend to be eliminated. Al-

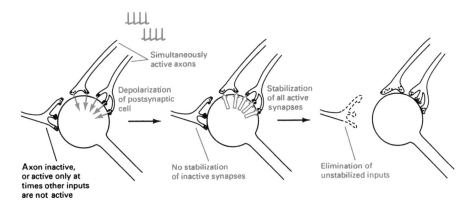

Figure 18–11. Hebb's rule. Excitatory synapses that successfully stimulate a postsynaptic neuron or are active when the postsynaptic neuron is depolarized are selectively stabilized (Hebb, 1949).

though the nature of the trophic factors involved is unknown, the general hypothesis that synapses are stabilized or eliminated on the basis of their patterns of activity can explain many different findings about synapse formation and remodeling.

Ocular dominance columns. In lower vertebrates including frogs, all the fibers from one retina cross the midline to innervate the contralateral tectum. Thus in the frog there is normally no competition between inputs from the two eyes in one tectum. It is possible, however, to implant a third eye into a tadpole. The fibers from this third eye grow normally into one of the tecta, where they must compete with axons from the normal eye for synaptic space on the tectal neurons. The final pathways that are established can be measured by injection of a radiactive amino acid into one of the eyes. The radiolabel is taken up by retinal cells and transported to their terminals in the tectum. The amount of radioactivity in these terminals can then be visualized directly by placing a piece of X-ray film against slices made from the tectum (Fig. 18–12). It is found that connections have

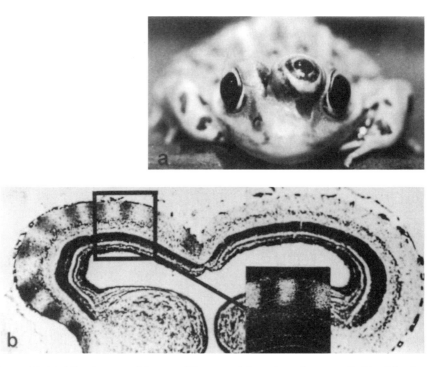

Figure 18–12. The three-eyed frog. *a*: Three-eyed frogs have been studied by Martha Constantine-Paton and her colleagues. *b*: Autoradiograph of the tectum shows the formation of stripes of inputs from the normal and the implanted eye. The *inset* shows an enlargement under dark-field illumination (Constantine-Paton and Law, 1978).

been established in a pattern of alternating columns, each of which contains inputs primarily from one eye. Under normal conditions, no such columns are observed in the tecta of frogs and other lower vertebrates.

The formation of such columns, termed *ocular dominance columns*, can be understood in terms of the resorting of synapses based on their electrical activity, a process that occurs during normal development (Fig. 18–13). Because all of the photoreceptor cells in one eye point toward one general region of visual space, the inputs in that one eye will tend to be activated approximately simultaneously. The other eye, however, covers a somewhat different visual field. Although the inputs from that eye generally will also be correlated with each other, they will tend not to be active at the same time as input from the competing eye. Thus a given small region of the tectum is innervated initially by inputs from both eyes. A small

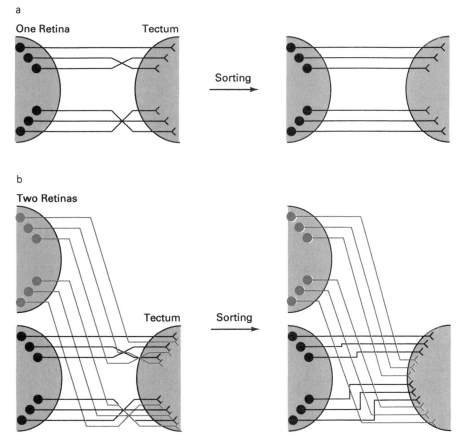

Figure 18–13. Segregation of retinal inputs to the tectum. *a*: Sorting of inputs from one eye only. *b*: Sorting in the presence of input from a second eye.

increase in the amount of input from one eye, however, tends to stabilize all of the approximately synchronously active synaptic inputs from that eye, at the expense of inputs from the other eye. Such stabilization leads to the formation of areas or columns that are preferentially innervated by one eye or the other.

Segregation of inputs from two eyes also occurs normally in the visual systems of mammals, in which each retina sends some fibers to both hemispheres of the brain. Indeed, it was the Nobel Prize–winning experiments of David Hubel and Torsten Wiesel on kittens and monkeys that first led to the idea that patterns of electrical activity shape synapse rearrangement. Sheets of cells that respond preferentially either to one eye or the other are found in the *lateral geniculate*, a visual relay station, of adult cats and monkeys. In the visual cortex, inputs from the two eyes are segregated into ocular dominance columns. The sorting of these inputs occurs by mechanisms that are similar to those in the three-eyed frogs. At first, geniculate and cortical cells are innervated relatively uniformly by incoming fibers carrying information from both eyes. At this early time many cells can be stimulated by inputs from either eye. However, as development proceeds, synapses are broken, reformed, and stabilized to produce the alternating ocular dominance columns.

The formation of these segregated patterns of synaptic connections is not programmed innately but depends on the electrical activity of the presynaptic fibers. This can be demonstrated in a number of ways. For example, tetrodotoxin can be introduced to block action potentials. This treatment does not interfere with the initial innervation itself but prevents the subsequent rearrangement into columns, leaving the presynaptic inputs from the two eyes relatively uniformly distributed. In other experiments the two eyes have been stimulated either synchronously or asynchronously. For example, if the two optic nerves of a cat are stimulated such that activity from the two eyes occurs at different times, then ocular dominance columns develop. If, however, the two nerves are stimulated simultaneously, such that the input from the two sets of presynaptic fibers is identical, then no segregation occurs.

We emphasized earlier in this book that many neurons are capable of generating spontaneous patterns of electrical activity in the absence of external inputs. Interestingly, such spontaneous activity may play a role in the sorting of synapses before the visual system is fully functional. In three-eyed frogs, as well as in other species, inputs from the two eyes can still segregate even when animals are reared in the dark or before visual inputs are functional. The ocular dominance columns formed in these circumstances are still blocked or reversed by treatment with tetrodotoxin, indicating that ongoing electrical activity is required for the segregation.

Activation of the NMDA type of glutamate receptor during development is involved in the selective stabilization of retinotectal projections in the frog and in related phenomena in higher vertebrates. One piece of evidence that implicates NMDA receptors in development is that treatment of tectal cells with the NMDA receptor antagonist APV does not prevent the stimulation of the tectal cells by retinal afferents, but reverses the segregation into ocular dominance columns in the three-eyed frog. As we saw in Chapter 11, the properties of the NMDA receptor make it particularly appropriate to induce biochemical changes in a cell when a set of inputs are synchronously active (see Fig. 18–11). For example, when several inputs that use glutamate as a transmitter are activated at the same time, the postsynaptic cell undergoes a depolarization. If NMDA receptors are present at these synapses, this depolarization allows calcium ions to enter the postsynaptic neurons. This calcium, in turn, is thought to activate some factor that acts back on the active presynaptic synaptic terminals, thereby stabilizing them (Fig. 18–14). According to this view, the synapses that are inactive do not respond to the factor and are subject to elimination. We shall discuss the possible actions of such retrograde factors later in this chapter.

Synaptic rearrangement at the neuromuscular junction and in other systems. This kind of remodeling of axonal and dendritic branches and synaptic connections occurs not only in visual pathways but also in many other regions of the nervous system of both vertebrates and invertebrates, and may be a very general phenomenon. Another well-studied example of this is found at neuromuscular junctions of vertebrates. When the axons of motor neurons first contact their skeletal muscle targets, the different branches of an axon contact several muscle fibers. Moreover, each muscle fiber is contacted by the terminals of several different motor neurons. This situation is termed *polyneuronal innervation*. Over a period of a few weeks, however, many of these branches are withdrawn. Eventually, in the adult, each muscle fiber comes to be innervated by only one motor neuron. This elimination of synapses can be observed both morphologically and electrophysiologically. As shown in Figure 18–15a, at the neuromuscular junction of the neonate, graded stimulation of a presynaptic nerve produces graded postsynaptic potentials in the muscle. This occurs because the postsynaptic response is made up of responses to several presynaptic axons, and graded stimuli to the nerve trigger action potentials in a progressively larger proportion of these presynaptic fibers. In the adult, however, different intensities of stimuli either trigger an action potential in the axon of the one motor neuron contacting the muscle or fail to excite this one axon, resulting in an all-or-none postsynaptic response.

Although the loss of polyneuronal innervation during development of the neuromuscular junction is produced by removal of axonal branches and their associated synapses from the muscle fiber, the number of individual synaptic terminals made by branches of the one axon whose inputs are stabilized actually increases (Fig. 18–15b). As in the retinotectal system, this restructuring of neuritic branches and synapses depends on the electrical activity of the presynaptic terminals. If electrical activity is abolished by pharmacological treatment of the presynaptic axons, for example, by using a local anesthetic, the elimination of synapses and the loss of polyneuronal innervation are greatly slowed. Direct stimulation of the presynaptic fibers, by contrast, substantially enhances the rate of synapse elimination.

As in the retinotectal system, the process of synapse stabilization and elimination at the neuromuscular junction is a Hebbian one. Insights into the role of electrical activity have come from studies using isolated neu-

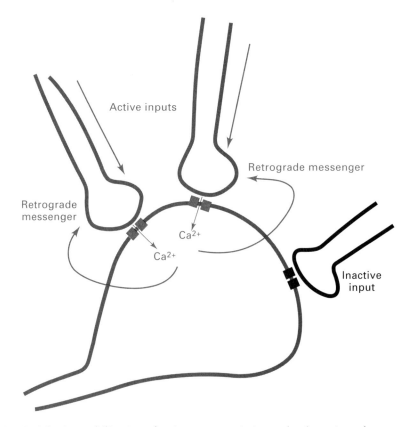

Figure 18–14. Selective stabilization of active presynaptic inputs by the action of a retrograde messenger.

rons and muscles in cell culture, where the activity of the presynaptic and postsynaptic cells can be controlled precisely. When an isolated embryonic muscle cell is innervated by two different motor neurons, stimulation of either neuron alone is, at first, sufficient to activate large postsynaptic currents in the muscle. Provided that stimulation to either neuron is applied only infrequently, both functional synapses may exist on the muscle for a prolonged period. If, however, one of the neurons is made to fire a rapid train of action potentials (a *tetanus*), the strength of the other synapse is immediately suppressed (Fig. 18–16a). This *heterosynaptic suppression* does not occur if the tetanus is applied to both motor neurons at the same time. The effect of a tetanus in one neuron to depress transmission in the

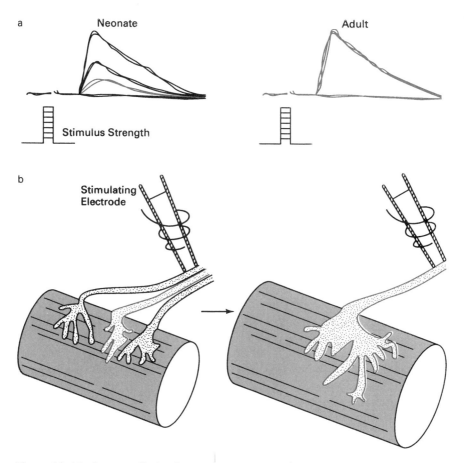

Figure 18–15. Synapse elimination at the neuromuscular junction. *a*: Postsynaptic potentials of varying sizes are recorded in the neonate, whereas stimulation of an adult junction gives an all-or-none postsynaptic potential. *b*: Elimination of synapses at the neuromuscular junction.

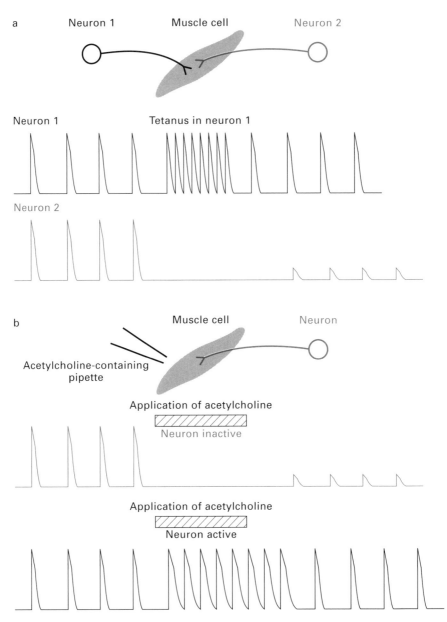

Figure 18–16. Experiments by Mu-Ming Poo and colleagues showing heterosynaptic suppression of synaptic inputs at the neuromuscular junction. *a*: A tetanus in one motor neuron causes a subsequent suppression of the inputs from a second neuron (Lo and Poo, 1992). *b*: Application of acetylcholine to a muscle cell causes suppression of synaptic inputs from a motor neuron if that neuron is inactive (*upper traces*), but does not suppress the synapse if the neuron is active at the time of exposure to the transmitter (Dan and Poo, 1992).

synapses of other inactive neurons can be mimicked by applying pulses of acetylcholine to the muscle from a nearby pipette (Fig. 18–16b). If such pulses are given while a presynaptic neuron is inactive, its synapses are immediately suppressed. Synapses are protected, however, from this suppression if the neuron is firing action potentials at the time of acetylcholine application.

This process of the rapid suppression of inactive synapses is likely to be the first step in the complete elimination of these synaptic junctions. One of the actions of acetylcholine pulses or tetanic stimulation on the muscle cell is to produce an elevation of intracellular calcium. This is known to be required for the suppression of inactive synapses and is believed to trigger the formation of a retrograde messenger that is released from the muscle cell. According to this line of thinking, the presynaptic terminals that are active during the release of this retrograde messenger are protected from elimination.

As we shall see in Chapter 20, this developmental stabilization of active synapses finds a parallel in schemes to account for plastic changes occurring in the adult brain. Restructuring of synapses during development has also been observed in many other parts of the nervous system, including the cerebellum, the cochlear nucleus, the superior cervical ganglion, the ciliary ganglion, and the submandibular gland of the rat. In each of these a progressive decrease in the number of axons that innervate a given postsynaptic cell is found during development, at times when little or no change occurs in the total number of pre- and postsynaptic cells. As in the retinotectal and neuromuscular systems, hypotheses can be invoked to explain these synaptic rearrangements based on the selective stabilization of active synapses. For example, in some cases a trophic factor could be released from the postsynaptic cell when it is activated, and such a factor may act only on the most recently active presynaptic terminals to stabilize them and to stimulate their growth. There is no reason to expect, however, that the detailed mechanisms of synaptic rearrangement are the same in all parts of the nervous system. For example, the retinotectal system requires activation of NMDA receptors, which are absent at the neuromuscular junction.

Although, as a result of competition, the number of presynaptic neurons that innervate a single postsynaptic cell may decrease during development, not all such competition leads to a single "winning" presynaptic cell. The competition may be localized to relatively small regions on the postsynaptic membrane. For example, on a cell that has a complex pattern of dendritic branches, competition may lead one cell to establish its terminals on one branch, at the expense of synapses from other cells. On another branch or a different region of the dendritic tree, the terminals of a different cell may gain precedence, and the mature postsynaptic cell will come to be innervated in different regions by different axons. As a general rule, it appears that cells that have limited dendritic branches, and in which all presynaptic inputs compete for postsynaptic membrane on the soma, become singly innervated. Cells with complex geometries remain multiply innervated.

Changes in Cell Properties Following Synapse Formation

The formation of a synaptic contact is usually followed by a sequence of changes in the properties of the postsynaptic cell. Receptors become reorganized in the postsynaptic membrane, and the types of proteins synthesized by the postsynaptic cell may alter dramatically. Some of these effects occur because the incoming axons induce new patterns of electrical activity in the postsynaptic cell. Other changes are the result of factors that do not depend directly on stimulation of the new input.

Receptor reorganization at the neuromuscular junction. Again, the neuromuscular junction of vertebrates has provided a classic preparation for the study of many of these effects. One of the first events observed following the arrival of the growth cone of a motor neuron at the muscle is the *clustering* of acetylcholine receptors under the newly formed presynaptic terminals. Even before the arrival of the motor neuron fibers, the immature muscle cells have an abundant concentration of acetylcholine receptors in the plasma membrane. These are distributed relatively uniformly over the surface of the cell. When the nerve arrives, however, it induces the appearance of new clusters of receptors under the newly formed presynaptic terminals (Fig. 18–17). These clusters appear to arise both because newly synthesized receptors are inserted preferentially into the membrane under the terminal and because preexisting receptors may be induced to aggregate at these sites (Fig. 18–18a).

The receptors under the terminals are termed *junctional* receptors, while those in the uninnervated parts of the membrane are termed *extrajunctional*. The extrajunctional receptors are synthesized and degraded at a higher rate than the receptors under the synaptic cleft, and in time the extrajunctional receptors disappear altogether. The formation of junctional clusters appears to depend not on the electrical activity of the presynaptic nerve or of the muscle itself but on factors that are released by the incoming nerve terminal.

Agrin: a signal for receptor clustering. The first step in the reorganization of postsynaptic receptors is the movement of preexisting receptors toward the site of synapse formation. A number of different factors, including basic fibroblast growth factor (bFGF) (see Chapter 16) are capable of inducing clustering of receptors. The key signal, however, appears to be agrin, which is made by the growing motor neurons. Agrin is transported to the

15 Day

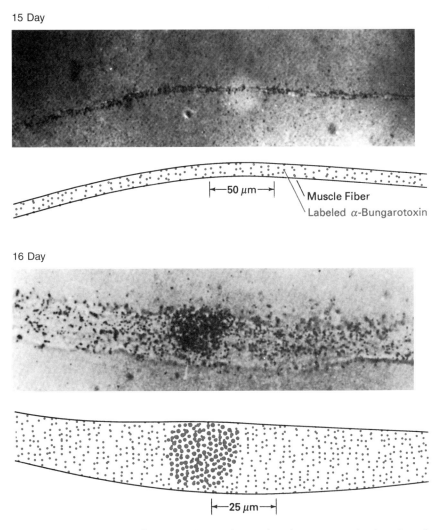

16 Day

Figure 18–17. Receptor clustering. Autoradiographs of neuromuscular junctions from 15- and 16-day rat embryos were made by Bevan and Steinbach (1977). The junctions were incubated with α-bungarotoxin, a ligand that binds to acetylcholine receptors. At the 16-day stage, clustering is apparent.

synaptic terminals and is then secreted into the basal lamina of the synaptic cleft. The basal lamina is an extracellular layer of proteins that surrounds the muscle, even at sites of synaptic contact, where it forms a thin permeable layer between the presynaptic and postsynaptic membranes. We shall encounter the basal lamina again when we discuss the phenomenon of regeneration.

Agrin has many of the features of other molecules that we have encountered that regulate the growth and differentiation of neurons (Fig. 18–18b). The molecule contains several EGF-like regions and a region that resembles laminin, and it also has a repeated sequence that resembles the active domain of certain protease inhibitors. A slightly different variant of the agrin protein is also synthesized by muscle cells, but the muscle form does not induce clustering. It is the form that is released by the neurons, termed the *z+ agrin* isoform, that produces receptor clustering.

Prior to the arrival of the nerve, acetylcholine receptors are relatively mobile and free to diffuse in the plane of the membrane. The recruitment of these extrajunctional receptors to the synaptic membrane depends on the binding of agrin to a receptor tyrosine kinase termed *MuSK* (for mus-

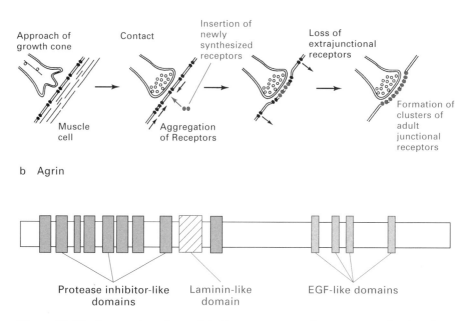

Figure 18–18. Aggregation of acetylcholine receptors at the neuromuscular junction. *a*: Scheme showing the onset of receptor clustering and the insertion of new species of receptors following innervation. *b*: The structure of agrin.

cle specific kinase) in the postsynaptic membrane. Other receptors in this family have been termed *Rors* (receptor orphans) and are present at high levels during development, although some neurons maintain high levels of these receptors even in adult animals. The MuSK receptor does not phosphorylate the acetylcholine receptor directly but probably acts by recruiting additional cytoplasmic kinases. The activation of this agrin receptor eventually leads to the phosphorylation of the acetylcholine receptors on tyrosine residues. This in turn appears to produce a tight and selective association of the receptors with the membrane under the synaptic cleft and with cytoskeletal components under this membrane, effectively immobilizing the receptors at this location. An important link in this association is *rapsyn*, a 43 kD protein that binds the acetylcholine receptor and couples it to other proteins at the synapse. One of these is an assembly of proteins termed the *dystrophin–glycoprotein complex* (Fig. 18–19).

The very large dystrophin–glycoprotein complex contains four transmembrane proteins, including adhalin and β-dystroglycan, an extracellular protein (α-dystroglycan), and several intracellular proteins such as syntrophin. This complex in turn, is able to bind other proteins in the synaptic cleft and the muscle cytoskeleton. On the extracellular side, two of the proteins that bind to the complex are laminin and agrin (although the

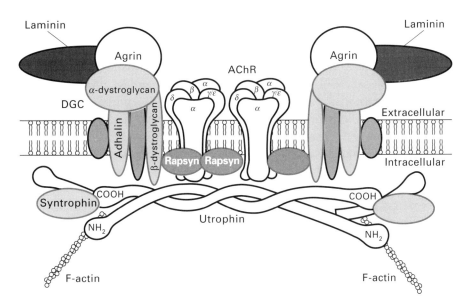

Figure 18–19. Immobilization of acetylcholine receptors (AChR) at the neuromuscular junction. The protein rapsyn links the receptors to the dystrophin–glycoprotein complex (DGC) (modified from Apel et al., 1995).

MuSK receptor is not part of this complex). On the intracellular side, the dystrophin–glycoprotein complex binds two cytoskeletal proteins, dystrophin, which is present at extrajunctional sites and the related protein, utrophin, which is found under the synaptic membrane. This protein scaffold that links the basal lamina to the cytoskeleton may thereby provide a firm anchor for proteins such as the acetylcholine receptors that associate with it.

Neuregulin: a signal for neuron-induced changes in receptor synthesis. After the initial clustering of preexisting acetylcholine receptors, there is an increase in synthesis of new receptors. In contrast to most types of cells, muscle cells have multiple nuclei, and some of these nuclei are strategically placed immediately under the sites of synapse formation. It is these subsynaptic nuclei that are dedicated to making mRNA for the acetylcholine receptor and other proteins of the postsynaptic membrane.

The signal that activates the synthesis of new acetylcholine receptors at the synapse is quite distinct from that which produces the clustering of preexisting receptors. It is yet another molecule that is released from the terminals of the incoming motor neurons into the synaptic part of the basal lamina, a synthesis-activating molecule called *neuregulin*. This molecule too bears EGF-like as well as immunoglobulin-like domains. By alternative splicing of messenger RNA from the neuregulin gene, a number of different growth factor–like molecules can be generated. These differ in the cells in which they are found and in characteristics, such as whether they are membrane proteins or are secreted into the external medium. Some of the neuregulins are capable of inducing cell division in Schwann cells and were therefore originally termed *glial growth factors*. The neuregulin that induces synthesis of acetylcholine receptors was first termed *ARIA* (for **A**cetylcholine **R**eceptor **I**nducing **A**ctivity). Like the other neuronal differentiation factors that we encountered in Chapter 16, the neuregulin at synaptic junctions interacts with a synaptic receptor tyrosine kinase that is closely related to the EGF receptor. This receptor, termed *erbB2*, undergoes autophosphorylation and may also bind to and phosphorylate a related receptor, *erbB3*. This in turn may trigger a cascade of signaling events leading to the increased transcription of the acetylcholine receptor gene in the subsynaptic nuclei.

Not only does the physical location and the amount of receptor change during maturation of the nerve–muscle contact, but the nature of the acetylcholine receptors themselves alters at this time. Patch clamp recordings have shown that the properties of the embryonic receptor channel are different from those of the adult. As we saw in Chapter 11, the fetal muscle receptor is made up of α, β, γ, and δ subunits. As the neuromuscular junction matures, the synthesis of the γ subunit ceases and synthesis of a new ϵ subunit begins. The change in channel properties can be attributed to this switch from the γ to the ϵ subunit.

Effects of electrical activity on the properties of a neuron or muscle cell. We have already encountered the fact that electrical activity within a neuron alters its response to growth factors and may of itself produce long-term changes in the properties of a neuron. In Chapter 16, for example, we saw that the action of cholinergic differentiation factor on neurons of the autonomic nervous system is blocked by electrical activity. In this chapter we have learned that electrical activity in one motor neuron can lead to the elimination of synapses from other neurons contacting the same muscle cell. The reader will not be surprised that the neuromuscular junction has provided a wealth of information on the role of electrical activity in shaping and maintaining the mature synaptic junction.

We have seen that the clustering and the synthesis of new acetylcholine receptors does not depend on electrical activity in the nerve or muscle but on the presence of specific factors in the basal lamina. The elimination of the remaining extrajunctional receptors, which occurs at the same time as these other developmental events, depends, however, directly on the stimulation that the presynaptic neuron provides. Thus, blocking the occurrence of action potentials in the motor neurons prevents the removal of these receptors. Even in the adult, block of the motor neurons produces an increase in the number of extrajunctional acetylcholine receptors, leading to supersensitivity of the muscle to acetylcholine. Direct electrical stimulation of the muscle itself can largely prevent these changes, indicating that continued activity in the muscle is required for its normal characteristics.

Two other proteins whose distribution and levels are altered by ongoing electrical activity are acetylcholinesterase, the enzyme that terminates the actions of acetylcholine, and the cell adhesion molecule N-CAM. Like the acetylcholine receptor, both of these molecules are initially distributed uniformly over the surface of the muscle. After innervation by the nerve terminal, however, both are lost from the extrajunctional regions but come to be clustered at high levels at the postsynaptic junction. Normal aggregation of these proteins at the synapse appears to require ongoing electrical activity in the muscle and is compromised by treatments that paralyze the muscle. Conversely, direct electrical stimulation of muscles promotes their aggregation at the synapses.

Finally, when the activity of the presynaptic axons is eliminated, either by denervation or by pharmacological block of the input to the muscle cells, there is a change in the properties of the voltage-dependent sodium channels in the muscle, which revert to a form that is insensitive to the

blocking agent tetrodotoxin. Such tetrodotoxin-insensitive sodium channels are normally found only early in development.

Fast and slow muscle fibers. A dramatic example of the way the pattern of
neuronal activity can influence a postsynaptic target comes from a finding by Sir John Eccles and his colleagues. Mammals have two forms of
skeletal muscle, fast and slow. The fibers that make up such *fast twitch*
and *slow twitch* muscles differ in a number of characteristic ways. For example, the fast and slow fibers possess different forms of the muscle contractile protein myosin. Furthermore, the fast muscle fibers, which are pale
in color, are used to produce rapid voluntary phasic movements. In contrast, slow muscle fibers, which are rich in the protein myoglobin and
hence reddish in color, are used in maintaining a fixed posture. The neurons that innervate these two different types of muscle fiber also have very
different electrophysiological properties. The motor neurons innervating
fast muscle typically fire intermittent bursts of rapid trains of action potentials. These action potentials are followed by only small afterhyperpo-
larizations, allowing these cells to fire at frequencies as high as 30–60
spikes/sec. In contrast, the neurons that innervate the slow muscle fibers
appear to have a slightly different set of ion channels that controls their
pattern of firing. These cells have a larger afterhyperpolarization following an action potential and fire at a slower, sustained rate of only about
10–20 spikes/sec (Fig. 18–20a).

The Eccles group found that if a nerve containing the axons of fast
motor neurons is forced to innervate a slow muscle, the muscle changes
its properties to those of a fast muscle. Conversely, the innervation of a
fast muscle by slow motor neurons causes the muscle to take on the properties of slow muscle (Fig. 18–20b). Subsequent work has confirmed that
it is the change in pattern of electrical activity that is responsible for the
shift in both the biochemical and contractile properties of the muscles. As
shown in Figure 18–20c, for example, when the nerve to a fast muscle is
forced to fire continually at a slow rate of about 10 spikes/sec for a period of several weeks, the muscle takes on the characteristics of a slow
muscle. But the pattern of incoming electrical activity may not be the sole
determinant of the response characteristics of a muscle. For example, very
early in development some myotubes, the precursors of mature muscle
fibers, differentiate as fast or slow fibers in the complete absence of neural input. Moreover, the role of patterned activity in the conversion of slow
to fast muscles is less clear than that for the fast-to-slow conversion.

Experiments have also been carried out on the effects of stimulation
on neurons in parts of the nervous system other than the neuromuscular
junction. One example has been provided by neurons of the sympathetic

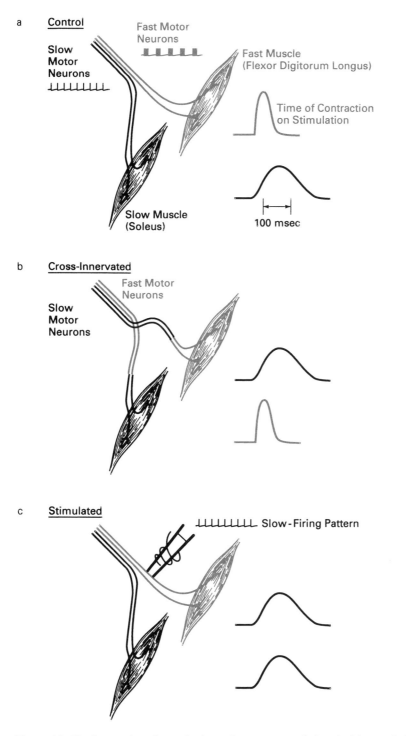

a **Control**

Slow
Motor
Neurons

Fast Motor
Neurons

Fast Muscle
(Flexor Digitorum Longus)

Time of Contraction
on Stimulation

Slow Muscle
(Soleus)

100 msec

b **Cross-Innervated**

Fast Motor
Neurons

Slow
Motor
Neurons

c **Stimulated**

Slow-Firing Pattern

Figure 18–20. Properties of muscle depend on pattern of electrical input. Buller et al. (1960) showed that innervation of a fast muscle with a slow motor neuron (*a, b*) causes the muscle to take on the properties of a slow muscle. Imposition of a slow pattern of firing on the fast motor neuron (*c*) has the same effect (Salmons and Streter, 1976).

ganglion. Electrical activity in these neurons is essential for maintaining levels of tyrosine hydroxylase, the rate-limiting enzyme in the synthesis of norepinephrine (see Chapter 10). Agents that block electrical activity cause levels of messenger RNA coding for this enzyme to fall, whereas stimulation of activity produces a prolonged increase in levels of this messenger RNA. Stimulation of the sympathetic ganglion also influences the levels of a neuropeptide, substance P. In this case, the effects are exactly the opposite of those on tyrosine hydroxylase. On blocking electrical activity, for example, by denervation of the ganglion, the levels of substance P rise, while stimulation prevents this rise.

Synaptic Plasticity in the Adult Nervous System

Sprouting in adult nerves. We have given an account of the extension of neurite branches and the making and breaking of synapses during the formation of the nervous system. It is clear that the adult nervous system retains nearly all of the machinery required for such synaptic plasticity. This can be demonstrated at the adult neuromuscular junction, where the stability of the synaptic connections depends on ongoing electrical activity in the muscles. Synaptic transmission can be blocked either by application of tetrodotoxin to the motor axons or by local injection of an agent such as α-bungarotoxin, which blocks the response of muscle cells to acetylcholine released at the synapses. When this occurs, new branches are formed at the synaptic terminals. They extend over the muscle fiber, forming new areas of synaptic contact.

Further evidence that adult axons are capable of sprouting new processes and forming new synapses comes from studies of recovery from injury of motor nerves at the neuromuscular junction. Following partial denervation of a muscle by cutting some of its incoming axons, the remaining intact motor neurons form new branches that extend toward the denervated region and establish new synapses (Fig. 18–21). These new *sprouts* may extend either from the terminals of motor neurons (terminal sprouts) or from the axons at the nodes of Ranvier (nodal sprouts). The sprouts that establish synapses on the denervated muscles become stabilized, perhaps through the action of some trophic factor from the muscle cells (see below). Sprouts that fail to reach a target, however, are eventually retracted. Sprouting can also be evoked by manipulations that do not sever axons or block their electrical activity entirely. For example, when axoplasmic transport is blocked in some motor axons by application of agents such as the microtubule-disrupting drug colchicine, sprouting is induced in the terminals of adjacent axons.

In addition to being able to generate sprouts near a terminal region, mature neurons are capable of regenerating full axons. In the case of the neuromuscular junction, when the axon of a motor neuron is severed, the distal part of the axon degenerates. The remaining part of the axon, which is attached to the soma, forms a new growth cone at its distal end and grows back to the denervated muscle. Biochemical changes characteristic of developing axons can be detected in the regenerating axons. For example, the concentration of the protein GAP-43 (see Chapter 17) increases dramatically at this time. When the growth cone reaches the muscle, new synapses are formed. If the original sites of synaptic contact have come to be filled by branch sprouts from neighboring terminals whose axons were not severed, then these sprouted branches may retract as a result of the reinnervation. In many respects, therefore, this restructuring of synaptic branches in the adult nervous system resembles what occurs during development.

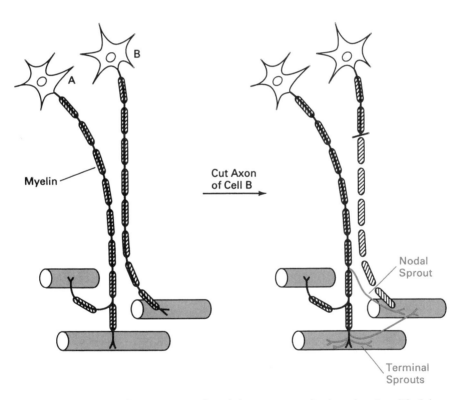

Figure 18–21. Axonal sprouting at the adult neuromuscular junction (modified from Brown, 1984).

Sites of synapse formation are marked by proteins in the basal lamina. The process by which a neuromuscular synapse is established by a regenerating axon may differ somewhat from synapse formation by the first axons of embryonic motor neurons. In particular, the first synapses of the embryonic axons may form at random locations on the muscle. Regenerating axons, by contrast, form synapses specifically at those sites where a synapse had previously existed. It appears that sites of former synaptic contact are marked by specific molecules that induce the growth cone to form a presynaptic structure. Interestingly, these molecules are not located on the surface of the muscle membrane. Instead, they are in the basal lamina, the extracellular layer of proteins that is secreted by the muscle cells and surrounds the muscle (Fig. 18–22).

The existence in the basal lamina of molecules that mark the sites of former synaptic contact can be demonstrated by severing both the motor axons and the muscle fibers, causing the latter to degenerate (Fig. 18–22). In this condition, only the basal lamina remains. The sites of former synaptic contact can be identified both morphologically and by the presence of the enzyme acetylcholinesterase. When the regenerating motor axons reach the basal lamina they form apparently normal synaptic terminals specifically at these sites. Thus it appears that some time after an initial synapse is established, muscle cells secrete a marker protein into the basal lamina at the synaptic cleft. Antibodies have been generated against various proteins of the basal lamina and some of these have been found to be localized selectively to the synaptic part of the basal lamina. One, termed *S-laminin* (for synaptic laminin; Fig. 17–8b), turns out to be a homolog of the B1 chain of the laminin protein that we discussed as a normal component of the extracellular matrix in Chapter 17.

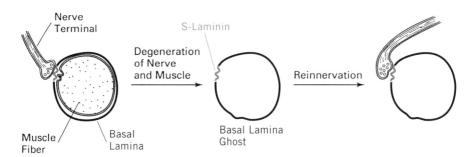

Figure 18–22. Basal lamina marks sites of synapse formation at the neuromuscular junction. This experiment, by Marshall et al. (1977), demonstrated that a regenerating motor axon specifically forms synapses at sites on basal lamina that had previously been occupied by a synapse.

Although the laminin trimer (see Fig. 17–8) is present throughout the basal lamina, the S-laminin chain is substituted for the normal B1 chain at synaptic sites. S-laminin differs from the normal B1 chain in an important way. The S-laminin molecule selectively binds the membrane of motor neurons. Interestingly, a sequence of only three amino acids (Leu-Arg-Glu) within S-laminin appears to be all that is required for this selective adhesion. Other proteins that are restricted to the synaptic basal lamina, such as agrin, also contain one or more repeats of this brief sequence. The binding of motor neuron membranes by S-laminin has a very important consequence for the growth of their axons. While motor neuron membranes grow well on the normal form of laminin, their outgrowth is actually inhibited by S-laminin. Thus the presence of S-laminin and other molecules containing the Leu-Arg-Glu sequence within the synaptic basal lamina may act as a signal to stop the growth of the axon prior to synapse formation. Another important function of S-laminin is to cause the repulsion of the processes of Schwann cells, which would impair access of the growing nerve onto the synaptic site.

Loss of presynaptic terminals after axotomy or interruption of axoplasmic transport. We have seen that cutting an axon or interrupting transport in an axon produces a restructuring of the synaptic contacts made by that axon and others that innervate the same target. These same procedures can also produce changes in the presynaptic contact onto the cell whose axon has been cut. For example, if the axons of neurons of the sympathetic ganglion are severed or exposed to colchicine, the synapses that they receive from other neurons retract (Fig. 18–23). As expected, this is accompanied by a substantial reduction in the synaptic potentials evoked in ganglionic neurons by stimulation of the preganglionic nerve. When transport is restored or the axons of the sympathetic ganglion cells are allowed to regrow and form new contacts, the branches of the presynaptic axons also extend to reestablish their full complement of synapses.

Such a loss of presynaptic terminals following interruption of an axon has been observed in many different pathways. It appears, therefore, that the normal maintenance of synaptic endings may depend on factors available only from an intact postsynaptic cell. In most cases the putative factor and its mode of action are unknown. For sympathetic neurons, however, nerve growth factor (NGF) may play an important role in this phenomenon. For example, application of NGF to the sympathetic ganglion following axotomy prevents the loss of presynaptic terminals illustrated in Figure 18–23. In addition, treatment of animals with an antiserum to NGF, which would be expected to bind to endogenous NGF and thereby prevent its uptake by cells, induces loss of synapses on sympathetic neurons even though their axons remain intact.

Does remodeling of synapses occur continually in the adult? Although the experiments described in this chapter indicate that the maintenance of synapses in mature neurons is dependent on ongoing electrical activity and that such neurons are fully capable of retracting their processes or establishing new synapses, the extent to which these processes occur in the absence of experimental manipulations is not easy to assess. Nevertheless, a variety of experiments have provided morphological evidence that such remodeling occurs normally, both at the neuromuscular junction and within the nervous system (e.g., Fig. 17–1). Some of these studies have examined changes in the structure of synapses as a function of the experiences to which an animal has been exposed. In addition, changes in the size of cell bodies, in the pattern of axonal branches, and in the number of synaptic contacts and of dendritic spines can be detected clearly in aged animals. Many of the biochemical pathways that initially regulate synapse formation, pathfinding, and even differentiation—for example, the Notch/Delta signaling pathway—continue to be present and active in mature neurons. The functional consequences of this substantial remodeling of neuronal

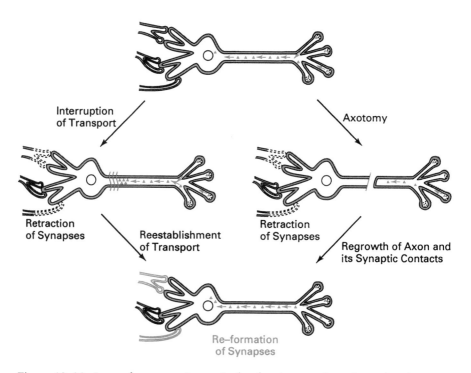

Figure 18–23. Loss of presynaptic terminals after interruption of axoplasmic transport or axotomy. Maintenance of presynaptic inputs may depend on a postsynaptic factor that is transported from the terminals back toward the soma.

structure in adult animals have yet to be discovered but are likely to reflect changes in learning and memory.

Transcription Factors are Activated by Neuronal Activity

This chapter has provided multiple examples of profound plastic changes
during development that are dependent on the ongoing electrical activity
of neurons. There exist biochemical pathways that transduce the external
signal—for example, calcium entry through calcium channels or the activation of a neurotransmitter receptor—into an intracellular message that
alters the expression of specific genes in the nucleus of a neuron or muscle cell. When any external stimulus switches a gene on or off, it acts
through transcription factors. These cellular switches control the synthesis of new sets of proteins, thereby effecting a change in the properties of
a cell. In Chapter 15, we alluded briefly to some of the transcription factors that contribute to neuronal differentiation. Some additional transcription factors are, however, of particular interest to the neurobiologist
because they can be activated rapidly by neuronal activity. Two such transcription factors are the fos and jun proteins. We shall encounter another
important transcription factor, cyclic AMP response element binding protein (CREB), in Chapter 20.

The *fos* and *jun* genes were first discovered as proto-oncogenes. An
oncogene is an aberrant gene that causes uncontrolled growth in a population of cells, while the term *proto-oncogene* is used to describe the normal cellular counterpart of the oncogene. At first one might think that,
although oncogenes should be of great interest to cancer researchers, they
may not be directly relevant to the study of neurons. However, it appears
that most oncogenes code for proteins that have counterparts in normal
cells, including neurons, and some of these normal gene products may have
specific roles in neuronal growth and in the response of neurons to external stimulation.

The fos and jun transcription factors belong to a large family of closely
related proteins. In many non-neuronal cells, exposure to growth factors
that stimulate cell division causes a very rapid synthesis of some of these
proteins (Fig. 18–24), which then move to the cell nucleus. For this reason, the genes for these transcription factors are sometimes termed
immediate-early genes, to reflect the fact that they are the first genes to
be activated in response to a stimulus to the cell. The fos and jun proteins
both contain a helical region in which the amino acid leucine is found at
every seventh position. This relatively common structural motif is known
as a *leucine zipper*. It tends to be involved in protein–protein interactions,

and its presence in the fos and jun proteins allows them to form a dimer. In fact the jun protein also exists as a dimer with other related transcription factors. The protein dimer then binds to certain sequences on DNA and thereby regulates the ability of nearby genes to be transcribed into messenger RNA. The fos–jun complex and its relatives can therefore be

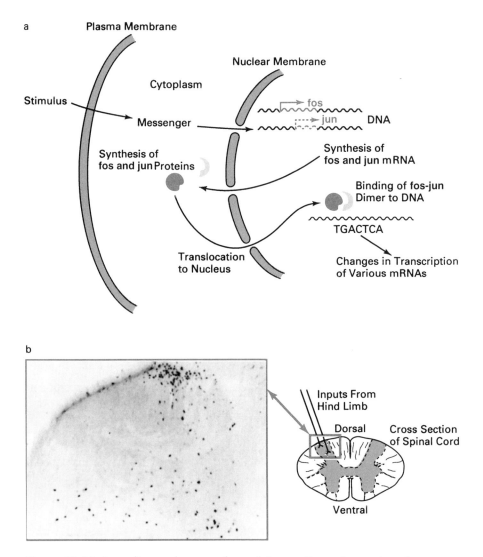

Figure 18–24. Immediate-early genes *fos* and *jun*. *a*: Formation and nuclear translocation of the fos and jun proteins after stimulation of a cell (Curran and Morgan, 1995). *b*: Steven Hunt and colleagues stained sections of spinal cord with antibodies to c-*fos*. This section came from an animal that had received noxious stimulation of a hind limb. Dark spots show the location of neuronal nuclei in which c-*fos* has been induced (Hunt et al., 1987).

thought of as messengers linking growth factor receptors to the synthesis of specific proteins. A variety of diverse factors including NGF, epidermal growth factor (EGF), insulin, and acetylcholine have been shown to induce *fos* expression as much as 100-fold in PC12 cells.

One particularly interesting aspect of the *fos* gene is that it can be induced by electrical activity alone, apparently as a result of calcium entry into cells. Even in certain adult neurons, synthesis of the fos protein can be evoked experimentally by manipulations such as direct electrical stimulation, application of convulsants or excitatory amino acids, and noxious sensory stimulation (Fig. 18–24). In fact, the localization of cells that begin to synthesize fos has been used as an anatomical tool to determine the neuronal pathways that are connected to a particular nerve or nucleus in the central nervous system. It has been suggested, therefore, that this transcription factor pathway allows short periods of neuronal stimulation to produce long-term changes in gene expression. Because there are families of regulatory proteins such as fos and jun, each family member may be evoked by a different stimulus to a neuron and in turn evoke a unique program of responses in the nucleus. It may be that such pathways contribute to long-term behavioral plasticity of the kind we shall discuss in Chapter 20.

Summary

When the developing axon reaches its appropriate postsynaptic target, it stops elongating. A series of characteristic morphological and biochemical changes, culminating in synapse formation, then occurs. Some of these are summarized in Table 18–1. Among the cues used by a neuron in choosing its correct postsynaptic partner are chemical labels that help to match appropriate pre- and postsynaptic cells. Not all synapses that form during development persist in the adult animal. Certain synapses are selectively stabilized, whereas others are lost. The pattern of electrical activity in the presynaptic neuron is important in the choice of synapses to be stabilized. It also regulates the properties of the postsynaptic cell.

Table 18–1 Some of the Steps in the Formation of a Chemical Synapse

1. Contact of the growth cone with an appropriate target
2. Increase in the release of neurotransmitter
3. Increase in the adhesion of the presynaptic terminal to the target
4. Elimination of other competing synapses by heterosynaptic suppression
5. Clustering of receptors at the postsynaptic membrane
6. Synthesis and insertion of new receptors at the postsynaptic membrane
7. Elimination of extrajunctional receptors

Synapses may also be broken and reformed continually in the adult animal. Some of the same mechanisms that govern synapse formation and stabilization during development contribute to this adult synaptic plasticity. This may be observed experimentally by severing presynaptic axons and allowing the synaptic terminals to degenerate. Neighboring undamaged axons come to occupy the vacated synaptic sites until the regenerating axon grows back to take them over again. Such connections may regenerate with sufficient specificity to allow recovery of appropriate synaptic function.

Molecular mechanisms involved in synapse formation and synaptic plasticity during development and in the adult are being vigorously pursued. Neurobiologists are still putting together a jigsaw puzzle in which ephrins, growth factors, receptor tyrosine kinases, neurotransmitters, and patterns of electrical activity are among the pieces. When the picture is complete, it should be possible to view the path by which an undifferentiated cell becomes a mature neuron, the involvement of electrical activity in determining the characteristics of the mature cell, and the role of various molecules in the plastic properties of the adult neuron.

19

Neural Networks and Behavior

*A*s cells go, neurons are not loners. Every function of the nervous system, from regulation of autonomic activities such as heartbeat to the control of complex animal behaviors such as dating and mating, reflects the coordinated action of a network of interacting neurons. A major challenge of neurobiology is to understand the nature of the interactions and computations that neural networks carry out. In this chapter, we describe a number of simple neural networks whose biological roles are known. These representative examples have been chosen to illustrate how specific cellular properties of different neurons in a network are essential to the function of the network as a whole.

Models of Neural Networks

It is evident that a network comprising many neurons may generate patterns of activity that could not have been predicted by the study of a single cell in isolation. These properties of a network that can be attributed to interactions between cells are referred to as its *emergent properties*. Over many years, attempts have been made to understand such emergent properties by analyzing simple mathematical or computer models of interacting units. Figure 19–1a illustrates a typical model network with a set of input units, some internal units, and a set of output units. The strength of a synaptic connection between one neuron and another, for example, neuron j and neuron k in the figure, is set by a parameter a_{jk} known as the *synaptic weight*. To make numerical calculation of the behavior of

507

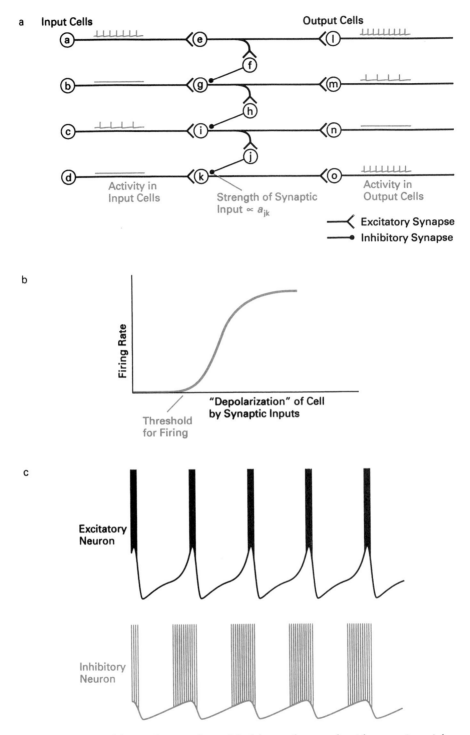

Figure 19–1. Model neural networks. *a*: Model neural network with synaptic weights assigned to each connection. *b*: Sigmoidal input–output function in a model neuron. *c*: Pattern of firing in a model neural network generating epileptiform activity (modified from Kaczmarek, 1976).

508

networks a practical proposition, it has usually been necessary to make highly simplified assumptions about the properties of single units in the network. For example, the earliest models assumed that a neuron has only two states: on when it fires an impulse and off when it is silent, much like elements in a digital computer. Many other models now assume a sigmoidal input–output function such as that shown in Figure 19–1b. In such cases the neuron fires as long as the balance of excitatory and inhibitory synaptic inputs from other cells in the network exceeds the threshold for firing. The firing frequency depends on the sum of the inputs at any given time.

The major lesson to be learned from such studies is that complex patterns of activity and relatively sophisticated computations can be carried out by networks of very simple units. For example, some networks can recognize patterns of inputs corresponding to letters of the alphabet. When stimuli in the shape of a letter *A* are applied to a two-dimensional array of input neurons, one set of output neurons will fire. A different set of output neurons fire when the shape *B* is applied. Other networks generate patterns of firing that very closely mimic pathological states, such as epileptic seizures (Fig. 19–1c). Still other networks tackle mathematical problems. In all cases, the responses of a network are in some way encoded in the pattern of activity of a set of output units. When the synaptic weights at individual connections are allowed to alter as a result of predetermined rules, the outputs of model networks may display features of learning.

The study of model networks is likely to have a profound influence in some engineering fields, for example, the design of computers, in years to come. Application to the understanding of real neurons and their interactions is also an emerging field, which will no doubt evolve as the advent of faster and more sophisticated computers accelerates the pace of theoretical modeling and allows the integration of what we learn about the properties of real neurons into the appropriate models. We shall now give an account of several real neural networks. Our goal is not to give an exhaustive review but rather to provide selected examples of how the intrinsic properties of neurons and their synaptic interactions shape the behavior of a network.

Networks Generating Rhythmic Movements

Central pattern generators. Many animal behaviors, such as walking or swimming, require the rhythmic contraction of muscles. We have already seen that a single neuron is capable of generating rhythmic bursts in the

absence of external stimulation. However, mos̲ ̲ ̲ ̲ic behaviors require that opposing groups of muscles be contra̲ ̲ ̲ ̲ ̲relaxed in a coordinated manner. This coordination can be carried out only by a network
in which different neurons innervate different muscles.

In theory, there are many ways to build a rhythmic network. For example, the generation and coordination of rhythmic movements could occur through a chain of reflexes in which receptors in the muscles signal
the state of extension or contraction of each muscle to the remainder of
the network, and this information would be essential for the network to
function rhythmically. If this were the case, the muscles themselves would
be integral components of the network. This, however, does not appear
to be the case for most rhythmic networks that have been examined in detail. Rather, the pattern of outputs to different muscles is generated by a
central pattern generator, a network of neurons that even in the absence
of direct feedback from the muscles themselves is capable of generating
the appropriate patterns of rhythmic excitation. (It is important to remember, however, that while sensory feedback is often not needed for the
basic rhythmic movements, it is required to shape these movements to the
needs of the animal in the real world.)

Rhythmic movements can be generated by networks with reciprocal inhibition. The
very simplest circuit that can generate alternating contraction and relaxation in two different muscles consists of only two neurons. Each neuron
makes an inhibitory synapse onto the other (Fig. 19–2a). For such a circuit to generate rhythmic output, it is not necessary that these neurons be
endogenously active in the absence of other synaptic inputs. However, it
is necessary for the neurons to display *postinhibitory rebound*. This simply means that after the membrane potential of the cell has been hyperpolarized for a short period of time, the cell becomes more excitable than
usual. When the membrane is then allowed to return to its normal resting potential, one or more action potentials may result. This is a relatively
common phenomenon in neurons, and when it follows an experimentally
applied hyperpolarizing current pulse as in Figure 19–2b, the action
potential is often termed an *anode break spike*. In some cases, the explanation for postinhibitory rebound is that an inward current, such as a
voltage-dependent sodium current or a T-type calcium current, is partly
inactivated at the resting potential. Transient hyperpolarization, for example, by an inhibitory input, removes some of this inactivation so that
the threshold for an action potential becomes more negative. As the cell
depolarizes toward the resting potential, the increased inward current triggers an action potential before inactivation again develops.

Networks based on the simple two-neuron circuit do indeed exist and contribute to locomotion in some species. Figure 19–2c illustrates the activity of two neurons in *Clione*, a small marine mollusc. This animal swims in the sea by moving a pair of wing-like structures (termed *parapodia*) that are alternately flexed in a dorsal and ventral direction. A major component of the central pattern generator for swimming appears to comprise four swim interneurons (Fig. 19–2c). One upswing neuron and one downswing neuron are found on each side of the nervous system. An action po-

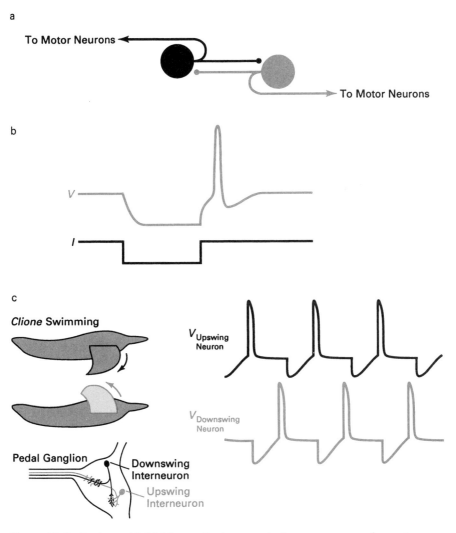

Figure 19–2. Reciprocal inhibition. *a*: Basic network that can generate alternating contraction and relaxation in two muscles. *b*: Anode break spike following a hyperpolarizing current pulse. (V, voltage I, current) *c*: Interneuron activity during swimming in *Clione* was studied by Satterlie (1985).

tential in an upswing neuron generates an inhibitory postsynaptic potential (IPSP) in a downswing neuron. Because of postinhibitory rebound, the downswing neuron generates an action potential at the end of the IPSP. This in turn triggers an IPSP in the upswing neuron. Thus a sustained ping-pong-like activity reverberates in this two-neuron network and is conveyed to the motor neurons that innervate the muscles in the parapodia, producing rhythmic swimming movements.

There is more than one way to design an oscillating network, even with only two neurons. For example, if individual neurons do not display postinhibitory rebound, but the firing of the individual neurons is subject to accommodation (see Fig. 3–13), a circuit such as that in Figure 19–2a can produce alternating bursts of action potentials provided that a source of maintained excitation is provided to the cells. The important point here is that the specific electrical properties of the individual neurons are the major factors that determine (1) whether the network oscillates, (2) the exact form of the oscillations (single action potentials, bursts, or some other pattern), and (3) the exact timing of the rhythm. The latter is particularly important as it translates directly into the behavior of the animal.

Multineuron networks allow flexibility. Central pattern generators in most nervous systems are substantially more elaborate and hence more versatile than simply two groups of mutually inhibitory neurons. The more complex the network, however, the more difficult it is for experimentalists to unravel the factors that make the system work. Table 19–1 lists some of the systems that have been used successfully to analyze the detailed neuronal interactions that control a variety of rhythmic behaviors. Many studies of this type have been carried out using invertebrates, primarily be-

Table 19–1 Examples of Some Oscillating Neural Networks That Have Been Analyzed

Species	Location of Oscillator	Behavior Controlled
Clione	Pedal ganglion	Swimming
Tritonia, sea slug	Cerebral and pleural ganglia	Swimming
Panuliris, spiny lobster *Homarus*, lobster *Cancer*, crab	Stomatogastric ganglion	Rhythmic stomach movements
Lobsters and crabs	Cardiac ganglion	Rhythmic contraction of heart muscle
Hirudo, leech	Segmental ganglia	Timing of heartbeat, swimming
Ichthyomyzon, lamprey	Spinal cord	Swimming

cause of the ease with which the intrinsic properties of invertebrate neurons can be analyzed and related to animal behaviors. Here, using the example of the crustacean stomatogastric ganglion, we shall summarize briefly some of the lessons that have been learned.

Rhythmic Neuronal Activity in Crustaceans

Although despised by gourmets, the stomachs of spiny lobsters and of crabs have provided pleasure to many neurobiologists. The stomach of such crustaceans is, like all of Gaul, divided into three parts: the cardiac sac, the gastric mill, and the pylorus (Fig. 19–3a). Food enters the stomach through the esophagus and is digested as it moves progressively through these three regions. Rhythmic contraction of muscles in all three regions contributes both to the physical disruption of the food and to movement through the stomach in a manner that resembles the chewing and swallowing of food by humans.

The stomatogastric ganglion. Muscles in the stomach are controlled by neurons in the stomatogastric ganglion, which contains 30 neurons. The three stomach regions are controlled by different sets of neurons. Initially, we shall consider only the central pattern generator for the pylorus, which consists of only 14 neurons. Synaptic connections between these are illustrated schematically in Figure 19–3b. The eight identical PY cells (lumped into a single neuron for simplicity in the figure), the two PD cells, and the VD, LP, and IC neurons are all motor neurons that directly innervate the pyloric muscles. Cell AB is an interneuron that makes connections only within the ganglion and sends information to the rest of the nervous system. Note that all the chemical synapses are inhibitory and that reciprocal inhibition between pairs of neurons is a dominant theme in the network. In addition, some pairs of neurons are coupled by electrical synapses.

As shown in Figure 19–4, the rhythmic output of the pyloric neurons may be recorded both by intracellular microelectrodes in individual neurons and by extracellular electrodes placed on the nerves containing axons from motor neurons such as LP and IC to different sets of muscles. Three different phases of bursting are recorded in the different nerves.

The first important lesson about the rhythm generated by the pyloric circuit is that it depends on the presence of inputs from other parts of the nervous system. Traces such as those of Figure 19–4 are recorded only when the inputs from two other ganglia are intact. When the nerve from these ganglia to the stomatogastric ganglion is blocked, rhythmic bursting ceases. This is not because the incoming inputs generate any rhythmic activity themselves. Instead, the neurotransmitters used by inputs from these other ganglia appear to act as local hormones (see Chapter 10). When the inputs are activated and release their hormones, the pyloric neurons acquire the specific electrical properties needed to generate rhythmic bursts. The repetitive bursts of action potentials in the AB neuron resemble those

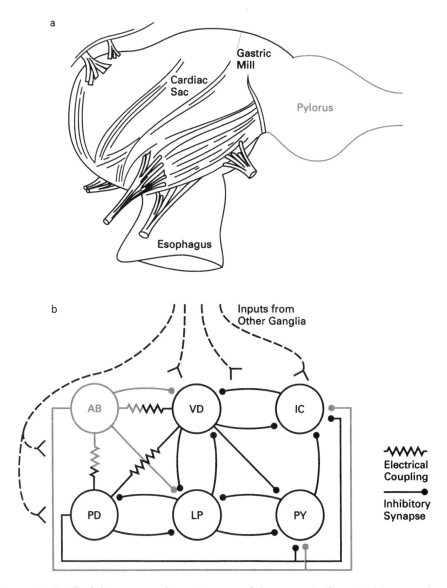

Figure 19–3. The lobster stomach. *a*: Diagram of the stomach (from Dickinson and Marder, 1989). *b*: Neuronal interactions in the pyloric network.

of *Aplysia* neuron R15, which was discussed in Chapter 13. In contrast to neuron R15, however, this pyloric neuron requires the presence of modulatory substances from the other ganglia to generate these bursts. This neuron can therefore be termed a *conditional burster*.

The other neurons of the pyloric network are not endogenously burst-

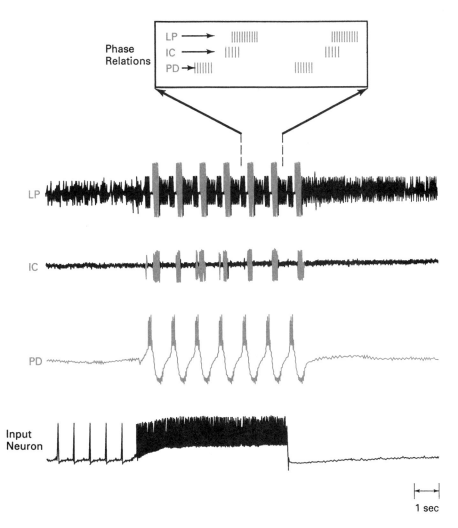

Figure 19–4. The pyloric rhythm. Recordings (made by Nusbaum and Marder, 1989) of rhythmic firing in three neurons (LP, IC, and PD) of the pyloric circuit during stimulation of a neuron with inputs to the ganglion. Because action potentials in the LP and IC neurons were detected with extracellular electrodes placed on nerves leading to the pyloric muscles, the activity of other neurons can also be seen in these recordings. The *inset* at the top shows phase relations among the three cells through two cycles.

ing neurons. In response to a brief depolarization, however, they can generate a single long burst of action potentials. This burst occurs because of a sustained, regenerative depolarization that outlasts the brief stimulus. This regenerative depolarization is sometimes termed a *plateau potential* or *driver potential* (Fig. 19–5). Again, this plateau depolarization occurs only when inputs from other ganglia have been activated.

Despite the fact that reciprocal inhibition can generate rhythmic activity, this is not the major factor that shapes the pyloric rhythm. Rather, it is the intrinsic burstiness of individual neurons that drives the network. The synaptic interactions and plateau potentials provide the appropriate phase relations and delays between the activities of different neurons. Only when the intrinsic electrical properties of the individual neurons in the network are considered is it possible to account for the timing and character of the bursts of action potentials that drive muscle contractions.

Modulatory neurotransmitters may "design" different networks. A period of dispassionate observation in a restaurant is sufficient to convince one that chewing and swallowing in humans are not simple processes but can take many different dynamic patterns, depending on the nature of the food and the psychological state of the diner. So it is with lobsters. The rhythmic output of the pyloric circuit does not always follow the very stereotyped pattern described above. When recorded in intact animals the phase, timing, and amount of activity in different motor neurons can vary with time and with the pattern of behavior of the animal.

In addition to simply maintaining the rhythm, inputs from other ganglia serve to fashion different patterns of activity. As we shall see, this may

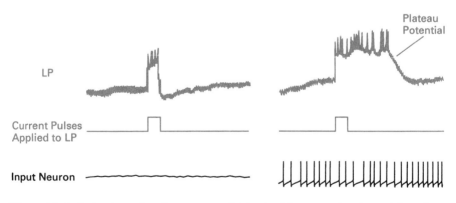

Figure 19–5. Induction of a plateau potential in the LP neuron by the activity of an input neuron (Moulins and Nagy, 1985).

occur because different transmitter substances act to effectively "rewire" the network into different configurations. A wealth of transmitters used by the inputs to the stomatogastric ganglion have been identified. These include acetylcholine, GABA, serotonin, dopamine, histamine, octopamine, and several neuropeptides including proctolin and an FMRFamide-like peptide. Because many of these act as local hormones, simple application of the transmitters to the external medium surrounding an isolated ganglion mimics the action of continuous firing in an input pathway. Here we shall compare the actions of two amines, serotonin and dopamine, when they are applied to the ganglion.

Figure 19–6a illustrates the effects of serotonin and dopamine on the properties of individual pyloric neurons when they are isolated from their synaptic inputs. Both of these agents induce endogenous bursting in interneuron AB. In contrast, PD motor neurons, which can fire at a low rate (but not burst) in the absence of synaptic input, are strongly inhibited by dopamine but not by serotonin. The VD neuron is strongly inhibited by both agents. LP and PY neurons are excited by dopamine but not by serotonin. Finally, neuron IC is excited by both agents. This inhibition or excitation of different neurons in the full network leads to a functional reorganization of the circuit. When either serotonin or dopamine is added to a stomatogastric ganglion that has been isolated from the neural inputs that would normally allow it to burst, they are able to reinstate the rhythm (Fig. 19–6b). The different amines, however, generate different rhythms. In fact, the two rhythms give the impression of being generated by very different networks, which, in a sense, they are.

This can be understood by a closer examination of the circuit. Neurons that are strongly inhibited, or simply not excited by serotonin, such as the VD, LP, and PY cells, are removed from the active circuit. Thus, in the presence of serotonin alone, the circuit is effectively driven by the endogenous activity of the AB–PD set of neurons (Fig. 19–6b). In the presence of dopamine, by contrast, both the endogenous bursting of AB and reciprocal inhibition between the LP and PY cells shape the output of the circuit. The influence on the pattern and timing of impulses from motor neurons to muscles is therefore different for serotonin and for dopamine. Other neuroactive amines and peptides have also been found to induce characteristic configurations of the circuit that differ from those of serotonin and dopamine. Each of these, in turn, differs from those observed when the combined spectrum of modulatory inputs from neurons in the other ganglia is allowed to tinker with the active pyloric circuit. Thus, by altering the excitability of specific neurons or the strength of individual connections, a wealth of different output patterns may be obtained.

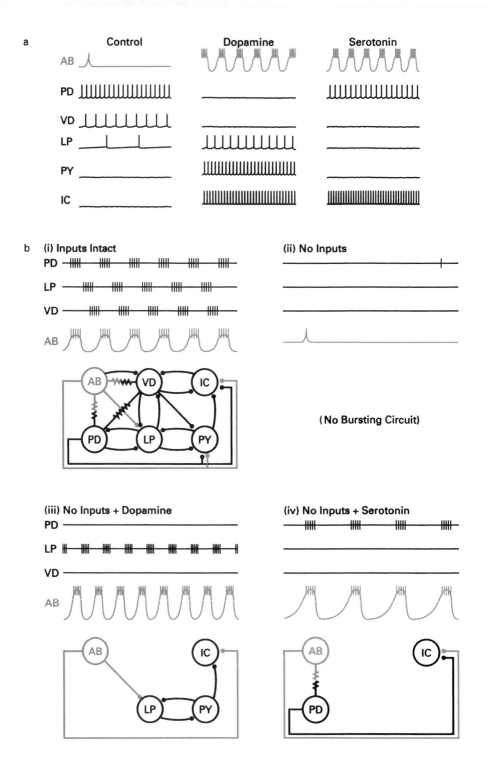

a   Control   Dopamine   Serotonin

AB

PD

VD

LP

PY

IC

b   (i) Inputs Intact   (ii) No Inputs

PD

LP

VD

AB

(No Bursting Circuit)

(iii) No Inputs + Dopamine   (iv) No Inputs + Serotonin

PD

LP

VD

AB

Overlapping networks. The neurotransmitter-induced insertion and excision of neurons into a circuit are not confined to a single network such as the pyloric. We have mentioned that the three different regions of the stomach are controlled by three different oscillating circuits in the stomatogastric ganglion. A neuron may participate in one or more of these circuits, depending on the state of inputs to the ganglion. For example, we have seen that neuron VD is an integral component of the pyloric network. It participates in the pyloric network, however, only when inputs from other ganglia allow this neuron to generate bursts driven by a plateau potential. These inputs are inhibited when certain sensory nerves are stimulated, and the VD neuron loses the ability to burst. When this happens, the change in its electrical properties allows it to become actively driven by neurons that generate the cardiac sac rhythm, a much slower oscillation than the pyloric. These remarkable examples of the flexibility that can occur in networks of very small numbers of neurons emphasize the importance of the endogenous properties of a cell in determining the behavior of a network. Moreover, they illustrate that modulatory changes in the electrical properties of neurons can produce changes in the output of a circuit that, at first glance, might be thought to require a physical rearrangement of synaptic connections. Some of the mechanisms of such modulation of neuronal electrical properties were covered in Chapter 13.

Command Systems of Neurons

Most animal behaviors do not persist day and night. Mechanisms must exist that allow activities such as walking, eating, swimming, and mating to be turned on and off. Furthermore, even relatively simple animal behaviors may require the coordinate activation or suppression of a number of apparently independent networks. These tasks are relegated to what are frequently termed *command systems* of neurons.

In some nervous systems, a single command neuron can exert control over relatively complex coordinated responses. The definition of a *command neuron* is that its activity should be both necessary and sufficient to

---

Figure 19–6. "Rewiring" the pyloric network. *a*: Actions of serotonin and dopamine on individual neurons in the pyloric circuit when synaptic connections with other cells have been eliminated. *b*: Actions of serotonin and dopamine on the intact pyloric circuit. Patterns of activity, together with the effective circuit diagram, are shown for four conditions: (*i*) "normal" rhythm with external inputs intact, (*ii*) no external inputs, (*iii*) no external inputs but with dopamine added to the ganglion, and (*iv*) no external inputs but with serotonin added (Harris-Warrick and Flamm, 1986).

trigger an entire coordinated behavior. For example, a flying cricket avoids high-pitched ultrasound, similar to that emitted by a bat, by contracting a set of muscles that causes the animal to fly away from the direction of the sound. Stimulation of a single identified neuron is able to trigger this behavior in a flying cricket. Moreover, when the neuron is hyperpolarized, the animal fails to respond to the sounds. In most animals, however, important behavioral decisions are not likely to be entrusted to a single neuron. Rather, command systems of neurons weigh the pros and cons of a given course of action before committing the animal to a specific choice. As in the case of rhythmic networks, a thorough analysis of such systems would be out of place in this book. We shall, however, describe three systems of neurons that preside over locomotor and reproductive behaviors, with an emphasis on the cellular properties of neurons in these command systems.

The swimming leech. The body of the medicinal leech *Hirudo medicinalis* is divided into segments (Fig. 19–7a). When it swims, it makes undulating motions with its body, in a manner generally similar to that of a fish or a snake. These movements result from the alternate contraction and relaxation of muscles in the body wall of the animal. In addition to neurons that control the head and tail of the animal, the ventral nerve cord comprises 21 ganglia, each of which innervates the muscles in one segment of the body. During swimming, rhythmic bursts of action potentials in motor neurons in each ganglion are carefully timed so that during one undulation a wave of contraction travels from the front to the rear of the animal.

Figure 19–7b presents a simplified scheme of the network that controls swimming. Numbers and letters have been given to identified neurons in the circuit. As in the examples described earlier, swimming in the leech results from the rhythmic output of a central pattern generator. Neurons that comprise the central pattern generator are found in each segmental ganglion, and the activity in each segment must be coordinated with that in adjacent segments. In part because of this greater complexity, the role of the intrinsic properties of different neurons and the extent to which they may be modified is not yet understood nearly as well as in the stomatogastric ganglion. However, reciprocal inhibition certainly is involved in generating the rhythmic bursts. The output of central pattern generator neurons is conveyed directly to motor neurons that innervate three sets of muscles.

A bout of swimming can be evoked by a brief, strong mechanical stimulus administered to the body of the animal. There appear to be at least two levels of neurons that act on the information from sensory neurons

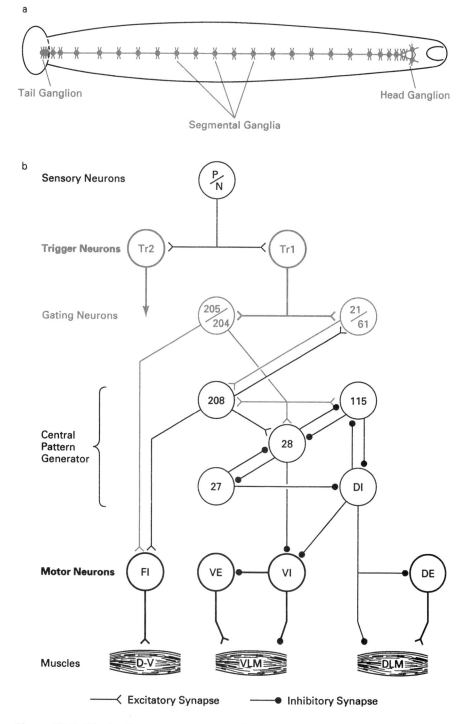

Figure 19–7. The leech nervous system. *a*: The nervous system of the leech comprises a chain of segmental ganglia. *b*: A simplified scheme of the network that controls swimming in the leech (modified from Friesen, 1989).

in the body wall before the central pattern generator can be set into motion. These are the *trigger* neurons and the *gating* neurons. Stimulation of the sensory pathway excites the trigger neurons, and experimental stimulation of the trigger neurons alone is sufficient to cause all of the neuronal activity that produces swimming. The duration of the swim that is induced, however, substantially outlasts the brief period during which the trigger neurons are active. This is because the transient stimulation of the trigger neurons leads to a more prolonged and sustained period of firing in the gating neurons (Fig. 19–8). The role of the gating neurons is, in some ways, similar to that of the inputs to the stomatogastric ganglion

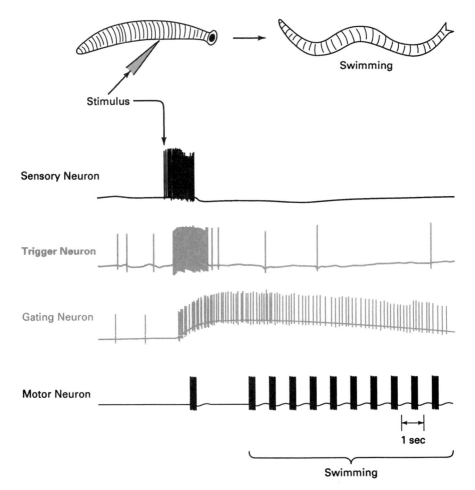

Figure 19–8. Trigger neurons. An experiment by Brodfuehrer and Friesen (1986) showed that transient activity in sensory neurons and in neuron Tr1 leads to a more prolonged and sustained period of firing in the gating neurons and motor output.

described earlier. The rhythmic activity of the central pattern generator is sustained only as long as the gating neurons are active. The gating neurons do not, however, provide the rhythm itself.

There are only a few trigger neurons, located in an anterior ganglion. They receive inputs from a large number of sensory neurons located along the length of the animal, and in turn project to a larger number of gating neurons, which are found in all of the segments. The trigger and gating neurons together may be considered to comprise the command system for swimming behavior.

A question that has yet to be answered is how the brief stimulation of trigger cells can lead to the sustained activity of the gating neurons. The answer is likely to lie in the actions of the neurotransmitters used in the synapses between the cells and in the membrane properties of the two types of cells. The cellular properties of these particular leech neurons have yet to yield their secrets, although it seems that long-term changes in membrane properties, of the kind discussed in Chapter 13, must occur. The beauty of leech swimming is that it provides a cellular explanation of how a transient behavioral stimulus can engage a more prolonged and relatively complex behavior, using a real network of neurons that can be identified at every level.

Locomotion in a "simpler" vertebrate. It is not by chance that, in this chapter, most of the examples of how the cellular properties of individual neurons shape the behavior of a network come from work with invertebrates. The relative ease with which individual neurons can be identified from animal to animal and the smaller numbers of cells in the networks have made invertebrate systems experimentally tractable. The complexity of the mammalian brain precludes this sort of detailed analysis. Nevertheless, lower vertebrates such as the lamprey have several orders of magnitude fewer neurons than mammals; through study of such animals, it has been possible to confirm that modulation of membrane properties determines how a network functions.

The eel-like lamprey swims by producing alternating contractions of the left and right sides of its body. The frequency of these contractions varies from one every five seconds, for slow movements, to ten per second for rapid swimming. Neurons that make up the pattern-generating circuit are found in each spinal segment, in a manner that resembles the leech nervous system. The principal components of these pattern-generating circuits are excitatory interneurons (E in Fig. 19–9a) and two types of inhibitory interneuron (L and C neurons). The C neurons on each side inhibit contralateral C neurons in the same spinal segment and in lower segments, providing the now familiar theme of reciprocal inhibition. This circuit can account for the basic alternating pattern of input to motor neurons. The pattern is shaped further by feedback from the muscles in the form of excitatory and inhibitory inputs from stretch receptor neurons (SR-E and SR-I in Fig. 19–9a).

The overall level of activity of the locomotor system is determined by neurons in the brain stem that are analogous to the gating neurons of the

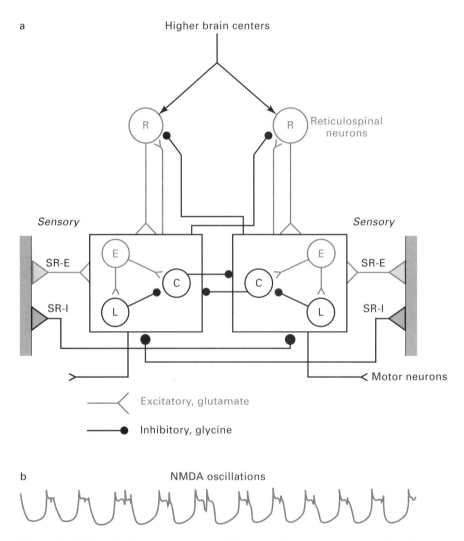

Figure 19–9. How the lamprey swims. *a*: Diagram of the pattern-generating circuit in one spinal segment and its input from the reticulospinal neurons, *b*: Oscillations of pacemaker potentials induced in pattern-generating neurons by treatment with NMDA (modified from Grillner et al., 1994). SR-E, excitatory stretch receptor; SR-I, inhibitory stretch receptor.

leech. The activity of these *reticulospinal neurons* (R neurons in Fig. 19–9a) both initiates the onset of swimming and controls the overall activity of the network. As their neurotransmitter the R neurons use glutamate, which activates both NMDA and KA/AMPA receptors on all of the neurons in the segmental networks. In addition to simply providing excitation to jump-start the pattern, this input from the R neurons induces plateau potentials in neurons of the pattern-generating network. We have already considered the importance of plateau potentials in generating the rhythmic behavior of the stomatogastric ganglion. For the lamprey, plateau potentials induced in the pattern-generating cells are particularly critical for slow movements, because they allow the network to maintain long-lasting stable bursts of action potentials.

The plateau potentials result from the activity of voltage-dependent ion channels in the plasma membrane. As in other cells with plateau potentials, voltage-dependent calcium channels contribute to the sustained depolarizing phase of the plateau potentials. In addition, the NMDA receptors play an important role in the lamprey pattern-generating neurons. In fact, the simple addition of NMDA to interneurons, in the presence of tetrodotoxin to block the connections between neurons in the network, is sufficient to induce repetitive plateau potentials (Fig. 19–9b). NMDA receptors are activated not only by the inputs from the R neurons but also by those from the E interneurons. In Chapter 11, we saw that NMDA receptors can be thought of as voltage-dependent cation channels that are gated by glutamate. Their voltage dependence arises because the channels are blocked by external magnesium ions at negative membrane potentials. At more positive potentials, the magnesium ions are expelled from the channel mouth, allowing sodium and calcium to flow through the channel, thereby depolarizing the cell (see Fig. 11–14). It is this voltage dependence that shapes the plateau potentials. Impulses from the R neurons, activating the KA/AMPA receptors, first produce a small depolarization in a pattern-generating interneuron. As the membrane depolarizes, however, the NMDA receptor channels begin to open. This, in turn, produces a larger depolarization, recruiting further NMDA receptor channels to produce the large sustained depolarizing phase of the plateau potential. Termination of each plateau phase is believed to occur because of calcium entry during the depolarization, which leads to the delayed activation of calcium-dependent potassium channels. These hyperpolarize the membrane back to rest so that the cycle may begin anew.

Many of the other lessons that we have learned about the role of intrinsic neuronal electrical properties from studying invertebrate networks also apply to the lamprey. For example, the amount of postinhibitory rebound and the rate of accommodation (see Fig. 3–13) in the pattern-generating neurons are key to generating specific outputs from the circuit. Moreover, as in the stomatogastric ganglion, such parameters are altered by inputs that use modulatory transmitters such as serotonin, dopamine, GABA, and somatostatin, which can reshape the network to generate a wide variety of frequencies and patterns of locomotion.

The bag cell neurons. We shall now turn to another command system of neurons, this time in the marine snail *Aplysia*. Two clusters of 200–400 cells each, located in the abdominal ganglion of this animal, control a sequence of very prolonged reproductive behaviors that lead to egg laying. Reproductive behaviors such as mating and egg laying are complex, even in *Aplysia*. For this reason the wiring diagram of the networks that control these behaviors is relatively poorly understood. In contrast, the cellular and molecular properties of the neurons in the command pathway for egg laying, termed the *bag cell neurons*, have been studied in substantial detail.

The bag cell neurons do not normally display any spontaneous electrical activity. In response to transient stimulation of an input from another ganglion, however, the cells depolarize and fire a long-lasting discharge of action potentials (Fig. 19–10a). Although the stimulus lasts only a few seconds, the evoked discharge usually persists for about 30 min. At the start of the discharge the neurons fire briskly for about 1 min, after which they settle down to a slower period of firing, during which the action potentials become enhanced in height and width (we have already discussed the molecular mechanisms of these changes in action potential shape in Chapter 13). When a discharge occurs in an intact animal, it is followed by a stereotyped sequence of behaviors. If the animal is feeding, it abandons its food. It then seeks out a vertical substrate such as the side of a rock, and begins a characteristic sequence of head movements before depositing its eggs on the rock. These behaviors occur because of the action of neuropeptides released from the bag cell neurons during the discharge.

In Chapter 8, we discussed the structure of the precursor protein from which the neuroactive peptides are cleaved in the bag cell neurons (Fig. 8–6b). The major neuroactive peptide released by the bag cell neurons is *egg-laying hormone* (ELH), which, when injected into animals, induces egg laying and its associated behaviors. During a discharge, ELH is released locally onto other neurons in the abdominal ganglion. There it induces a change in the electrical properties of several identified neurons (Fig. 19–10a). This peptide is also released directly into the blood from which it reaches peripheral targets and neurons in other ganglia, to influence the electrical properties of neurons in networks controlling activities such as feeding. In this way, ELH orchestrates changes in neural circuits that control different components of the evoked behaviors. In addition to

ELH, several smaller peptides (*bag cell peptides*, or BCPs) are cleaved from the precursor protein (Fig. 8–6b). These also act as neurotransmitters and alter the activity of other neurons in the abdominal ganglion. Moreover, the BCPs act at *autoreceptors* on the bag cell neurons to further influence their excitability. Interestingly, during the production of neurotransmitter-filled secretory granules, the BCPs are not packaged into the same populations of granules as those containing ELH. It is possible, therefore, that the BCPs are released at different times or at different sites from those of ELH. The role of the BCPs in the behaviors is, however, not known.

At the end of the 30 minute discharge, it is not possible to stimulate another long-lasting discharge, although intense electrical stimulation can

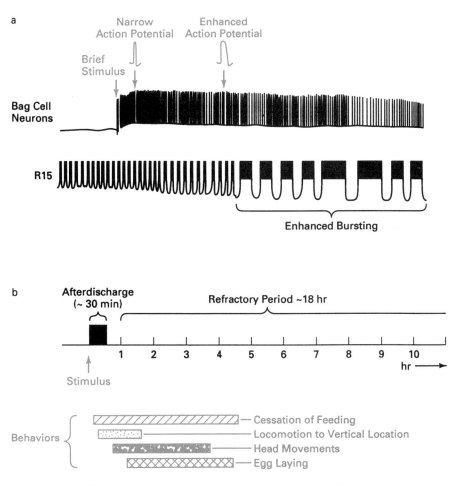

Figure 19–10. The bag cell neurons. *a*: Afterdischarge in bag cell neurons and the effects of egg-laying hormone (ELH) on neuron R15. *b*: Time scale of changes in excitability of the bag cell neurons (Conn and Kaczmarek, 1990).

sometimes trigger short discharges. Recovery from this period of inhibition, sometimes termed the *refractory period* (not to be confused with the action potential refractory period described in Chapter 3), occurs gradually over about 18 hours. As the sequence of behaviors triggered by a discharge can last for several hours, the bag cell neurons are in the refractory state during these behaviors (Fig. 19–10b). Thus, the prolonged refractory period may prevent the reinitiation of the behavioral sequence once it is underway and also serve to limit the frequency with which the behaviors can be evoked. Thus, by undergoing a sequence of changes in their endogenous properties by the mechanisms discussed in Chapter 13, the bag cell neurons act as a sophisticated master switch for the sequence of behaviors leading to egg laying.

Cellular Specializations for Rapid Communication of Sensory Information

The outputs of each of the networks that we have discussed thus far have been honed through evolution to generate different patterns of motor output. In such cases, it is easy to see that the intrinsic electrical properties, such as the ability to generate patterned bursts of action potentials, can be adapted to shape the eventual behavior of an animal. Having the right types of channels, receptors, and synaptic structures can, however, be equally important for the transmission and analysis of sensory information. We shall now consider a network within the auditory system that rapidly computes facts about the outside world. It does so thanks to very specific characteristics of the neurons within the network.

Action potential timing in auditory brain stem networks. For some neural networks, both real and theoretical, the exact timing of action potentials is not critical. For example, in the bag cell neurons described above, the occurrence of a train of action potentials triggers a behavior, but individual action potentials hold no significance. In other networks, however, the precision with which an action potential fires is of the utmost importance. One of the clearest examples of this occurs in neurons in the brain stem that calculate differences in the sounds that arrive at the two ears. In Chapter 14, we emphasized that while most sensory systems use relatively slow second messenger pathways for transduction, the mechanics of hair cells in the cochlea allows them to respond to sounds very rapidly. The neurons that receive this information must also respond equally rapidly.

Transmitter release from the cochlear hair cells activates neurons in the *spiral ganglion* located in the cochlea itself. These, in turn, send their axons into the brain where they terminate on a variety of neurons in the *cochlear nucleus* (Fig. 19–11a,b). Among these is a class of neurons termed *bushy cells*, which have the ability to *phase-lock* their action potentials to a sound stimulus. When a sinusoidal sound with a frequency of several hundred Hz is presented to the cochlea, these neurons follow the stimulus, firing their action potentials at a very precise point during each sine wave (Fig. 19–11c). Our ability to hear accurately requires two things of these cells. First, they must be capable of firing at extremely high rates (up to 500–1000 Hz). Secondly, the timing of each action potential must be accurate to within a few microseconds. This accuracy of timing is required even at higher frequencies of sound, when the neurons fire action potentials during only some of the individual waves.

Probably much of what we hear and interpret, such as speech and music, requires this degree of accuracy. A particularly clear example, however, is our ability to determine the source of a sound in space. This is accomplished by neuronal networks that compare the difference in time of arrival of sounds at the two ears (Fig. 19–11c), as well as their relative intensities. Phase-locking neurons are essential for this. For example, one component of the network is the *medial superior olive* (MSO), which receives excitatory input from bushy cells on both sides of the brain, i.e., from both ears (Fig. 19–11a). A neuron in the MSO may fire when, and only when, the timing of excitatory inputs it receives from each ear is exactly balanced. Thus some MSO neurons will fire only when a sound stimulus occurs directly in front of a subject. Because axonal conduction to individual neurons in the nucleus takes a finite time, however, each MSO neuron receives inputs a little earlier or later than its neighbor. Thus, for some MSO neurons, the timing of inputs is balanced only when a sound arrives earlier at the right ear, while for others, simultaneous activation of its two inputs occurs when a sound originates on the left. In fact, there appears to be an orderly anatomical arrangement of "delay lines" such that the position of a sound stimulus can be mapped to specific locations in the MSO (Fig. 19–11a).

Another comparison of inputs from left and right occurs in another auditory nucleus, the *lateral superior olive* (LSO) (Fig. 19–11b). As with the MSO, the LSO receives an excitatory input from bushy cells on the same side of the brain. The input from the contralateral side, however, is an inhibitory one. Rather than sending their axons directly to LSO neurons on the opposite side, the bushy cells make a connection onto neurons in the *medial nucleus of the trapezoid body* (MNTB). These neurons, which use the inhibitory neurotransmitter glycine, then continue the signal to the LSO. This integration of the excitatory inputs from one side and inhibitory inputs from the other is again thought to compute the direction of a sound stimulus, using both the intensity and timing of sounds as cues.

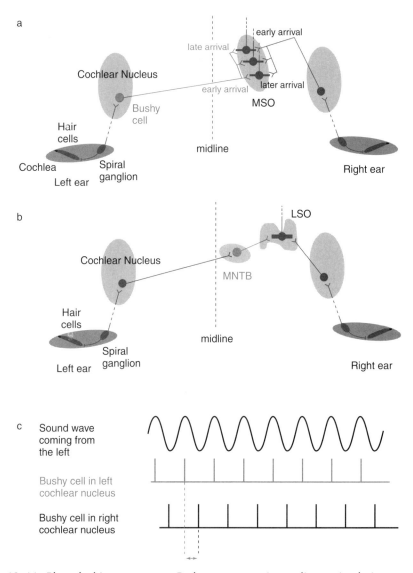

Figure 19–11. Phase-locking neurons. *a*: Pathways connecting auditory stimulation to the medial superior olive (MSO). *b*: Connections to the lateral superior olive (LSO) are from excitatory bushy cells on one side and inhibitory medial nucleus of the trapezoid body (MNTB) neurons from the other. *c*: Many auditory neurons lock their action potentials to a specific phase of a sinusoidal sound stimulus. The delay between two phase-locked action potentials in different neurons can be used to compute parameters such as the direction of a sound source.

What are the cellular specializations that allow these networks to function? The specific types of potassium channels and synaptic receptors within the bushy cells and neurons of the MNTB are essential for the rapid responses of these cells. Potassium channels that are open near the resting potential ensure that the membrane time constant is very small (see Chapter 3), allowing the cells to respond very rapidly to stimulation. Potassium channels also ensure that only a single action potential is evoked by each synaptic stimulus. A specific type of delayed rectifier potassium channel allows the cells to fire at very high rates with little or no relative refractory period (see Fig. 3–6). Without this particular channel, the cells are unable to follow high-frequency stimuli (Fig. 19–12a). A specific form of

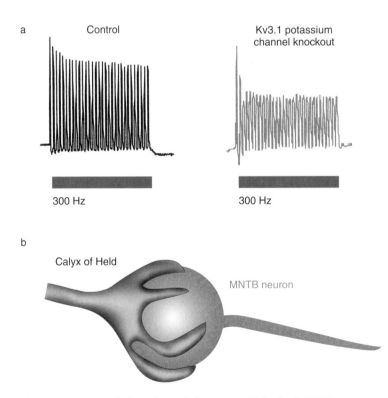

Figure 19–12. Medial nucleus of the trapezoid body (MNTB) neurons. *a*: Firing pattern of a control MNTB neuron and one in which a delayed rectifier potassium channel, termed the Kv3.1 channel, has been deleted by genetic manipulation. When stimulated at 300 Hz, the control neuron responds to every stimulus, while in the knockout, full action potentials are generated only at the onset of stimulation (Macica et al., 2000). *b*: A calyx of Held synaptic ending, which is at the terminal of a Bushy cell, surrounds the cell body of an MNTB neuron.

glutamate receptor of the AMPA subclass (see Table 11–4), which activates and inactivates very rapidly, is used in the excitatory synapses onto bushy cells and MNTB neurons.

Finally, the structure of the synaptic connections between these auditory neurons is exquisitely adapted to their activity. To achieve the rapidity and accuracy of transmission that is required, enormous excitatory postsynaptic currents are generated in the postsynaptic bushy cells and MNTB neurons. These large currents ensure that a presynaptic action potential produces an almost immediate depolarization of the postsynaptic cells to the threshold for firing. Enormous currents require enormous synapses. The synaptic endings onto the bushy cells (termed the *end-bulbs of Held*) and those onto the MNTB neurons (termed the *calyces of Held*) are the largest synapses in the central nervous system. A single synaptic ending on an MNTB neuron is shaped much like a baseball glove and completely envelops its cell body (Fig. 19–12b). Indeed, because of the ease of recording from these large endings, the calyx of Held is becoming a favored preparation for investigators of the mechanisms of synaptic transmission.

The electrical and morphological characteristics of the bushy cells and MNTB neurons are essential for their ability to transmit auditory information. The system simply would not work the same way if one were to substitute a different set of channels and synaptic components into these neurons. Nevertheless, modulation of excitability and secretion occurs in these neurons, and probably adapts them to different patterns of auditory stimuli and ambient acoustic environments.

Clocks in the Brain: The Generation of Circadian Rhythms

As we stated at the outset of this chapter, we have chosen examples of neuronal networks in which specific cellular properties of neurons within the network are essential for the function of the entire network. Another particularly clear example of this is found in neurons that control cyclic behaviors such as waking and sleeping. In all animals, there are neurons that fire with a *circadian rhythm*, a 24-hr cycle during which the neurons fire at a relatively high rate for about 12 hr and then are silent or much less active for the remainder of the cycle. The activity of these neurons controls the sleep–wake cycle. These rhythms of firing are entirely intrinsic to individual neurons, which can manifest these slow cycles even when isolated in a culture dish. As anyone who has recovered from jet lag can attest, however, their activity in an intact brain can slowly be reset by a change in the light–dark cycle.

In many invertebrates, these neurons are located in the retina. Although mammals also have cells in the retina that display a circadian rhythm, the master switch for the circadian behavior of the entire animal is located in the *suprachiasmatic nucleus*, a small nucleus of the hypothalamus. During a normal day, the firing rate of these neurons is highest at about noon, and is lowest during the night. These neurons receive inputs from the retina and project to other regions of the hypothalamus and to the thalamus. Their activity produces the circadian oscillations that occur in the levels of many hormones and also indirectly controls the different motor patterns that are associated with nighttime and daytime.

How is this slow rhythm generated? This question is not unique to neurons. Internal biological clocks that regulate rhythmic behaviors are found in many different organisms, including cyanobacteria. In all cases, although the circadian rhythms can be synchronized to the light–dark cycle, they can also persist with a similar period in the complete absence of environmental cues. Clues to the molecular basis for the clock have arisen from detailed genetic and molecular analyses of a variety of simple systems, including our old friend, the fruit fly *Drosophila*, which exhibits circadian rhythmicity in locomotion and other behaviors.

The circadian clock in *Drosophila* and other organisms is composed of a number of genes (so-called clock genes), the protein products of which can feed back to regulate their own synthesis. Some of these genes [with colorful names such as *period* (*per*), *timeless* (*tim*), *doubletime* (*dbt*), *clock* (*clk*), and *cycle* (*cyc*)] and the interactions among their protein products are illustrated in Figure 19–13a. It will be evident that these various components form what can be thought of as a *molecular feedback network* within neurons (and other cell types) that can generate regular oscillations in the cellular levels of the clock gene mRNA and protein products (Fig. 19–13b). These oscillations are in turn used by the organism, by mechanisms that remain largely unknown, to produce rhythms in various physiological processes and behaviors (Fig. 19–13c). It is interesting that very similar molecular players seem to be involved in the circadian clocks of many different organisms, for example, in flies and in mice, but the interactions among them may not be the same in all cases. The general idea of a molecular network in which clock genes regulate the synthesis of components such as ion channels or neurohormones is likely to apply to the neurons of the suprachiasmatic nucleus.

Although there has been enormous progress in identifying the molecular components of circadian clocks, many features that contribute to making biological clocks tick, for example, how light regulates the circadian cycle and how the molecular oscillations are converted to rhythmic behavioral outputs, are not yet completely understood. Because of wide-

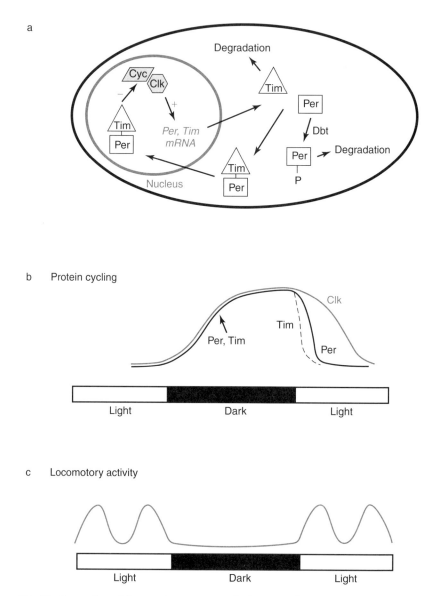

Figure 19–13. Examples of interactions among clock genes that participate in circadian rhythmicity. *a*: Tim and Per proteins dimerize and enter the nucleus, where they feed back and inhibit transcription of their own mRNAs by inhibiting the Cyc and Clk transcription factors. In the cytoplasm, Per degradation is promoted by its phosphorylation, via the protein kinase Dbt. *b*: Stable rhythms result from the fact that different clock gene mRNA and protein products have different half-lives. *c*: The molecular rhythms give rise to behavioral rhythms by mechanisms that are still being elucidated.

spread interest in the large array of circadian behaviors exhibited by creatures throughout the phylogenetic scale, this can be characterized as a growth area of modern cellular and molecular neurobiology, and it seems reasonable to expect continued rapid progress on these questions in the future.

Networks with Electrical Synapses

In the networks that we have described, many of the interactions among neurons occur through chemical synapses or local hormonal actions. Another important category that must not be overlooked is networks in which the cells interact via electrical synapses, mediated by gap junctions (see Chapter 8). In such networks, neurons are coupled electrically such that an action potential may propagate from one cell to the next with no chemical intermediary. In fact, some of the cells discussed above, for example, cells AB and PD in the stomatogastric ganglion, are electrically coupled and therefore tend to fire together during bursts. Electrical synapses among individual bag cell neurons act to preserve synchrony of firing in this population of neurons. Gap junctions between the reticulospinal neurons and the pattern-generating cells of the lamprey also contribute to excitation of these cells.

It is important to realize, however, that the role of electrical coupling may be more than simply to make two cells behave as one. Many groups of neurons that do not fire in synchrony have been found to be connected by electrical synapses, both in vertebrates and invertebrates. In some electrically coupled networks, action potentials can reverberate through the network, producing a sustained burst, which terminates when full synchrony is achieved. Such a burst has been found to underlie the activity of neurons in the command system for escape swimming in the sea slug *Tritonia*, for example. Other changes in the mode of operation of a network can occur when electrical synapses between neurons are subject to modulation by chemical synaptic inputs. For example, in the retina of vertebrates such as fishes and turtles, a class of neurons known as *horizontal cells* is coupled electrically. The neurotransmitter dopamine, acting through the second messenger cyclic AMP in these cells, produces a strong decrease in the strength of this coupling. This in turn causes a decrease in the area of the visual field to which an individual horizontal cell responds. Such modulatory effects of neurotransmitters on synaptic networks are likely to have profound effects on the way the network processes incoming information.

Summary

In previous chapters we discussed the properties of individual neurons or pairs of neurons connected by a single synapse. However, complex interactions, involving both chemical and electrical synaptic connections among larger numbers of neurons, are required to generate most behaviors. Mathematical models, as well as studies in biological model systems, have provided insights concerning the organization of neurons into the neural networks that underlie particular behaviors. Some neurons can participate simultaneously in more than a single network, and the properties of a network may be modulated by the actions of neurotransmitters and hormones. In some cases the activation of a single command neuron or command system of neurons can trigger a complicated and long-lasting behavior. Intracellular molecular feedback networks are also important for generating complex patterns of behavior. In the next chapter we shall consider some neuronal properties that may be involved in the phenomena of learning and memory.

20

Learning and Memory

We saw in the previous chapter that animals exhibit different kinds of behavior. There are, for example, *fixed-action patterns*, behaviors that always occur in a fixed and stereotyped manner once they are triggered. The trigger for a particular fixed-action pattern may arise from within the animal, as, for example, in the case of a chemical cue that appears at a certain time during development. Alternatively, fixed-action patterns may be triggered by a specific set of environmental conditions. It is thought that the neural circuitry underlying these invariant behaviors is more-or-less hard wired, that it is specified by the genome and is only to a limited extent subject to modulation. Many, but by no means all, behaviors in invertebrates and lower vertebrates tend to fall into this hard-wired category. We have seen, however, that modulation by neurotransmitters allows a considerable variety of behavioral outputs to be generated by a single hard-wired circuit.

This pattern changes as we move up the phylogenetic tree. Although many behaviors, particularly rhythmic ones such as breathing and locomotion, remain essentially hard wired in higher vertebrates including humans, many more examples of adaptive behavior begin to appear. In this chapter we will consider two closely related behavioral phenomena that are crucial for animals to survive: learning and memory. We may define *learning* in very broad terms as a change in behavior as a result of experience, and *memory* as the ability to store and recall learned experiences.

How the brain encodes, stores, and retrieves memories has fascinated not only scientists but the lay public for thousands of years. There is good reason for this wide interest in learning and memory. They are essential

537

ingredients in defining an animal (or human being) as an individual. In addition, the complexity of the nervous system makes the understanding of such higher functions a challenging and exciting intellectual goal. Accordingly, many scientists from different disciplines have devoted their careers to the study of learning and memory, including the search for the *engram*, the physical memory trace in the brain; and technical and conceptual advances during the last few decades have produced substantial and exciting progress. An in-depth treatment of the various forms of learning and memory that have been defined and characterized by neuropsychologists is well beyond the scope of this book. We will focus here on several simple kinds of behavioral phenomena, the mechanisms of which are beginning to be clarified with the techniques of cell and molecular biology.

Different Kinds of Learning and Memory

Before proceeding further we must define several different classes of behavioral modification exhibited by nervous systems. Historically, it has been useful to divide both learning and memory into two categories: *nonassociative* and *associative* learning and *short-term* and *long-term* memory (Fig. 20–1).

Nonassociative learning: habituation and sensitization. Habituation and sensitization are two simple forms of learning that involve a change in the intensity of response to a stimulus. *Habituation* can be defined simply as a decrement in the behavioral response during repeated presentations of the same stimulus. It is a form of learning that is observed in invertebrates and in all vertebrate species including humans. An example might be the diligent student of cellular and molecular neurobiology who is trying to study when the student is interrupted by some distracting noise, for example, a radio playing in the next room. Although initially the stimulus—the noise—interferes with the ability to concentrate, after many repetitions

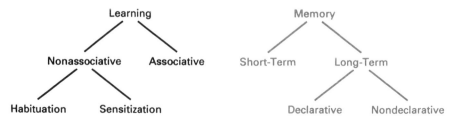

Figure 20–1. Categories of learning and memory.

of the noise the nervous system for all intents and purposes stops responding, and the contemplation of ion channels can resume.

Sensitization is functionally the opposite of habituation, in that it can be defined as the enhancement of a reflex response by the introduction of a strong or noxious stimulus. It also differs from habituation in that the sensitizing stimulus is different from the stimulus that elicits the reflex. Furthermore there is no specificity—there is a general arousal of the nervous system, and all reflex pathways are strengthened. To carry our analogy further, if the diligent student is startled by the loud ringing of a telephone, the student may subsequently be more distracted by the radio than when it was first turned on. Sensitization has important adaptive value; it allows a novel stimulus to alert an animal to possible predators and other potentially harmful stimuli in its environment.

Associative learning. Associative learning is more complex than habituation or sensitization, in that two stimuli must be closely associated in time for learning to occur. When a normally ineffective or neutral conditioned stimulus is paired temporally with a meaningful unconditioned stimulus, the animal learns to respond to the former as if it were the latter. The archetypal example of such *classical conditioning* is that of Pavlov's dogs, who learned to associate the ringing of a bell (the conditioned stimulus) with the presentation of food (the unconditioned stimulus), and would salivate in response to the bell alone. The unconditioned stimulus might be *reinforcing*, as in the example above, or *aversive*, for example, an electric shock, in which case the animal will take the conditioned stimulus as a cue and attempt to escape the aversive unconditioned stimulus associated with it. In contrast with nonassociative learning, which does not involve any temporal relationship between stimuli, associative conditioning allows the animal to draw conclusions about causal relationships in its environment. There is another category of conditioning with different characteristics, called *operant conditioning*, which we will not consider here.

Short-term and long-term memories: different mechanisms. Another important concept that has arisen from studies in invertebrates and a variety of vertebrates including humans is that there are at least two temporally distinct forms of memory (Fig. 20–1). *Short-term memory* is the ability to acquire new information and retain it for periods of time ranging from a few seconds to some minutes. In contrast, *long-term memory* can involve retention for hours, days, years, or even a lifetime. Both associative and nonassociative learning can exhibit these two temporal components. An example of this distinction in real life involves looking up a new telephone number and retaining it in short-term memory (often with rehearsal, for example, by repeating it continuously) long enough to dial it. A few minutes after dialing, the number will no longer be available in memory. Only those few numbers that are dialed (and hence rehearsed) often eventually find their way into long-term memory storage.

The finding that certain localized brain lesions disrupt long-term but not short-term memory suggests that different brain regions are involved in storage and retrieval in these two categories of memory. This will be discussed in more detail later in this chapter. Other experiments suggest that the molecular mechanisms that underlie short- and long-term memory are also different. For example, electroconvulsive shock selectively prevents the setting down of long-term memory traces. In addition, as we shall see below, inhibition of protein synthesis has no effect on the acquisition and short-term retrieval of a new behavior, but does inhibit long-term memory.

Organization of Memory in the Brain: The Search for the Engram

To explore the biophysical and molecular mechanisms that contribute to learning and memory, it is necessary to identify the cells that participate in the memory trace. In fact, the difficulty in locating the memory trace has been the greatest barrier to progress in understanding molecular mechanisms of learning and memory. The quest for the physical basis of the memory trace can be pursued at many levels of organization. The first step is localizing the engram to a particular organ. Although we take it for granted now that the brain is the right organ, there is evidence that the early Egyptians thought the heart and liver were the seat of human emotions and behavior. This conclusion was based on simple kinds of experiments: for example, if you remove the heart from an animal, it stops behaving. By the time of Hippocrates a millennium later, it was recognized by many that organs like the heart are necessary simply to keep the brain alive (cardiac chauvinists may object to this simplification), and at the end of the nineteenth century Santiago Ramón y Cajal expressed the central role of the brain in lyrical and eloquent terms:

> To know the brain is the same thing as knowing the material course of thought and will, the same thing as discovering the intimate history of life in its perpetual duel with eternal forces, a history summarized and literally engraved in the defensive nervous coordination of the reflex, the instinct, and the association of ideas.

But localization of the memory trace to the brain was only the beginning. We shall see that narrowing things down further to a particular brain region, and to individual neurons within that region, has proven to be a much more formidable task. However, there are several behavioral paradigms in vertebrate and invertebrate animals for which cellular correlates are now available, and we are learning much about the cellular, biophysical, and molecular mechanisms that may be responsible for some elementary forms of learning in these neural circuits. In new in vivo imaging techniques, now in widespread use in clinical medicine, measures of local blood flow are used to define brain regions in which neuronal electrical activity is changing (see Plate 10). In addition to their clinical utility, these techniques have been enormously useful in studying memory localization and other cognitive functions in humans and nonhuman primates.

Where in the brain is the memory trace? The great neuropsychologist Karl Lashley spent some three decades during the first half of the 20th century trying to locate the engram in rodents. The basic approach was to train animals in a particular task, then to make lesions of the nervous system and ask whether the animals could still remember how to perform the task. The consistent result was that no single part of the brain was essential for long-term memory; impaired performance was proportional to the extent of the lesion but was not dependent on its location. In an influential 1950 paper entitled "In Search of the Engram," Lashley summarized his career-long search by concluding (somewhat plaintively) that there is no discrete memory trace, but that memories are distributed diffusely throughout the brain:

> This series of experiments has yielded much information about what and where the memory trace is *not*. It has discovered nothing directly of the real nature of the memory trace. I sometimes feel, in reviewing evidence on localization of the memory trace, that the necessary conclusion is that learning is just not possible. Nevertheless, in spite of such evidence against it, learning does sometimes occur.

We now have a good idea why Lashley's efforts were unsuccessful. The maze learning task that he used depends on many kinds of sensory information and cognitive functions that are processed and stored separately in different parts of the brain. Localized lesions may eliminate part of this information, but what remains is sufficient to allow the animals to perform the task, albeit less proficiently.

In thinking about the engram, it is important to distinguish among different kinds of long-term memory that have been elucidated (Fig. 20–1). Some of these distinctions have come from the study of human subjects who are amnesic as a result of accidental or surgical brain damage. *Nondeclarative* knowledge includes memory for skills and procedures—

knowing *how*—for example, the rules of a game. Such knowledge depends on many different kinds of information that are processed and localized separately in different brain regions. It can be acquired even by severely amnesic human subjects. In contrast, *declarative* knowledge involves the memory of specific facts or events—knowing *that*—and new long-term memories of this class cannot be acquired by the amnesic patients. Some of the most striking evidence in support of these concepts comes from studies with amnesic patients who can remember new factual information for only a very short time and cannot store new long-term declarative memories. However, when such patients are taught to read words in a mirror, they learn at a normal rate to carry out this complex task and they retain the mirror-reading skill when retested months later. Interestingly, the (nondeclarative) skill is retained, although they do not remember the specific words themselves or even the (declarative) fact that they have ever been trained to perform the task. When asked why they are able to perform so well they may reply that they are "just good at that sort of thing."

It is now evident from anatomical studies, either at autopsy or using in vivo imaging techniques, that many of these amnesic patients have suffered damage to the *limbic system*, a group of cortical structures that includes the amygdala, the hippocampus, and anatomically related structures (Fig. 20–2). When similar lesions are produced surgically in non-

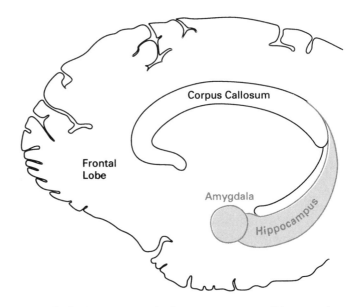

Figure 20–2. Structures in the brain important for long-term memory. Diagram after one drawn by Larry Squire depicting the medial aspect of the human brain to illustrate structures important in the setting down of long-term memories.

human primates, similar defects in declarative (but not in nondeclarative) memory tasks are observed. A wide variety of other animal studies have also implicated the hippocampus in certain kinds of learning and memory. It is believed that the long-term memory traces themselves are not stored there, but rather that the hippocampus participates in memory acquisition and in establishing an enduring and retrievable memory elsewhere. Furthermore, the role of the hippocampus is limited to the acquisition and storage of declarative knowledge.

Other studies have suggested that the cerebellum is involved in certain kinds of learned behaviors. One analysis has been carried out on a learned eyeblink response in the rabbit. Through lesioning studies it has been found that a portion of the cerebellum, on the opposite side of the brain from the trained eye, is essential for the learning and retrieval of the response. Another kind of learning that has been localized to the cerebellum is adaptation of the *vestibuloocular reflex*, a compensatory eye motion in response to head turn. The relevant neuronal pathways involved in this example of *motor learning* are now sufficiently well defined that cellular changes in the circuit, associated with the learning, can be explored. Finally, there is an important category of short-term memory called *working memory*, in which representations are formed from the combination of immediate sensory information and stored memories. These representations are stored transiently in cortical regions, most notably the frontal lobe (Fig. 20–2).

Molecular Mechanisms of Memory

Even without detailed information about the localization of the memory trace, it is still possible to ask general questions about the molecular mechanisms that may be involved in learning and memory. Two distinct approaches to this question, the interference approach and the correlation approach, have been important historically. More recently, a powerful genetic approach has also been exploited. We will consider each of these approaches in turn.

The interference approach. The interference approach requires one to make a reasonable guess about the involvement of a particular molecular mechanism in learning and memory, and then use pharmacological agents that interfere with that mechanism to see whether acquisition and/or retrieval are affected. In the 1950s and 1960s a popular guess was that protein synthesis is required for long-term memory. As reasonably specific inhibitors of protein synthesis became available, investigators administered the inhibitors to animals subjected to several different training paradigms. Let us examine, as a typical example of this approach, an avoidance response to an aversive stimulus in goldfish or mice.

Creatures such as goldfish or mice can be trained to avoid an electric shock by pairing the shock with light. In one classic example of a *conditioned avoidance response*, the fish (or mice) learn to associate a light at one end of the their tank (or cage) with the subsequent shock, and escape from the shock by moving to the opposite side of the tank (or cage) whenever they see the light. As shown in Figure 20–3a, the animals acquire the behavior rapidly and retain it for many hours and even days after the training has ended. At various times before, during, or after training, the animals can be injected with puromycin or cycloheximide, inhibitors that block protein synthesis in their brains by more than 90%. If the inhibitor is injected immediately prior to testing of the already trained animals, it is without effect, demonstrating that inhibition of protein synthesis does not alter recall or performance (Fig. 20–3b; compare with Fig. 20–3a). On the other hand, if the inhibitor is injected immediately after training, the memory (as tested hours or days later) is inhibited completely (Fig. 20–3c). Injections at progressively later times within the first hour following training produce progressively less of an impairment. These results demonstrate that the laying down of the long-term memory trace requires protein synthesis during the first hour or so following training. Finally, if the inhibitor is injected immediately prior to training, the acquisition is completely normal, but again the long-term memory is blocked (Fig. 20–3d). Thus these experiments point to protein synthesis as being necessary for the establishment of long-term memory, but not for the short-term memory that is required during acquisition.

Although the precise timing of the short- and long-term components of memory differs from one experimental system to another, these general conclusions hold for studies in a variety of different creatures in addition

---

Figure 20–3. Protein synthesis during or immediately after training is required for long-term memory of a conditioned avoidance response in goldfish. Bernard Agranoff and colleagues found that when the turning on of a light is followed invariably by an electric shock, goldfish will swim over a barrier in response to the light and hence avoid the shock. *a*: Acquisition and long-term memory of the light–shock association. *b*: If the protein synthesis inhibitor puromycin is injected into the goldfish brain immediately prior to retesting, the performance of the animal is normal, indicating that protein synthesis is not required for retrieval of existing memories (compare with *a*). *c*: In contrast, if puromycin is injected immediately after the training period, there is no long-term memory. *d*: If puromycin is injected immediately prior to training, acquisition is normal, but again there is no long-term memory (see Agranoff et al., 1965).

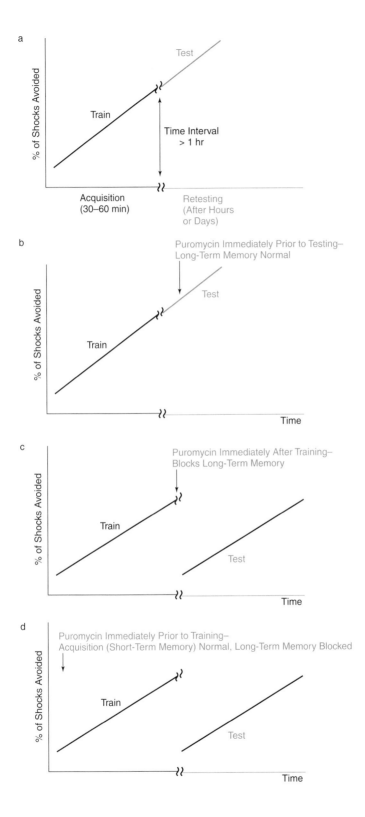

a

% of Shocks Avoided

Test

Train

Time Interval
> 1 hr

Acquisition
(30–60 min)

Retesting
(After Hours
or Days)

b

% of Shocks Avoided

Puromycin Immediately Prior to Testing–
Long-Term Memory Normal

Test

Train

Time

c

% of Shocks Avoided

Puromycin Immediately After Training–
Blocks Long-Term Memory

Train

Test

Time

d

% of Shocks Avoided

Puromycin Immediately Prior to Training–
Acquisition (Short-Term Memory) Normal, Long-Term Memory Blocked

Train

Test

Time

545

to fish and mice. Indeed, these experiments provide one of the most convincing pieces of evidence that short- and long-term memory are distinct processes with different properties. Although inhibitors of protein synthesis almost certainly will produce side effects in addition to inhibiting protein synthesis, it is reassuring that the same results are obtained with several different kinds of inhibitor that work through different molecular mechanisms. Since the side effects are likely to be different for the different inhibitors, it is reasonable to attribute their actions on memory to the one effect they are known to have in common, namely disruption of protein synthesis. As we shall see later in this chapter, more recent variants of the interference approach have been used to confirm this general conclusion and to begin to identify some of the key proteins whose synthesis is necessary for learning to occur.

The correlation approach. A complementary approach is to ask what molecular changes in the brain accompany learning and memory. Again, this requires a guess about appropriate molecular mechanisms, and protein synthesis has again been a popular guess. This, of course, is very reasonable given the findings we have described above, and many investigators have measured patterns of protein (and RNA) synthesis in the brains of animals during and at various times following training. For the most part, this approach has not been fruitful. One might expect the changes in protein synthesis that accompany the learning of a discrete behavioral task to be subtle and accordingly difficult or perhaps impossible to measure against the large background of protein synthesis that occurs normally in the brain. Surprisingly enough, large changes in the incorporation of radioactive amino acids into proteins, as a function of training, are often observed in such experiments. It seems likely that these changes result from some epiphenomenon associated with the training, but do not provide any clues to the molecular basis of the memory trace itself.

The central conclusion drawn from the interference approach, that protein synthesis is required for many kinds of long-term learning to occur, has not been seriously challenged. However, we do not know the identities or roles of the proteins that are required. It is interesting that these classical approaches to the molecular underpinnings of learning and memory have enjoyed a revival in recent years. As we shall see below, there are several experimental systems in which the cellular correlates of certain behaviors have been identified, and both interference and correlation are being used to probe the details of the molecular mechanisms involved. Once again, protein synthesis is one mechanism that has been implicated, but it is not the only one.

The genetic approach. The rationale for investigating the genetics of behavior is simple and straightforward: if one can generate mutants that exhibit aberrant patterns of behavior, an examination of the mutated gene might provide clues to the molecular mechanisms underlying the behavior. Again, this approach is valid even if the precise location of the engram is not known. Such genetic studies of memory have focused on the fruit fly *Drosophila* and the nematode worm *Caenorhabditis elegans*, because their genetics are better understood than those of any other multicellular organism. We shall focus here on *Drosophila*, which can undergo both associative and nonassociative forms of learning, because a large and growing series of behavioral mutants of different types exist (Table 20–1). As an example we will discuss the first of these behavioral mutants to be isolated, a stupid fly called *dunce*.

Fruit flies can learn to associate a particular odorant with an electric shock and avoid the odorant in subsequent tests. *dunce* was isolated when flies were treated with a chemical mutagen and their offspring screened in this behavioral assay. *dunce* has normal sensory and motor capacities, but its learning is impaired. When the time course of memory decay is examined (Fig. 20–4), it is found that its short-term memory decays unusually rapidly, and there is little sign of long-term memory. However, when some low level of residual long-term memory is detected, it appears to decay at the same rate as in normal flies. This suggests that the primary effect of the *dunce* mutation is to severely attenuate short-term memory, and the loss of long-term memory may be a secondary effect.

What is the protein encoded by the *dunce* genetic locus? The *dunce* gene codes for a form of the enzyme cyclic AMP phosphodiesterase (see

Table 20–1 Selected Examples of *Drosophila* Mutants That Exhibit Defects in Learning and Memory

Mutant	Behavioral Phenotype	Gene Product or Affected Pathway
dunce	Rapid decay of short-term memory	cAMP phosphodiesterase
rutabaga	Rapid decay of short-term memory	Adenylate cyclase
amnesiac	Defective memory	Neuropeptide modulator of adenylate cyclase
turnip	Defective acquisition and retention	Modulator of PKC
CREB	Defective long-term memory	Transcription factor
Leonardo	Defective Pavlovian learning	14-3-3, a signaling protein scaffold

Fig. 12–9), which contributes a large percentage of the cyclic AMP hydrolyzing activity in *Drosophila*. The levels of cyclic AMP in *dunce* are as much as sixfold higher than those in normal flies, which suggests that cyclic AMP may in some way be linked to memory formation. This suggestion is reinforced by the finding that another memory mutant, *rutabaga* (Table 20–1), is also defective in cyclic AMP metabolism. Like *dunce* flies, *rutabaga* flies exhibit an abnormally rapid decay of short-term memory in various associative conditioning paradigms. However, in this mutant the phosphodiesterase activity is normal. Instead, *rutabaga* exhibits a defect in a calcium/calmodulin-dependent subpopulation of the enzyme adenylate cyclase, which is responsible for the synthesis of cyclic AMP (see Chapter 12).

These findings contribute to the emerging picture that cyclic AMP plays an important role in learning and memory in the fruit fly (and, we shall see, in other organisms). What, precisely, is this role? Recent molecular genetic experiments indicate that regulation of gene expression by cyclic AMP is critical for learning. It is known that cyclic AMP–dependent protein kinase phosphorylates a transcription factor called the *cyclic AMP response element binding protein* (CREB; Fig. 20–5a) at a specific serine residue. Phosphorylated CREB in turn binds to an eight base pair sequence,

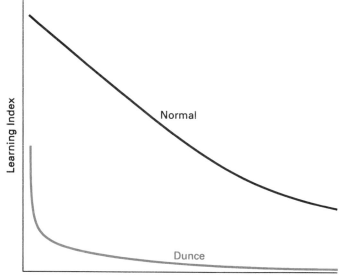

Figure 20–4. Odorant-based shock avoidance in *Drosophila*. Decay of memory as a function of time after training, in normal flies and those carrying the *dunce* mutation. (After a drawing by Tully, 1987.)

called the *cyclic AMP response element* (CRE), that is present in the regulatory region of a variety of genes whose transcription is regulated by cyclic AMP (Fig. 20–5a). Transcription of these genes is turned on only when CREB binds to the CRE, and CREB binds only when elevated levels of intracellular cyclic AMP cause it to be phosphorylated. In flies that have been genetically engineered to express a blocker of CREB function, long-term memory is specifically disrupted (Fig. 20–5b). This finding suggests that CREB-regulated gene expression may act as a molecular switch for certain kinds of long-term memory. These kinds of results confirm and extend the conclusions from the interference approach—indeed, targeted disruption of CREB function can be thought of as a sophisticated way of

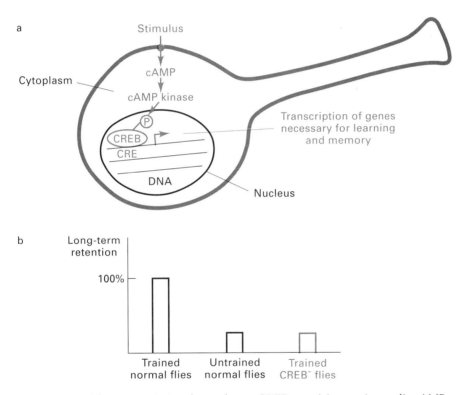

Figure 20–5. The transcriptional regulator CREB participates in cyclic AMP–dependent learning and memory. *a*: A stimulus generates cyclic AMP, which in turn activates cyclic AMP–dependent protein kinase (cAMP kinase), among whose substrates is CREB. Phosphorylated CREB binds to the CRE, activating the transcription of genes that have the CRE sequence in their regulatory domains. The protein products of some of these genes are essential for learning and memory. *b*: Fruit flies in which CREB is disrupted by genetic manipulation (CREB⁻ flies) exhibit impaired long-term retention (from an experiment by Tim Tully and colleagues; see DeZazzo and Tully, 1995).

inhibiting protein synthesis—but the critical proteins whose synthesis is required are still to be identified.

Other fly learning and memory mutants exist, and not all of them involve defects in the cyclic AMP pathway. As summarized in Table 20–1, interruption of other signaling pathways can also disrupt various features of memory acquisition, consolidation, and recall. This list emphasizes the diversity of molecular mechanisms that participate in even simple forms of behavior.

Model Systems for the Cellular and Molecular Analysis of Learning and Memory

Since the time of Ramón y Cajal and Sherrington it has been widely accepted that the synapse must be an important site of neuronal plasticity and that plastic changes in synaptic efficacy might contribute to behavioral plasticity. It has been known for more than 50 years that certain synapses in the peripheral nervous system can undergo changes in synaptic efficacy that can last for seconds or minutes (see Chapter 9). Such changes, in sympathetic ganglia and at the neuromuscular junction, have been thoroughly studied and are fairly well understood. But what does this have to do with learning and memory? One cannot claim that the neuromuscular junction or the sympathetic ganglion has the capacity to "behave." In this case the synapse that is modulated is accessible for study, but there is no behavioral correlate.

Workers interested in mechanisms of learning and memory are faced with a dilemma. The ideal model system would be a two-neuron/one-synapse organism with the behavioral repertoire of humans. Needless to say, this is not available. Accordingly, many investigators have compromised on both sides of the issue and have chosen model systems that exhibit reasonably sophisticated behavioral plasticity yet have reasonably accessible nervous systems. We shall now discuss one of these models, the gastropod mollusc, in some depth. Finally, we shall consider an increasingly popular model for long-term learning in mammals: long-lasting changes in synaptic strength in the hippocampus and other parts of the brain.

Model Systems I: The Gastropod Mollusc Aplysia

The advantages of molluscan nervous systems for cellular neurobiology have already been emphasized in different contexts throughout this book. The gastropod molluscs not only provide highly accessible nervous systems with a relatively small number of large, identifiable neurons but they also exhibit a surprisingly varied repertoire of behaviors, including both nonassociative and associative learning. In Chapter 19 we saw how patterns of synaptic connections between identified neurons could explain the control of a variety of behaviors in different creatures. Now we shall discuss the cellular and molecular analysis of short- and long-term memory in the marine snail *Aplysia* (Fig. 20–6). This work was pioneered by Eric Kandel and colleagues, and has been honored by a Nobel Prize to Kandel.

Defensive withdrawal reflexes in Aplysia. *Aplysia* can withdraw from strong tactile stimuli, an effect that is analogous to reflex escape and withdrawal observed in vertebrates. The tail withdrawal reflex is a contraction of the tail musculature in response to a stimulus to the skin on the posterior portion of the animal. The gill and siphon withdrawal is a reflex evoked by touching the siphon or mantle shelf (these are external organs of the mantle cavity, a respiratory chamber that contains and protects the gill; Fig. 20–6). An analogous reflex response in humans would be the rapid withdrawal of the arm and hand from a hot stove. Both of the *Aplysia* withdrawal reflexes can be modified by experience, and they appear to be similar with respect to cellular and molecular mechanisms of the behavioral modifications. We focus here on the gill and siphon withdrawal.

The essential neuronal circuitry that underlies the gill and siphon withdrawal reflex has been more or less identified (Fig. 20–7). There are approximately 50 sensory neurons (SN) that have their sensory receptive fields in the skin of the siphon and mantle shelf. These sensory neurons make both monosynaptic and polysynaptic connections (the latter via interneurons, or IN) with a group of motor neurons (MN). The latter in turn synapse directly onto the gill and siphon musculature, which contracts to produce the reflex withdrawal. The cell bodies of all of these neurons are within the *Aplysia* abdominal ganglion, but these identified central neurons do not tell the entire story. There is also a peripheral circuit that participates in the gill and siphon withdrawal, but the extent of its contribution to the reflex and to the behavioral plasticity is not known.

Nonassociative plasticity in the gill withdrawal reflex: habituation and sensitization. This simple form of behavior can undergo both habituation and sensitization as well as associative conditioning. When a weak tactile stimulus to the siphon is presented repeatedly, the reflex withdrawal is initially robust but becomes weaker with each subsequent stimulus (Fig. 20–8a); that is, the response habituates. An examination of the wiring diagram for the reflex (Fig. 20–7) reveals several potential loci for cellular plasticity that might account for this behavioral habituation. In principle, the cellular change might lie in (1) the sensitivity of the sensory neurons to the stimulus; (2) the sensory or motor neuron firing patterns, spike amplitudes, or durations; or (3) the efficacy of the sensory neuron-to-motor neuron or motor neuron-to-muscle synapses. By surveying the various components of the circuit in the behaving animal, Kandel and colleagues found that a decrement in synaptic transmission from the sensory to the motor neuron accompanies and might account for the habituation (Fig. 20–8b). This *synaptic depression*, the cellular correlate of behavioral habituation, ap-

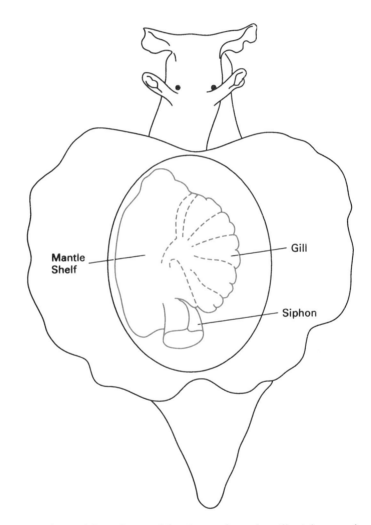

Mantle
Shelf

Gill

Siphon

Figure 20–6. Drawing of an adult *Aplysia californica* to show the gill, siphon, and mantle shelf. A tactile stimulus to the mantle or siphon area results in contraction and withdrawal of the gill. (After a drawing by Kandel, 1979.)

pears to be *homosynaptic*; that is, it is a property of the sensory–motor
pathway itself and can be evoked simply by repeated stimulation of the
presynaptic sensory neuron. It is possible that there are also changes in
the interneurons in the polysynaptic pathway. In fact, simultaneous recording of the membrane potentials of many of the neurons in the abdominal
ganglion, using optical techniques and voltage-sensitive dyes, reveals
changes in the electrical activity of as many as 300 neurons upon sensory
stimulation.

When one delivers a strong noxious stimulus such as an electric shock
to the animal's head or tail, a large increase in the gill and siphon withdrawal reflex occurs. Depending on the conditions of stimulation, this increase is termed either *sensitization* or *dishabituation*. As shown in Figure
20–8a, the reflex response is markedly enhanced, and this is accompanied
by an increase in transmission at the sensory–to–motor neuron synapse
(Fig. 20–8b). The *synaptic facilitation*, the cellular correlate of the en-

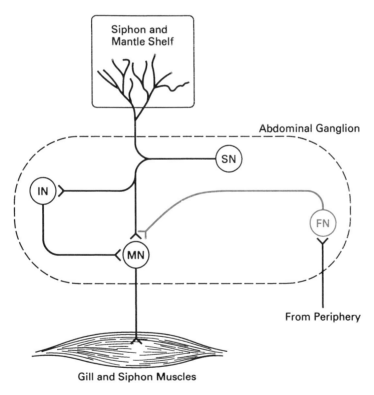

Figure 20–7. Wiring diagram for the gill withdrawal response. Sensory neurons (SN)
synapse either directly, or indirectly via interneurons (IN), with the motor neurons
(MN) that innervate the gill and siphon musculature. Facilitatory neurons (FN) receive
synaptic input from the periphery and influence the SN-to-MN synapse.

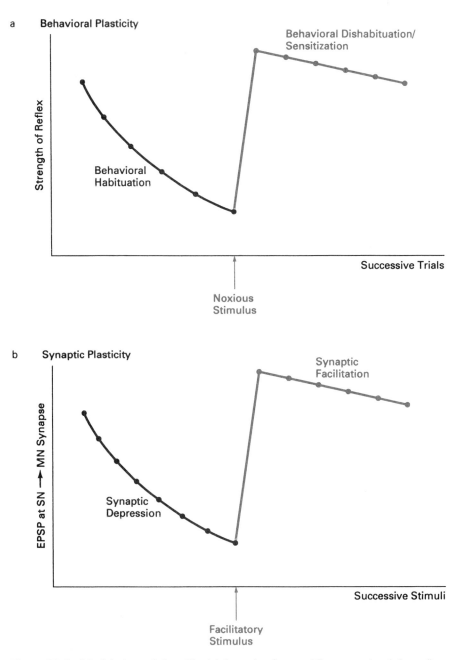

Figure 20–8. Modulation of the gill withdrawal reflex. *a*: The strength of the reflex can be measured by determining the amount of time the gill remains withdrawn following a stimulus. *b*: A change in the efficacy of the sensory neuron (SN)-to-motor neuron (MN) synapse accompanies behavioral habituation and dishabituation/sensitization (see Kandel and Schwartz, 1982). EPSP, excitatory postsynaptic potential.

hanced reflex, is *heterosynaptic*. It results from the activation by the noxious stimulus of facilitatory neurons (FN) that synapse on the sensory neurons (Fig. 20–7), thereby altering the properties of the sensory–to–motor neuron synapse. Both depression and facilitation of the synapse can be observed in the isolated abdominal ganglion, the former by repeated stimulation of the sensory neurons with an intracellular electrode and the latter by stimulation of a nerve trunk that contains the axons of the facilitatory neurons (Fig. 20–8b). With appropriately spaced stimuli, both the enhancement of the behavioral reflex and the heterosynaptic facilitation can be made to last for 24 hr or longer. In other words, the animal exhibits long-term memory for this nonassociative behavioral modification, and the accompanying synaptic plasticity can also last for a very long time.

Associative plasticity in the gill withdrawal reflex: classical conditioning. The gill and siphon withdrawal reflex can be enhanced not only by nonassociative sensitization but also by associative conditioning. The conditioning is carried out by pairing a mild tactile stimulus to the siphon, the conditioned stimulus, with a strong electric shock to the tail, the unconditioned stimulus. Prior to conditioning, the conditioned stimulus elicits a weak withdrawal response and the unconditioned stimulus elicits a powerful one. After the stimuli have been paired in time, the conditioned stimulus elicits a powerful response and the conditioning can persist for days (Fig. 20–9a).

What are the cellular correlates of this associative behavioral plasticity? Again, there is an increase in the efficacy of the sensory–to–motor neuron synapse and a similar associative change in synaptic efficacy can be elicited in the isolated nervous system (Fig. 20–9b). When action potentials in one sensory neuron (SN_1, the conditioned stimulus) are paired temporally with stimulation of nerves from the tail (FN, the unconditioned stimulus), after several trials there is a dramatic increase in the excitatory postsynaptic potential, in the motor neuron, that is evoked by the conditioned stimulus SN_1. However, the response to stimulation of all the other sensory neurons, which have not been paired with the unconditioned stimulus, remains unchanged (represented by SN_2 in Fig. 20–9b). A very similar result is observed in neurons that participate in the tail withdrawal reflex.

A mechanism for synaptic plasticity: modulation of transmitter release. All of these plastic changes in synaptic strength involve a change in the amount of excitatory neurotransmitter released from the sensory neuron. Earlier classical work on mammalian and crustacean neuromuscular junctions by Bernard Katz and Stephen Kuffler, respectively, had pointed to modulation

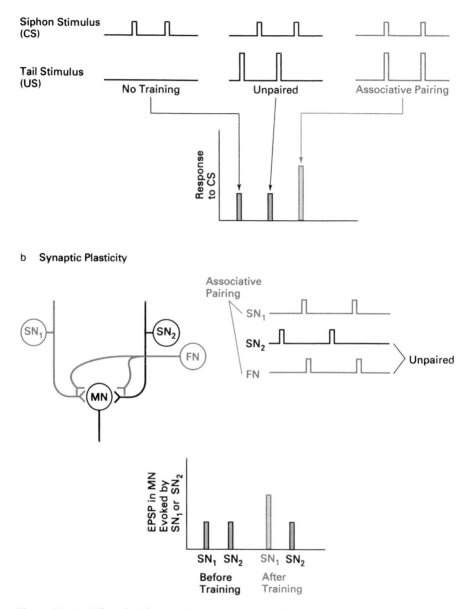

a   Behavioral Plasticity

Siphon Stimulus
(CS)

Tail Stimulus
(US)

No Training   Unpaired   Associative Pairing

Response to CS

b   Synaptic Plasticity

Associative
Pairing

SN₁

SN₂

FN

Unpaired

SN₁   SN₂   FN   MN

EPSP in MN
Evoked by
SN₁ or SN₂

SN₁ SN₂   SN₁ SN₂
Before   After
Training   Training

Figure 20–9. Gill and siphon withdrawal can be enhanced by associative condition-ing. *a*: When a conditioned stimulus (CS) to the siphon is paired in time with an un-conditioned stimulus (US) to the tail, the response to the conditioned stimulus is en-hanced. *b*: An associative change in synaptic strength accompanies this behavioral response (see Kandel and Schwartz, 1982). EPSP, excitatory postsynaptic potential; FN, facilitatory neuron; MN, motor neuron; SN₁, SN₂, sensory neurons.

of transmitter release as an important mechanism of synaptic plasticity. The technique of quantal analysis, pioneered by Katz (see Chapter 9), was used by Kandel and colleagues to demonstrate that the synaptic depression that underlies short- and long-term behavioral habituation of the gill withdrawal reflex is accompanied by a decrement in transmitter release. Conversely, the synaptic facilitation that is responsible for short- and long-term sensitization results from an enhancement of transmitter release.

The increase in transmitter release from the sensory neurons during facilitation results in part from modulation of action potential duration by mechanisms discussed in Chapter 13. The transmitter released by the facilitatory neurons increases sensory neuron action potential duration, in part via a cyclic AMP–mediated decrease in the S potassium current (see Fig. 13–11). However, other second messenger systems and other ion channels are also involved in modulating transmitter release from the sensory neurons.

Long-term facilitation requires protein synthesis. Short-term (lasting minutes) and long-term (lasting hours or days) facilitation of the sensory–to–motor neuron synapse share a common cellular mechanism: both involve an increase in the release of the sensory neuron neurotransmitter. Thus it might be expected that the details of the underlying molecular mechanisms would also be similar. However, the use of the interference approach, described above, reveals an important difference: the long-term facilitation of synaptic transmission, produced by application of a facilitatory transmitter, is blocked by inhibitors of RNA and protein synthesis, whereas the short-term facilitation is unaffected.

Several kinds of experiments suggest a role for CREB in long-term facilitation. One experiment involves injecting into the nucleus of the sensory neuron an excess of an oligonucleotide corresponding in sequence to the CRE. This treatment blocks long-term facilitation, presumably because the excess free CRE binds all the phosphorylated CREB and prevents transcription of the genes necessary for the synaptic plasticity. A complementary experiment involves injecting into the sensory neurons a *reporter gene*, whose transcription is under the control of a CRE sequence in the regulatory region of the gene. The reporter gene encodes an enzyme that catalyzes the formation of a colored reaction product. When such injected sensory neurons are treated with serotonin under conditions that produce long-term synaptic facilitation, the cells produce the colored reaction product. This response indicates that transcription of the reporter gene and presumably other genes controlled by the CRE can be activated by serotonin. Thus the initial increase in cyclic AMP in sensory neurons, induced by serotonin, gives rise to both short- and long-term facilitation, but via different molecular pathways (Fig. 20–10). This finding is in agreement with the *Drosophila* results described above, and with the classical earlier studies in vertebrates that suggested an essential role for protein synthesis in long-term but not short-term memory.

Model Systems II: Long-Term Potentiation and Long-Term Depression

Can these kinds of cellular and molecular analyses be carried out in vertebrates? To recapitulate a point that we have already emphasized, the

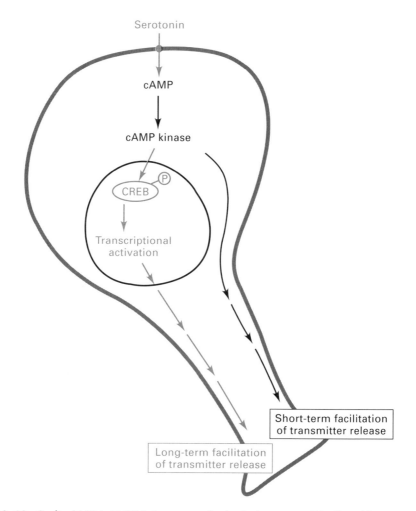

Figure 20–10. Cyclic AMP (cAMP) is important for both short-term (*black*) and long-term (*blue*) synaptic facilitation (modified from Stevens and Verma, 1994).

complexity of the vertebrate central nervous system and the lack of read-ily identifiable neurons present a formidable barrier to identifying the ap-propriate neurons to analyze. In only a very few experimental systems is the identification of the essential memory trace circuits at all within reach. Thus there has been an ongoing search for a system in vertebrate brain in which long-term changes in synaptic efficacy, evoked by experience, can be investigated. *Long-term potentiation* (LTP), a phenomenon that occurs at several different kinds of central and peripheral synapses but has been investigated most thoroughly in the hippocampus, is amenable to this kind of investigation. Although hippocampal LTP is not clearly and unequivo-cally associated with any known behavioral modification, it is a long-term increase in synaptic strength in a brain region known to be important for learning and memory. In addition it has an associative component, and hence provides a model for the kinds of synaptic modulation that might be involved in long-term associative learning. More recently a related phe-nomenon, long-term depression (LTD), has also been investigated in some detail.

What is long-term potentiation? It is worth noting in passing that although the synaptic organization of the vertebrate brain may appear at first glance to be hopelessly complex, certain structures, including the cerebellum and hippocampus, actually exhibit an exquisitely precise organization. One cannot identify single cells as unique individuals as can be done in the gastropod molluscs. Nevertheless, particular classes of neurons and the synapses between them can indeed be recognized reliably. As shown in Figure 20–11a, there are three major synapses in the hippocampus at which LTP has been investigated. In 1973 it was shown in the rabbit that the strength of one of these synaptic connections, between the (presynaptic) perforant fibers and (postsynaptic) granule cell neurons, can be markedly potentiated following a brief high-frequency (tetanic) stimulus to the presy-naptic axons (Fig. 20–11b). This potentiation, which can last as long as several weeks in intact animals, was subsequently demonstrated at the other two synapses as well.

The study of LTP became much easier (and hence much more popu-lar) with the development of the in vitro hippocampal slice, a cross sec-tion through the hippocampus in which the pathways and synaptic orga-nization depicted in Figure 20–11a remain intact. Long-term potentiation can also be elicited in the slice and, although it cannot last for weeks be-cause the slice dies within a matter of hours, it can persist as long as the slice does. In this preparation it is relatively easy to carry out intracellu-lar recording (and even voltage clamp), thus LTP can be examined in in-dividual postsynaptic neurons as well as in populations of postsynaptic neurons via an extracellular electrode. This and other technical advances have made it possible to investigate the mechanisms of several temporally distinct components of LTP: initiation, storage, and expression.

Initiation of long-term potentiation. From the earliest experiments it was evident that the induction of LTP requires high-frequency stimulation of the

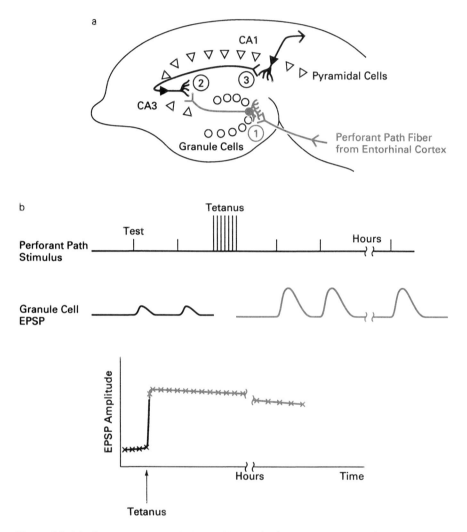

Figure 20–11. Long-term potentiation (LTP) in the hippocampus. *a*: Schematic drawing of a hippocampal slice. Fibers from the entorhinal cortex enter the hippocampus via the perforant path and synapse on dendrites of granule cell neurons (*1*). These in turn synapse on pyramidal cell neurons in the CA3 region of the hippocampus (*2*). The CA3 pyramidal cells synapse on other pyramidal cell neurons in the CA1 region (*3*). *b*: LTP of the perforant path to granule cell neuron synapse. EPSP, excitatory postsynaptic potential. (Modified from Nicoll et al., 1988; see also Bliss and Lomo, 1973.)

presynaptic fibers at a stimulus intensity that is above a certain threshold. Both the high frequency and the strong stimulus (which activates a large number of presynaptic axons) are essential. Weak stimuli do not produce LTP even following tetanic stimulation, nor do strong stimuli if they are given at low frequency (Fig. 20–12a). It is known now that these conditions reflect the requirement for a large depolarization of the postsynaptic cell for LTP to be initiated. For example, LTP induction by a strong tetanic stimulus can be prevented by voltage clamping the postsynaptic cell to prevent the depolarization (Fig. 20–12b). However, although the postsynaptic depolarization is necessary, it is not in itself sufficient. For example, injection of depolarizing current via an intracellular electrode in the postsynaptic neuron can induce LTP, but only when it is paired with a weak synaptic input. Thus concurrent stimulation of the synaptic input, together with postsynaptic depolarization, is required for LTP induction.

The requirement for synaptic activation coupled with depolarization can be understood when we consider the neurotransmitter at the excitatory synapses that undergo LTP. There is substantial evidence that glutamate is the transmitter at these synapses, and this is not surprising when we recall (see Chapter 10) that glutamate is the major excitatory neurotransmitter in the mammalian brain. Remember also from Chapter 11 that glutamate binds to several different classes of postsynaptic receptor and that the excitatory postsynaptic potential evoked by a weak stimulus is normally mediated by glutamate binding to the KA/AMPA class of receptor. Only the pronounced depolarization produced by a strong tetanic stimulus can relieve the magnesium block of the NMDA class of receptor and allow calcium to flow through the NMDA receptor channel into the cell (see Fig. 11–14). This requirement then explains why both depolarization and synaptic activation are required; neither alone can activate the NMDA receptor channel, and calcium entry through this channel is necessary for the initiation of LTP.

The key role of NMDA receptor channels in LTP is underscored by targeted gene knockout experiments in mice, of the sort described in earlier chapters. Recall that gene knockout can be thought of as a sophisticated version of the interference approach for studying synaptic and behavioral plasticity, in which the interference is limited to a specific protein whose role can then be assessed. As indicated in Table 20–2, targeted disruption of genes encoding NMDA receptor channel subunits eliminates LTP. Learning and synaptic plasticity are not always affected in parallel in mutant mice lacking one or another key modulator or ion channel protein (Table 20–2), which suggests that LTP and at least some forms of learning and memory may not be tightly correlated.

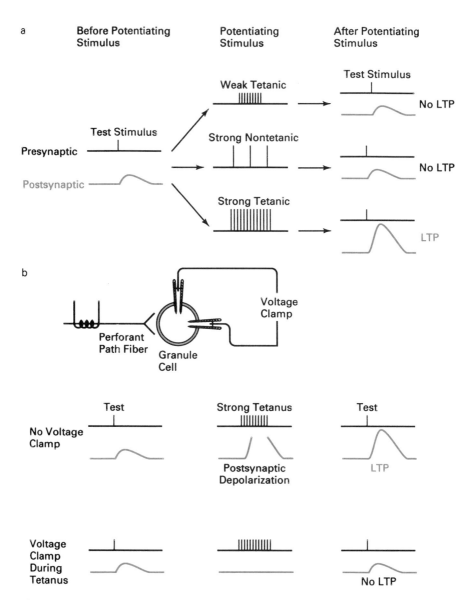

Figure 20–12. Presynaptic transmitter release together with postsynaptic depolarization is required for long-term potentiation (LTP). *a*: Neither a weak tetanic stimulus nor a strong nontetanic stimulus is capable of producing LTP. Only following a strong tetanic stimulus is enhancement of the excitatory postsynaptic potential (EPSP) amplitude seen. *b*: When the postsynaptic cell is voltage clamped to prevent depolarization during the tetanus, even a strong tetanic stimulus does not produce LTP. See Nicoll et al. (1988).

Associative long-term potentiation: Hebb's postulate. As we discussed in Chapter 18 in the context of synapse stabilization during development, Donald Hebb suggested that synaptic strength might be enhanced by concurrent activity in the pre- and postsynaptic neurons. He postulated further that this might provide a mechanism for associative learning. This idea has enjoyed a revival in recent years, in particular in the context of LTP. From the discussion above we can see that homosynaptic LTP fulfills the requirements of Hebb's postulate, in that simultaneous presynaptic activity (which results in glutamate release) and postsynaptic activity (in the form of membrane depolarization) are necessary for the long-lasting change in synaptic strength. There is also an associative form of LTP, in which activity at one synapse can contribute to the generation of LTP at another. Consider the situation illustrated in Figure 20–13a, in which a weak and a strong input synapse on the same target neuron. We know from Figure 20–12a that stimulation of the weak input, even tetanic stimulation of this input, does not produce LTP, whereas tetanic stimulation of the strong input will generate homosynaptic LTP (Fig. 20–13b). Suppose now that the two inputs are tetanized simultaneously. The strong input can depolarize the postsynaptic cell, and this depolarization can spread to the site of the weak input. Since the latter is active and releasing glutamate at the time of the depolarization, both criteria necessary for producing LTP have been satisfied, and the result is LTP at the weak input (as well as at the strong; see Fig. 20–13c). The requirements for temporal pairing of the two stimuli are identical to those required for associative learning paradigms.

Table 20–2 Selected Examples of Effects of Targeted Gene Disruption in Mice on Synaptic Placticity and Behavior

Gene Disrupted	Synaptic Phenotype	Behavioral Phenotype
NMDA receptor channel	Loss of LTP	Impaired memory formation and consolidation
AMPA receptor channel	Loss of LTP	Spatial memory intact
TrkB neurotrophin receptor	Impaired LTP	Passive avoidance learning intact, more complex learning impaired
Potassium channel β subunit Kvβ1.1	Normal LTP	Spatial learning impaired
CaMKII	Loss of LTP	Learning impaired

Molecular mechanisms of long-term potentiation induction: what does the calcium do? Simply knowing that calcium entry into the postsynaptic neuron is necessary for the induction of LTP does not provide us with a detailed molecular mechanism, since calcium does many things in cells (see Fig.

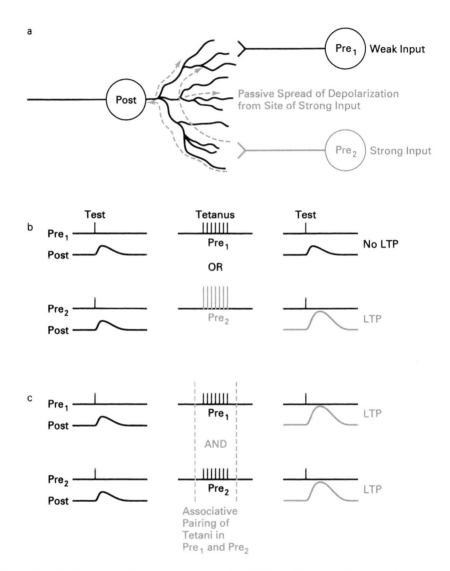

Figure 20–13. Associative long-term potentiation (LTP). *a*: Diagram depicting the spatial relationships between a strong and a weak presynaptic input. *b*: Stimulation of the strong input produces LTP, but stimulation of the weak input alone does not. *c*: When the strong and the weak inputs are paired, the depolarization produced by the strong input spreads to the site of the weak input and contributes to the induction of LTP. See Nicoll et al. (1988).

12–16). Protein kinase C translocation and activation accompany LTP, and inhibitor experiments suggest an essential role for protein kinase C. It is intriguing that protein-kinase-C–mediated phosphorylation of the protein GAP-43 (see Chapter 17) has been reported to accompany LTP, which suggests that events similar to those occurring during neurite outgrowth may contribute to synaptic plasticity. Structural modifications have also been hypothesized to play a role in LTP. Among the ultrastructural changes that have been reported to occur, within minutes after induction of LTP, are increases in the numbers of dendritic spines and of both spine and dendritic shaft synapses (recall from Fig. 1–5 and Plate 1 that spines are highly dynamic structures). Interestingly, changes in these parameters have also been associated with other models of learning and memory discussed in this chapter, including the rabbit eyeblink reflex and long-term sensitization of the gill withdrawal reflex in *Aplysia*.

As indicated in Figure 12–16, calmodulin is central in mediating the effects of calcium in cells. There is evidence from the use of pharmacological inhibitors that the actions of calcium during LTP induction require its interaction with calmodulin. One attractive hypothesis for the role of calmodulin in LTP induction is that it activates the multifunctional Ca^{2+}/Cam kinase II. This enzyme is highly concentrated in postsynaptic densities, so it is in the right location to contribute to the modulation of synaptic efficacy. In addition, as shown in Chapter 9, the enzyme can undergo autophosphorylation in the presence of calcium, after which time its activity becomes independent of calcium. Thus it provides a mechanism whereby a transient rise in postsynaptic calcium could trigger a long-lasting change in the properties of the postsynaptic cell.

Support for the involvement of the Ca^{2+}/Cam kinase II in LTP induction comes from targeted gene knockout experiments. Mutant mice that lack the α-isoform of the Ca^{2+}/Cam kinase II exhibit little or no LTP and are also unable to learn certain behavioral tasks (Table 20–2). However, they do not have any gross anatomical abnormalities in their brains, and they can exhibit a brief form of synaptic plasticity, post-tetanic potentiation (PTP; see Chapter 9). These findings suggest that the activity of Ca^{2+}/Cam kinase II is necessary for LTP induction, but is it also sufficient? Probably not, because knockouts of other kinds of protein kinases are also able to disrupt LTP.

Long-term depression. Can synaptic strength also be decreased for long periods of time? A phenomenon known as *long-term depression* (LTD), a long-lasting decrease in synaptic strength in response to a particular pattern of stimulation (Fig. 20–14a), has been described at synapses in various regions of the mammalian brain, including the cerebellum, where it may be involved in motor learning. One form of homosynaptic (nonasso-ciative) LTD can be evoked in the CA1 region of the hippocampus (see Fig. 20–11a), a favorite system for the study of LTP. In contrast to LTP, which requires a tetanus for its induction, homosynaptic LTD is induced by low-frequency stimulation, usually several hundred stimuli delivered at a frequency of 1–3 Hz (compare Figs. 20–11b and 20–14a).

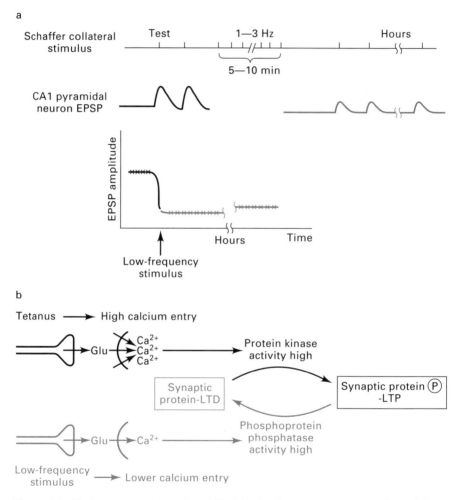

Figure 20–14. Long-term depression (LTD) in the hippocampus. *a*: Prolonged low-frequency stimulation of the Schaffer collateral pathway from region CA3 to region CA1 (Fig. 20–11a) produces a long-lasting, NMDA receptor–dependent depression of the synaptic response in the CA1 pyramidal neurons (compare with Fig. 20–11b). *b*: A model to account for production of long-term potentiation (LTP) and LTD in the same cell (modified from Bear and Malenka, 1994).

Interestingly, many of the same molecular players seem to be involved in both LTP and LTD. Like LTP, LTD can last for many hours in hippocampal slices in vitro and can be blocked by preventing calcium entry through NMDA receptor/channels with NMDA receptor antagonists. In addition, LTD cannot be evoked in the Ca^{2+}/Cam kinase II-deficient mice discussed above, which suggests that this enzyme is a critical participant in both forms of synaptic plasticity. How can the same inducing signal, calcium entry through NMDA receptor/channels, trigger both LTP and LTD, and how can the same kinase be required for both processes? One model (Fig. 20–14b) suggests that the amount of calcium that accumulates in the postsynaptic dendritic spine is critical. According to this model, the state of the synapse—potentiated or depressed—depends on the state of phosphorylation of some yet-to-be identified synaptic protein. High-frequency stimulation leads to a high concentration of calcium in the spine, activation of the Ca^{2+}/Cam kinase II, phosphorylation of the synaptic protein, and LTP. In contrast, low-frequency stimulation leads to lower levels of calcium in the spine, and this leads preferentially to activation of phosphoprotein phosphatase(s), dephosphorylation of the synaptic protein, and LTD (Fig. 20–14b). Consistent with this model is the finding that inhibitors of phosphoprotein phosphatases can block homosynaptic LTD in the CA1 region of the hippocampus. Although it is not yet known what kinase/phosphatase substrate(s) is (are) involved in synaptic plasticity, recall from Chapter 13 that glutamate receptor subunits are good substrates for various protein kinases, and that phosphorylation can modulate glutamate receptor/channel function.

Expression of long-term potentiation: presynaptic or postsynaptic? There is widespread agreement that the onset of LTP (and LTD) is triggered by events occurring in the postsynaptic neuron. What about storage and expression? Is there a long-lasting change in the release of the neurotransmitter glutamate from the presynaptic cell, a change in the responsiveness of the postsynaptic target neuron, or perhaps both? This issue remained unresolved and rather contentious for a long time, but a consensus is finally beginning to emerge.

Recall that, because of the magnesium block of NMDA receptor channels, it is the AMPA receptor channels that are largely responsible for the ongoing glutamatergic transmission at normal, potentiated, or depressed synapses. It is now evident that many excitatory synapses in the brain may be *silent* (Fig. 20–15a) because they have few or no AMPA receptor channels in their postsynaptic membrane (the NMDA receptor channels that are present at such synapses contribute little to ongoing synaptic transmission). After induction of LTP (for which the NMDA receptor channels are of course essential), new AMPA receptor channels appear rapidly in the membrane (Fig. 20–15a), concurrent with the increase in amplitude of the synaptic response. In contrast, LTD may be correlated with a rapid removal of AMPA receptor channels from synapses that were not silent previously (Fig. 20–15b). These findings suggest that AMPA receptor chan-

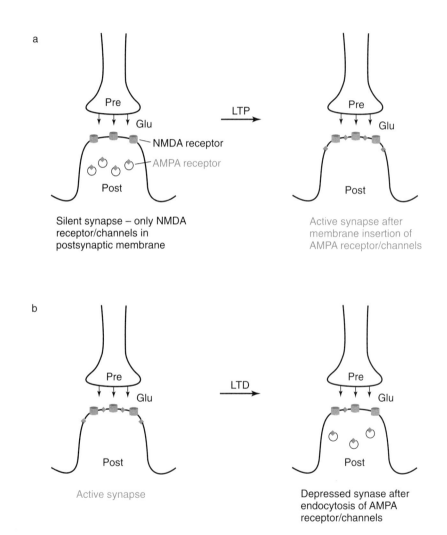

Figure 20–15. The silent synapse concept and synaptic plasticity. *a:* Many glutamatergic synapses are "silent" because they do not contain postsynaptic AMPA receptors. Long-term potentiation (LTP) may result from the membrane insertion of AMPA receptors (*right*) from a readily available store of receptor-containing membrane vesicles. *b:* Long-term depression (LTD) may result from the opposite process, removal of AMPA receptors from previously active synapses.

nels may cycle in and out of the postsynaptic plasma membrane at a rate unexpectedly high for intrinsic membrane proteins and that the neuron may take advantage of this high turnover rate by regulating it to stably modulate synaptic strength.

Although this postsynaptic receptor trafficking hypothesis is an attractive one for which considerable evidence exists, a number of features of LTP and LTD expression have not yet been explained. For example, it remains possible that glutamate release from the presynaptic terminals is also modulated, and this would require some mechanism of communicating information from the postsynaptic induction site back to the presynaptic neuron. Such communication might be mediated by a retrograde messenger molecule, released from the postsynaptic neuron, or by direct intercellular contacts via adhesion molecules or other extracellular proteins of the sort we have discussed in the context of neuronal development. The roles of other factors that influence synaptic plasticity also remain to be explored in depth. For example, it is known that the neurotrophin brain-derived neurotrophic factor (BDNF) has both short- and long-term effects on synaptic plasticity (as well as on intrinsic excitability; see Fig. 13–9), and targeted gene knockout experiments in mice demonstrate that the TrkB receptors for BDNF are required for LTP (Table 20–2). It may well be that the roles of BDNF and other molecular players in the plasticity game can be explained in terms of the silent synapse concept, but we emphasize that much remains to be done before such phenomena as LTP and LTD can be said to be thoroughly understood.

Summary

The goal of neurobiologists, whether their experimental system is the single ion channel or the behaving human, is to understand how the brain works. One aspect of brain function that has most fascinated scientists and the lay public alike is learning and memory. Psychologists have described different kinds of learning and memory, and there is an ongoing search for the physical basis of these distinctions and for the cellular and molecular mechanisms responsible. Because of the complexity of most nervous systems, the search has focused to a large extent on animals with relatively simple nervous systems and on reduced preparations. In such systems it is sometimes possible to locate the neuronal pathways that participate in particular behaviors and to identify changes in synaptic efficacy or neuronal membrane properties that are associated with learning and memory. A variety of approaches can also be used to obtain clues about the molecular changes that underlie the modulation of synaptic strength and membrane characteristics. Much in this area of study remains to be understood. We can anticipate that the search for the cellular and molecular underpinnings of learning and memory will occupy neurobiologists for a long time to come.

Bibliography

Chapter 1

Recommended reading

A. Matus. Actin-based plasticity in dendritic spines. *Science* 290:754–758 (2000).

A. McAllister. Cellular and molecular mechanisms of dendrite growth. *Cereb. Cortex* 10:963–973 (2000).

A. Peters, S. L. Palay, and H. De F. Webster. *The Fine Structure of the Nervous System: The Neurons and Supporting Cells*. Philadelphia: W. B. Saunders (1976).

S. Ramón y Cajal. Croonian Lecture. La fine structure des centres nerveux. *Proc. R. Soc. Lond.* 55:444–468 (1894).

C. Sherrington. *The Integrative Action of the Nervous System*. Cambridge: Cambridge University Press (1948).

References

M. Fischer, S. Kaech, D. Knutti, and A. Matus. Rapid actin-based plasticity in dendritic spines. *Neuron* 20:847–854 (1998).

L. K. Kaczmarek, M. Finbow, J.-P. Revel, and F. Strumwasser. The morphology and coupling of Aplysia bag cells within the abdominal ganglion and in cell culture. *J. Neurobiol.* 10:525–550 (1979).

M. D. Landis. Initial junctions between developing parallel fibers and Purkinje cells are different from mature synaptic junctions. *J. Comp. Neurol.* 260:513–525 (1987).

O. Loewi. Uber humorale Ubertragbarkeit der Herznervenwirkung. *Pflugers Arch.* 189:239–242 (1921).

Chapter 2

Recommended reading

S. T. Brady and A. O. Sperry. Biochemical and functional diversity of microtubule motors in the nervous system. *Curr. Opin. Neurobiol.* 5:551–558 (1995).

P. G. Haydon. Neuroglial networks: neurons and glia talk to each other. *Curr. Biol.* 10:R712–R714 (2000).

A. D. Mehta, M. Rief, and J. A. Spudich. Biomechanics: one molecule at a time. *J. Biol. Chem.* 274:14517–14520 (1999).

S. J Smith. Glia help synapses form and function. *Curr. Biol.* 8:R158–R160 (1998).

J. A. Spudich. How molecular motors work. *Nature* 372:515–518 (1994).

J. Travis. Glia: the brain's other cells. *Science* 266:970–972 (1994).

References

J. W. Dani, A. Chernjavsky, and S. J Smith. Neuronal activity triggers calcium waves in hippocampal astrocyte networks. *Neuron* 8:429–440 (1992).

A. Peters, S. L. Palay, and H. De F. Webster. *The Fine Structure of the Nervous System: The Neurons and Supporting Cells.* Philadelphia: W. B. Saunders (1976).

M. P. Sheetz, E. R. Steuer, and T. A. Schroer. The mechanism and regulation of fast axonal transport. *Trends Neurosci.* 12:474–478 (1989).

Chapter 3

Recommended reading

B. Hille. *Ionic Channels of Excitable Membranes,* 3rd ed. Sunderland, MA: Sinauer Associates (2001).

B. Katz. *Nerve, Muscle and Synapse.* New York: McGraw-Hill (1966).

C. F. Stevens. *Neurophysiology: A Primer.* New York: John Wiley & Sons (1966).

References

M. N. Rasband and J. S. Trimmer. Subunit composition and novel localization of K^+ channels in spinal cord. *J. Comp. Neurol.* 429:166–176 (2001).

M. N. Rasband, J. S. Trimmer, E. Peles, S. R. Levinson, and P. Shrager. K^+ channel distribution and clustering in developing and hypomyelinated axons of the optic nerve. *J. Neurocytol.* 28:319–331 (1999).

Chapter 4

Recommended reading

B. Hille. *Ionic Channels of Excitable Membranes,* 3rd ed. Sunderland, MA: Sinauer Associates (2001).

C. Miller. How ion channel proteins work. In *Neuromodulation: The Biochemical Control of Neuronal Excitability,* L. K. Kaczmarek and I. B. Levitan (Eds.). New York: Oxford University Press, pp. 39–63 (1987).

B. Sakmann and E. Neher (Eds.). *Single-Channel Recording*, 2nd ed. New York: Plenum (1995).

References
O. P. Hamill, A. Marty, E. Neher, B. Sakmann, and F. J. Sigworth. Improved patch-clamp techniques for high-resolution current recording from cells and cell-free membrane patches. *Pflugers Arch. 391*:85–100 (1981).

Chapter 5

Recommended reading
W. A. Catterall. From ionic currents to molecular mechanisms: the structure and function of voltage-gated sodium channels. *Neuron 26*:13–25 (2000).
B. Hille. *Ionic Channels of Excitable Membranes*, 3rd ed. Sunderland, MA: Sinauer Associates (2001).
L. Y. Jan and Y. N. Jan. Cloned potassium channels from eukaryotes and prokaryotes. *Annu. Rev. Neurosci. 20*:91–123 (1997)

References
C. M. Armstrong. Sodium channels and gating currents. *Physiol. Rev. 61*:644–683 (1981).
C. M. Armstrong, F. Bezanilla, and E. Rojas. Destruction of sodium conductance inactivation in squid axons perfused with pronase. *J. Gen. Physiol. 62*:375–391 (1973).
W. A. Catterall. Molecular properties of voltage-sensitive sodium channels. *Annu. Rev. Biochem. 55*:953–985 (1986).
D. A. Doyle, J. Morais Cabral, R. A. Pfuetzner, A. Kuo, J. M. Gulbis, S. L. Cohen, B. T. Chait, and R. MacKinnon. The structure of the potassium channel: molecular basis of K^+ conduction and selectivity. *Science 280*:69–77 (1998).
T. Hoshi, W. N. Zagotta, and R. W. Aldrich. Biophysical and molecular mechanisms of Shaker potassium channel inactivation. *Science 250*:533–538 (1990).
M. Li, N. Unwin, K. Stauffer, Y. N. Jan, and L. Y. Jan. Images of purified Shaker potassium channels. *Curr. Biol. 4*:110–115 (1994).
T. L. Schwarz, B. L. Tempel, D. M. Papazian, Y. N. Jan, and L. Y. Jan. Multiple potassium-channel components are produced by alternative splicing at the Shaker locus in *Drosophila*. *Nature 331*:137–142 (1988).

Chapter 6

Recommended reading
B. Hille. *Ionic Channels of Excitable Membranes*, 3rd ed. Sunderland, MA: Sinauer Associates (2001).

References

A. L. Hodgkin and A. F. Huxley. Currents carried by sodium and potassium ions through the membrane of the giant axon of Loligo. *J. Physiol. (Lond.) 116*: 449–472 (1952a).

A. L. Hodgkin and A. F. Huxley. The components of membrane conductance in the giant axon of Loligo. *J. Physiol. (Lond.) 116*:473–496 (1952b).

A. L. Hodgkin and A. F. Huxley. The dual effect of membrane potential on sodium conductance in the giant axon of Loligo. *J. Physiol. (Lond.): 116*: 497–506 (1952c).

A. L. Hodgkin and A. F. Huxley. A quantitative description of membrane current and its application to conduction and excitation in nerve. *J. Physiol. (Lond.) 117*:500–544 (1952d).

A. L. Hodgkin, A. F. Huxley, and B. Katz. Measurements of current-voltage relations in the membrane of the giant axon of Loligo. *J. Physiol. (Lond.) 116*: 424–448 (1952).

Chapter 7

Recommended reading

W. A. Catterall. Structure and function of neuronal Ca^{2+} channels and their role in neurotransmitter release. *Cell Calcium 24*:307–323 (1998).

L. L. Isom, K. S. De Jongh, and W. A. Catterall. Auxiliary subunits of voltage-gated ion channels. *Neuron 12*:1183–1194 (1994).

L. Y. Jan and Y. N. Jan. Cloned potassium channels from eukaryotes and prokaryotes. *Annu. Rev. Neurosci. 20*:91–123 (1997).

F. Lehmann-Horn and K. Jurkat-Rott. Voltage-gated ion channels and hereditary disease. *Physiol. Rev. 79*:1317–1372 (1999).

O. Pongs, T. Leicher, M. Berger, J. Roeper, R. Bahring, D. Wray, K. P. Giese, A. J. Silva, and J. F. Storm. Functional and molecular aspects of voltage-gated K^+ channel beta subunits. *Ann N Y Acad Sci 868*:344–355 (1999).

References

J. P. Adelman, K.-Z. Shen, M. P. Kavanaugh, R. A. Warren, Y.-N. Wu, A. Lagrutta, C. T. Bond, and R. A. North. Calcium-activated potassium channels expressed from cloned complementary DNAs. *Neuron 9*:209–216 (1992).

K. Dunlap, J. I. Luebke, and T. J. Turner. Exocytotic calcium channels in mammalian central neurons. *Trends Neurosci. 18*:89–98 (1995).

E. A. Ertel, K. P. Campbell, M. M. Harpold, F. Hofmann, Y. Mori, E. Perez-Reyes, A. Schwartz, T. P. Snutch, T. Tanabe, L. Birnbaumer, R. W. Tsien, and W. A. Catterall. Nomenclature of voltage-gated calcium channels. *Neuron 25*:533–535 (2000).

J. M. Gulbis, M. Zhou, S. Mann, and R. MacKinnon. Structure of the cytoplasmic β subunit—T1 assembly of voltage-dependent K^+ channels. *Science 289*: 123–127 (2000)

R. W. Meech and N. B. Standen. Potassium activation in Helix aspersa neurons under voltage clamp: a component mediated by calcium influx. *J. Physiol. (Lond.)* 249:211–239 (1975).

P. H. Reinhart, S. Chung, and I. B. Levitan. A family of calcium-dependent potassium channels from rat brain. *Neuron* 2:1031–1041 (1989).

J. Rettig, S. H. Heinemann, F. Wunder, C. Lorra, D. N. Parcej, J. O. Dolly, and O. Pongs. Inactivation properties of voltage-gated K^+ channels altered by presence of β subunit. *Nature* 369:289–294 (1994).

A. Wei, T. Jegla, and L. Salkoff. Eight potassium channel families revealed by the *C. elegans* genome project. *Neuropharmacology* 35:805–829 (1996).

Chapter 8

Recommended reading

G. J. Augustine, M. E. Burns, W. M. DeBello, S. Hilfiker, J. M. Morgan, F. E. Schweizer, H. Tokumaru, and K. Umayahara. Proteins involved in synaptic vesicle trafficking. *J. Physiol.* 520:33–41 (1999).

L. Brodin, P. Löw, and O. Shupliakov. Sequential steps in clathrin-mediated synaptic vesicle endocytosis. *Curr. Opin. Neurobiol.* 10:312–320 (2000).

S. Mochida. Protein-protein interactions in neurotransmitter release. *Neurosci. Res.* 36:175–182 (2000).

J. E. Rothman. Mechanisms of intracellular protein transport. *Nature* 372:55–63 (1994).

T. C. Südhof. The synaptic vesicle cycle: a cascade of protein-protein interactions. *Nature* 375:645–653 (1995).

T. C. Südhof and R. Jahn. Proteins of synaptic vesicles involved in exocytosis and membrane recycling. *Neuron* 6:665–677 (1991).

References

L. J. Breckenridge and W. Almers. Current through the fusion pore that forms during exocytosis of a secretory vesicle. *Nature* 328:814–817 (1987).

N. Brose, C. Rosenmund, and J. Rettig. Regulation of transmitter release by Unc-13 and its homologues. *Curr. Opin. Neurobiol.* 10:303–311 (2000).

J. M. Burt and D. C. Spray. Single channel events and gating behavior of the cardiac gap junction channel. *Proc. Natl. Acad. Sci. U.S.A.* 85:3431–3434 (1988).

A. J. Cochilla, J. K. Angleson, and W. J. Betz. Monitoring secretory membrane with FM1–43 fluorescence. *Annu. Rev. Neurosci.* 22:1–10 (1999).

P. I. Hanson, R. Roth, H. Morisaki, R. Jahn, and J. E. Heuser. Structural and conformational changes in NSF and its membrane receptor complexes visualized by quick-freeze/deep-etch electron microscopy. *Cell* 90:523–535 (1997).

T. M. Hohl, F. Paralti, C. Wimmer, J. E. Rothman, T. H. Söllner, and H. Engelhardt. Arrangement of subunits in 20S particles consisting of NSF, SNAPs and SNARE complexes. *Mol. Cell* 2:539–548 (1998).

L. K. Kaczmarek, M. Finbow, J.-P. Revel, and F. Strumwasser. The morphology and coupling of Aplysia bag cells within the abdominal ganglion and in cell culture. *J. Neurobiol. 10*:525–550 (1979).

L. Makowski, D. L. D. Caspar, W. C. Phillips, and D. A. Goodenough. Gap junction structures. II. Analysis of the X-ray diffraction data. *J. Cell Biol. 74*:629–645 (1977).

R. B. Sutton, D. Fasshauer, R. Jahn, and A.T. Brunger. Crystal structure of a SNARE complex involved in synaptic exocytosis at 2.4 Angstrom resolution. *Nature 395*:347–353 (1998).

Chapter 9

Recommended reading

P. Greengard, F. Valtorta, A. J. Czernik, and F. Benfenati. Synaptic vesicle phosphoproteins and regulation of synaptic function. *Science 259*:780–785 (1993).

S. Hilfiker, V. A. Pieribone, A. J. Czernik, H.-T. Kao, G. J. Augustine, and P. Greengard. Synapsins as regulators of neurotransmitter release. *Phil. Trans. R. Soc. Lond. B 354*:269–279 (1999)

R. Llinas. Calcium in synaptic transmission. *Sci. Am. 247(4)*:56–65 (1982).

V. O'Connor, G. J. Augustine, and H. Betz. Synaptic vesicle exocytosis: molecules and models. *Cell 76*:785–787 (1994).

S. J Smith and G. J. Augustine. Calcium ions, active zones and synaptic transmitter release. *Trends Neurosci. 11*:458–464 (1988).

A.M. Thomson. Facilitation, augmentation and potentiation at central synapses. *Trends Neurosci. 23*:305–312 (2000).

K. M. Turner, R. D. Burgoyne, and A. Morgan. Protein phosphorylation and the regulation of synaptic membrane traffic. *Trends Neurosci. 22*: 459–464 (1999).

R. S. Zucker. Neurotransmitter release and its modulation. In *Neuromodulation: The Biochemical Control of Neuronal Excitability*, L. K. Kaczmarek and I. B. Levitan (Eds.). New York: Oxford University Press, pp. 243–263 (1987).

References

G. J. Augustine, M. P. Charlton, and S. J. Smith. Calcium entry and transmitter release at voltage-clamped nerve terminals of squid. *J. Physiol. 369*:163–181 (1985).

I. A. Boyd and A. R. Martin. The end-plate potential in mammalian muscle. *J. Physiol. 132*:74–91 (1956).

M. Geppert, V. Y. Bolshakov, S. A. Siegelbaum, K. Takel, P. DeCamilli, R. E. Hammer, and T. C. Südhof. The role of Rab3A in neurotransmitter release. *Nature 369*:493–497 (1994).

G. Grynkiewicz, M. Poemie, and R. Y. Tsien. A new generation of Ca^{2+} indicators with greatly improved fluorescence properties. *J. Biol. Chem. 260*:3440–3450 (1985).

J. E. Heuser, T. S. Reese, M. J. Dennis, Y. Jan, L. Jan, and L. Evans. Synaptic vesicle exocytosis captured by quick freezing and correlated with quantal transmitter release. *J. Cell Biol. 81*:275–300 (1979).

R. Llinas, T. L. McGuinness, C. S. Leonard, M. Sugimori, and P. Greengard. Intraterminal injection of synapsin I or calcium/calmodulin-dependent protein kinase II alters neurotransmitter release at the squid giant synapse. *Proc. Natl. Acad. Sci. U.S.A. 82*:3035–3039 (1985).

S. J. Smith, J. Buchanan, L. R. Osses, M. P. Charleton, and G. Augustine. The spatial distribution of calcium signals in squid presynaptic terminals. *J. Physiol. 472*:573–593 (1993).

Y.-G. Tang and R. S. Zucker. Mitochondrial involvement in post-tetanic potentiation of synaptic transmission. *Neuron 18*:483–491 (1997).

Chapter 10

Recommended reading

J. R. Cooper, F. E. Bloom, and R. H. Roth. *The Biochemical Basis of Neuropharmacology*, 7th ed. New York: Oxford University Press (1996).

R. P. Seal and S. G. Amara. Excitatory amino acid transporters: a family in flux. *Annu. Rev. Pharmacol. Toxicol. 39*:431–456 (1999).

S. H. Snyder and C. D. Ferris. Novel neurotransmitters and their neuropsychiatric relevance. *Am. J. Psychiatry 157*:1738–1751 (2000).

D. G. Trist. Excitatory amino acid agonists and antagonists: pharmacology and therapeutic applications. *Pharm. Acta Helv. 74*:221–229 (2000).

References

B. Giros, Y.-M. Wang, S. Suter, S. B. McLeskey, C. Pifl, and M. G. Caron. Delineation of discrete domains for substrate, cocaine, and tricyclic antidepressant interactions using chimeric dopamine-norepinephrine transporters. *J. Biol. Chem. 269*:15985–15988 (1994).

S. W. Kuffler. Slow synaptic responses in autonomic ganglia and the pursuit of a peptidergic transmitter. *J. Exp. Biol. 89*:257–286 (1980).

A.-J. Silverman and E. A. Zimmerman. Magnocellular neurosecretory system. *Annu. Rev. Neurosci. 6*:357–380 (1983).

Chapter 11

Recommended reading

J. A. Dani and M. L. Mayer. Structure and function of glutamate and nicotinic acetylcholine receptors. *Curr. Opin. Neurobiol. 5*:310–317 (1995).

C. C. Garner, J. Nash, and R. L. Huganir. PDZ domains in synapse assembly and signalling. *Trends Cell Biol. 10*:274–280 (2000).

T. Kuner, L. P. Wollmuth, and B. Sakmann. The ion-conducting pore of glutamate receptor channels. *Handbook Exp. Pharmacol.* 141:219–249 (1999)

J. Lindstrom. Nicotinic acetylcholine receptors in health and disease. *Mol. Neurobiol.* 15:193–222 (1997).

S. Nakanishi and M. Masu. Molecular diversity and functions of glutamate receptors. *Annu. Rev. Biophys. Biomol. Struct.* 23:319–348 (1994).

M. Sheng and D. T. Pak. Ligand-gated ion channel interactions with cytoskeletal and signaling proteins. *Annu. Rev. Physiol.* 62:755–778 (2000).

References

E. A. Barnard, R. Miledi, and K. Sumikawa. Translation of exogenous messenger RNA coding for nicotinic acetylcholine receptors produces functional receptors in *Xenopus* oocytes. *Proc. R. Soc. Lond. Ser. B. Biol. Sci.* 215:241–246 (1982).

G.-Q. Chen, C. Cui, M. L. Mayer, and E. Gouaux. Functional characterization of a potassium-selective prokaryotic glutamate receptor. *Nature* 402:817–821 (1999).

A. V. Maricq, A. S. Peterson, A. J. Brake, R. M. Meyers, and D. Julius. Primary structure and functional expression of the $5HT_3$ receptor, a serotonin-gated ion channel. *Science* 254:432–437 (1991).

M. L. Mayer, G. L. Westbrook, and P. B. Guthrie. Voltage-dependent block by Mg^{2+} of NMDA responses in spinal cord neurones. *Nature* 309:261–263 (1984).

D. S. McGehee and L. W. Role. Physiological diversity of nicotine acetylcholine receptors expressed by vertebrate neurons. *Ann. Rev. Physiol.* 57:521–546 (1995).

L. Nowak, P. Bregestovski, P. Ascher, A. Herbet, and A. Prochiantz. Magnesium gates glutamate-activated channels in mouse central neurones. *Nature* 307:462–465 (1984).

B. Sakmann, C. Methfessel, M. Mishina, T. Takahashi, T. Takai, M. Kurasaki, K. Fukuda, and S. Numa. Role of acetylcholine receptor subunits in gating of the channel. *Nature* 318:538–543 (1985).

N. Unwin. Nicotinic acetylcholine receptor at 9 Å resolution. *J. Mol. Biol.* 229:1101–1124 (1993).

N. Unwin. Acetylcholine receptor channel imaged in the open state. *Nature* 373:37–43 (1995).

Chapter 12

Recommended reading

M. J. Berridge. Inositol trisphosphate and calcium: two interacting second messengers. *Am. J. Nephrol.* 17:1–11 (1997).

M. J. Berridge. Neuronal calcium signaling. *Neuron* 21:13–26 (1998).

D. E. Clapham and E. J. Neer. G protein beta gamma subunits. *Annu. Rev. Pharmacol. Toxicol.* 37:167–203 (1997).

B. E. Ehrlich. Functional properties of intracellular calcium release channels. *Curr. Opin. Neurobiol.* 5:304–309 (1995).

L. Fagni, P. Chavis, F. Ango and J. Bockaert. Complex interactions between mGluRs, intracellular Ca^{2+} stores and ion channels in neurons. *Trends Neurosci.* 23:80–88 (2000).

H. W. Fu and P. J. Casey. Enzymology and biology of CaaX protein prenylation. *Recent Prog. Horm. Res.* 54:315–342 (1999).

L. Y. Jan and Y. N. Jan. Voltage-gated and inwardly rectifying potassium channels. *J. Physiol.* 505:267–282 (1997).

E. J. Neer. Heterotrimeric G proteins: organizers of transmembrane signals. *Cell* 80:249–257 (1995).

S. H. Snyder, S. R. Jaffrey, and R. Zakhary. Nitric oxide and carbon monoxide: parallel roles as neural messengers. *Brain Res. Rev.* 26:167–175 (1998).

References

G. E. Breitwieser and G. Szabo. Uncoupling of cardiac muscarinic and β-adrenergic receptors from ion channels by a guanine nucleotide analogue. *Nature* 317:538–540 (1985).

N. Divecha and R. F. Irvine. Phospholipid signaling. *Cell* 80:269–278 (1995).

T. Furuichi, K. Kohda, A. Miyawaki, and K. Mikoshiba. Intracellular channels. *Curr. Opin. Neurobiol.* 4:294–303 (1994).

M. B. Kennedy. Regulation of neuronal function by calcium. *Trends Neurosci.* 12:417–420 (1989).

I. B. Levitan. It is calmodulin after all! Mediator of the calcium modulation of multiple ion channels. *Neuron* 22:645–648 (1999).

D. E. Logothetis, Y. Kurachi, J. Galper, E. J. Neer, and D. E. Clapham. The β subunits of GTP-binding proteins activate the muscarinic K^+ channel in heart. *Nature* 325:321–326 (1987).

P. J. Pfaffinger, J. M. Martin, D. D. Hunter, N. M. Nathanson, and B. Hille. GTP-binding proteins couple cardiac muscarinic receptors to a K^+ channel. *Nature* 317:536–538 (1985).

Chapter 13

Recommended reading

L. K. Kaczmarek and I. B. Levitan. *Neuromodulation: The Biochemical Control of Neuronal Excitability*. New York: Oxford University Press (1987).

I. B. Levitan. Modulation of ion channels by protein phosphorylation and dephosphorylation. *Annu. Rev. Physiol.* 56:193–212 (1994).

I. B. Levitan. Modulation of ion channels by protein phosphorylation. How the brain works. *Adv. Second Messenger Phosphoprotein Res.* 33:3–22 (1999).

G. G. Turrigiano and S. B. Nelson. Hebb and homeostasis in neuronal plasticity. *Curr. Opin. Neurobiol.* 10:358–364 (2000).

References

S. A. DeRiemer, J. A. Strong, K. A. Albert, P. Greengard, and L. K. Kaczmarek. Enhancement of calcium current in Aplysia neurones by phorbol ester and protein kinase C. *Nature 313*:313–316 (1985).

N. S. Desai, L. C. Rutherford, and G. G. Turrigiano. Plasticity in the intrinsic excitability of cortical pyramidal neurons. *Nat. Neurosci. 2*:515–520 (1999a).

N. S. Desai, L. C. Rutherford, and G. G. Turrigiano. BDNF regulates the intrinsic excitability of cortical neurons. *Learning and Memory 6*:284–291 (1999b).

K. Dunlap and G. D. Fischbach. Neurotransmitters decrease the Ca component of sensory neurone action potentials. *Nature 276*:837–838 (1978).

S. W. Jones and P. R. Adams. The M-current and other potassium currents of vertebrate neurons. In *Neuromodulation: The Biochemical Control of Neuronal Excitability*, L. K. Kaczmarek and I. B. Levitan (Eds.). New York: Oxford University Press, pp. 159–186 (1987).

E. R. Kandel. *Cellular Basis of Behavior: An Introduction to Behavioral Neurobiology*. San Francisco: Freeman (1976).

E. S. Levitan and I. B. Levitan. Serotonin acting via cyclic AMP enhances both the hyperpolarizing and depolarizing phases of bursting pacemaker activity in the *Aplysia* neuron R15. *J. Neurosci. 8*:1152–1161 (1988).

K. J. Loechner and L. K. Kaczmarek. Control of potassium currents and cyclic AMP levels by autoactive neuropeptides in *Aplysia* neurons. *Brain Res. 532*: 1–6 (1990).

R. Numann, W. A. Catterall, and T. Scheuer. Functional modulation of brain sodium channels by protein kinase C phosphorylation. *Science 254*:115–118 (1991).

L. A. Raymond, C. D. Blackstone, and R. L. Huganir. Phosphorylation and modulation of recombinant gluR6 glutamate receptors by cAMP dependent protein kinase. *Nature 361*:637–641 (1993).

J. A. Strong, A. P. Fox, R. W. Tsien, and L. K. Kaczmarek. Stimulation of protein kinase C recruits covert calcium channels in Aplysia bag cell neurons. *Nature 325*:714–717 (1987).

R. W. Tsien. Calcium currents in heart cells and neurons. In *Neuromodulation: The Biochemical Control of Neuronal Excitability*, L. K. Kaczmarek and I. B. Levitan (Eds.). New York: Oxford University Press, pp. 206–242 (1987).

J. W. West, R. Numann, B. J. Murphy, T. Scheuer, and W. A. Catterall. A phosphorylation site in the sodium channel required for modulation by protein kinase C. *Science 254*:866–868 (1991).

Chapter 14

Recommended reading

L. B. Buck. The molecular architecture of odor and pheromone sensing in mammals. *Cell 100*:611–618 (2000).

G. L. Fain, H. R. Matthews, and M. C. Cornwall. Dark adaptation in vertebrate photoreceptors. *Trends Neurosci. 19*:502–507 (1996).

T. A. Gilbertson. The physiology of vertebrate taste reception. *Curr. Opin. Neurobiol.* 3:532–539 (1993).

P. Mombaerts. Seven-transmembrane proteins as odorant and chemosensory proteins. *Science* 286:707–711 (1999).

J. O. Pickles. *An Introduction to the Physiology of Hearing*. London: Academic Press (1988).

References

J. J. Art and R. Fettiplace. Variation of membrane properties in hair cells isolated from the turtle cochlea. *J. Physiol.* 385:207–242 (1987).

I. A. Belyantseva, H. J. Adler, R. Curi, G. I. Frolenkov, and B. Kachar. Expression and localization of prestin and the sugar transporter GLUT-5 during development of electromotility in cochlear outer hair cells. *J. Neurosci.* 20:RC116 (1–5) (2000).

E. F. Fesenko, S. S. Kolesnikov, and A. L. Lyubarsky. Induction by cyclic GMP of cationic conductance in plasma membrane of retinal rod outer segments. *Nature* 313:310–313 (1985).

L. W. Haynes, A. R. Kay, and K.-W. Yau. Single cyclic GMP-activated channel activity in excised patches of rod outer segment membrane. *Nature* 321:66–70 (1986).

A. J. Hudspeth and R. S. Lewis. A model for electrical resonance and frequency tuning in saccular hair cells of the bull-frog, *Rana catesbeina*. *J. Physiol.* 400:275–297 (1988).

S. Kinnamon. Taste transduction: a diversity of mechanisms. *Trends Neurosci.* 11:491–496 (1988).

T. D. Lamb. Transduction in vertebrate photoreceptors: the roles of cyclic GMP and calcium. *Trends Neurosci.* 9:224–228 (1986).

R. S. Lewis and A. J. Hudspeth. Voltage- and ion-dependent conductances in solitary vertebrate hair cells. *Nature* 304:538–541 (1983).

J. H. Martin. Somatic sensory system I: receptor physiology and submodality coding. In *Principles of Neural Science*, E. R. Kandel and J. H. Schwartz (Eds.). New York: Elsevier North Holland, pp. 157–169 (1981).

K. Palczewski, T. Kumasaka, T. Hori, C. A. Behnke, H. Motoshima, B. A. Fox, I. Le Trong, D. C. Teller, T. Okada, R. E. Stenkamp, M. Yamamoto, and M. Miyano. Crystal structure of rhodopsin: A G Protein–coupled receptor. *Science* 289:739–745, 2000.

K. J. Ressler, S. L. Sullivan, and L. B. Buck. A molecular dissection of spatial patterning in the olfactory system. *Curr. Opin. Neurobiol.* 4:588–596 (1994).

Chapter 15

Recommended reading

C. Chang and A. Hemmati-Brivanlou. Cell fate determination in embryonic ectoderm. *J. Neurobiol.* 36:128–151 (1998).

D. R. Green and J. C. Reed. Mitochondria and apoptosis. *Science* 28:1309–1312 (1998).

J.-M. Lee, G. J. Zipfel, and D. W. Choi. The changing landscape of ischaemic brain injury mechanisms. *Nature* 399:A7–A14 (1999).

M. F. Mehler, P. C. Mabie, D. Zhang, and J. C. Kessler. Bone morphogenetic proteins in the nervous system. *Trends Neurosci.* 20:309–317 (1997).

D. Purves and J. W. Lichtman. *Principles of Neural Development.* Sunderland, MA: Sinauer Associates (1985).

References

F. H. Gage. Mammalian neural stem sells. *Science* 287:1433–1438, (2000).

M. Jacobson. *Developmental Neurobiology.* New York: Plenum (1978).

P. Rakic. Neuron–glia relationship during ganglion cell migration in developing cerebellar cortex. A Golgi and electron microscopic study in Macacus rhesus. *J. Comp. Neurol.* 141:283–312 (1971).

R. Sattler and M. Tymianski. Molecular mechanisms of calcium-dependent excitotoxicity. *J. Mol. Med.* 78:3–13 (2000).

D. van der Kooy and S. Weiss. Why stem cells? *Science* 287:1439–1441, (2000).

Chapter 16

Recommended reading

D. J. Anderson, A. Groves, L. Lo, Q. Ma, M. Rao, N. M. Shah, and L. Sommer. Cell lineage determination and the control of neuronal identity in the neural crest. *Cold Spring Harb. Symp. Quant. Biol.* 62:493–504 (1997).

S. Artavanis-Tsakonas, K. Matsuno, and M. E. Fortini. Notch signaling. *Science* 268:225–232 (1995).

E. Cattaneo, L. Conti, and C. De-Fraja. Signalling through the JAK-STAT pathway in the developing brain. *Trends Neurosci.* 22:365–369 (1999).

L. J. Klesse and L. F. Parada. Trks: signal transduction and intracellular pathways. *Microsc. Res. Tech.* 45:210–216 (1999).

R. M. Lindsay, S. J. Wiegant, C. A. Altar, and P. S. DiStefano. Neurotrophic factors: from molecules to man. *Trends Neurosci.* 17:182–190 (1994).

M. Perron and W. A. Harris. Determination of vertebrate retinal progenitor cell fate by the Notch pathway and basic helix-loop-helix transcription factors. *Cell. Mol. Life Sci.* 57:215–223 (2000).

T. Raabe. The Sevenless signaling pathway: variations of a common theme. *Biochim. Biophys. Acta* 1496:151–163 (2000).

C. J. Tabin and A. P. McMahon. Recent advances in Hedgehog signalling. *Trends Cell Biol.* 7:442–446 (1997).

M. Uusitalo, M. Heikkila, and S. Vainio. Molecular genetic studies of Wnt signaling in the mouse. *Exp. Cell Res.* 253:336–348 (1999).

References

G. L. Barrett. The p75 neurotrophin receptor and neuronal apoptosis. *Prog. Neurobiol.* 61:205–229 (2000).

D. Bar-Sagi and J. R. Feramisco. Microinjection of the ras oncogene protein into PC12 cells induces morphological differentiation. *Cell* 42:841–848 (1985).

T. J. DeVoogt. Androgens can affect the morphology of mammalian CNS neurons in adulthood. *Trends Neurosci.* 10:341–342 (1987).

R. M. Evans. The steroid and thyroid hormone receptor superfamily. *Science* 240:889–895 (1988).

S. A. Goldman and M. B. Luskin. Strategies utilized by migrating neurons of the postnatal vertebrate forebrain. *Trends Neurosci.* 21:107–113 (1998).

R. A. Gorski. Structural sex differences in the brain: their origin and significance. In *Neural Control of Reproductive Function*, J. M. Lakoski, J. R. Perez-Polo, and D. K. Rassin (Eds.). New York: Alan R. Liss, pp. 33–44 (1989).

M. E. Gurney. Hormonal control of cell form and number in the zebra finch song system. *J. Neurosci.* 1:658–673 (1981).

P. McCaffery and U. C. Drager. Regulation of retinoic acid signaling in the embryonic nervous system: a master differentiation factor. *Cytokine Growth Factor Rev.* 11:233–249 (2000).

R. Nishi. Neurotrophic factors: two are better than one. *Science* 265:1052–1053 (1994).

F. Nottebohm. From bird song to neurogenesis. *Sci. Am.* 260:74–79 (1989).

J. R. Sanes. Roles of extracellular matrix in neural development. *Annu. Rev. Physiol.* 45:581–600 (1983).

Chapter 17

Recommended reading

E. A. Clark and J. S. Brugge. Integrins and signal transduction pathways: the road taken. *Science* 268:233–239 (1995).

C.-H. Lin, C. A. Thompson, and P. Forscher. Cytoskeletal reorganization underlying growth cone motility. *Curr. Opin. Neurobiol.* 4:640–647 (1994).

B. K. Mueller. Growth cone guidance: first steps towards a deeper understanding. *Annu. Rev. Neurosci.* 22:351–388 (1999).

D. D. M. O'Leary. Attractive guides for axons. *Nature* 371:15–16 (1994).

M. Takeichi, T. Uemura, Y. Iwai, N. Uchida, T. Inoue, T. Tanaka, and S. C. Suzuki. Cadherins in brain patterning and neural network formation. *Cold Spring Harb. Symp. Quant. Biol.* 62:505–509 (1997).

D. Van Vactor and L. J. Lorenz. Neural development: the semantics of axon guidance. *Curr. Biol.* 9:R201–R204 (1999).

References

L. I. Benowitz and A. Routtenberg. A membrane phosphoprotein associated with neural development, axonal regeneration, phospholipid metabolism and synaptic plasticity. *Trends Neurosci.* 10:527–532 (1987).

P. Forscher and S. J Smith. Actions of cytochalasins on the organization of actin filaments and microtubules in a neuronal growth cone. *J. Cell Biol.* 107:1505–1516 (1988).

D. Frey, T. Laux, L. Xu, C. Schneider, and P. Caroni. Shared and unique roles of CAP23 and GAP43 in actin regulation, neurite outgrowth and anatomical plasticity. *J. Cell Biol.* 149:1442–1453 (2000).

J. L. Goldberg and B.A. Barres, Nogo in nerve regeneration. *Nature* 403:369–370 (2000).

A. L. Harrelson and C. S. Goodman. Growth cone guidance in insects: fasciclin II is a member of the immunoglobulin superfamily. *Science* 242:700–708 (1988).

P. G. Haydon, D. P. McCobb, and S. B. Kater. Serotonin selectively inhibits growth cone dynamics and synaptogenesis of specific identified neurons. *Science* 226:561–564 (1984).

M. Hiromoto, Y. Hiromi, E. Giniger, and Y. Hotta. The *Drosophila* Netrin receptor *Frazzled* guides axons by controlling Netrin distribution. *Nature* 406:886–889 (2000).

A. L. Kolodkin, D. M. Matthes, and C. S. Goodman. The semaphorin genes encode a family of transmembrane and secreted growth cone guidance molecules. *Cell* 75:1389–1399 (1993).

M. Matsunaga, K. Hatta, A. Nagafuchi, and M. Takeichi. Guidance of optic nerve fibers by N-cadherin cell adhesion molecules. *Nature* 334:62–64 (1988a).

M. Matsunaga, K. Hatta, and M. Takeichi. Role of N-cadherin cell adhesion molecules in the histogenesis of neural retina. *Neuron* 1:289–295 (1988b).

F. Polleux, T. Morrow, and A. Ghosh. Semaphorin 3A is a chemoattractant for cortical apical dendrites. *Nature* 404:567–573 (2000).

D. Purves and R. D. Hadley. Changes in the dendritic branching of adult mammalian neurones revealed by repeated imaging in situ. *Nature* 315:404–406 (1985).

T. Serafini, T. E. Kennedy, M. J. Galko, C. Mirzayan, T. M. Jessell, and M. Tessier-Lavigne. The netrins define a family of axon outgrowth-promoting proteins homologous to C. *elegans* UNC-6. *Cell* 78:409–424 (1994).

H.-J. Song, G.-L.-Ming, Z. He, M. Lehmann, K. McKerracher, M. Tessier-Lavigne, and M.-M. Poo. Conversion of neuronal growth cone responses from repulsion to attraction by cyclic nucleotides. *Science* 281:1515–1518 (1998).

S. M. Strittmatter. Dendrites go up, axons go down. *Nature* 404:557–559 (2000).

M. Westerfield and J. S. Eisen. Neuromuscular specificity: pathfinding by identified motor growth cones in a vertebrate embryo. *Trends Neurosci.* 11:18–22, 1988.

Chapter 18

Recommended reading

M. Constantine-Paton, H. T. Cline, and E. Debski. Patterned activity, synaptic convergence, and the NMDA receptor in developing visual pathways. *Annu. Rev. Neurosci. 13*:129–154 (1990).

M. C. Crair. Neuronal activity during development: permissive or instructive. *Curr. Opin. Neurobiol. 9*:88–93 (1999).

T. Curran and J. I. Morgan. Fos: an immediate-early transcription factor in neurons. *J. Neurobiol. 26*:403–412 (1995).

C. S. Goodman and C. J. Shatz. Developmental mechanisms that generate precise patterns of neuronal connectivity. *Cell 71/Neuron* 10(Suppl.):77–98 (1993).

D. G. Herrera and H. A. Robertson. Activation of *c-fos* in the brain. *Prog. Neurobiol. 50*:83–107 (1996).

G. Mellitzer, Q. Xu, and D. G. Wilkinson. Control of cell behavior by signalling through Eph receptors and ephrins. *Curr. Opin. Neurobiol. 10*:400–408 (2000).

M. Nakamoto. Eph receptors and ephrins. *Int. J. Biochem. Cell Biol. 32*:7–12 (2000).

J. R. Sanes and J. W. Lichtman. Development of the vertebrate neuromuscular junction. *Annu. Rev. Neurosci. 22*:389–442 (1999).

References

E. D. Apel, S. L. Roberds, K. P. Campbell, and J. P. Merlie. Rapsyn may function as a link between the acetylcholine receptor and the agrin-binding dystrophin-associated glycoprotein complex. *Neuron 15*:115–126 (1995).

S. Bevan and J. H. Steinbach. The distribution of γ-bungarotoxin binding sites on mammalian skeletal muscle developing in vivo. *J. Physiol. 267*:195–213 (1977).

M. C. Brown. Sprouting of motor nerves in adult muscles. A recapitulation of ontogeny. *Trends Neurosci. 7*:10–14 (1984).

A. J. Buller, J. C. Eccles, and R. M. Eccles. Interactions between motoneurons and muscles in respect of the characteristic speed of their responses. *J. Physiol. 150*:417–439 (1960).

M. Constantine-Paton and M. I. Law. Eye-specific termination bands in tecta of three-eyed frogs. *Science 202*:639–641 (1978).

Y. Dan and M.-M. Poo. Hebbian depression of isolated neuromuscular synapses in vitro. *Science 256*:1570–1573 (1992).

U. Drescher. Excitation at the synapse: Eph receptors team up with NMDA receptors. *Cell 103*:1005–1008 (2000).

P. Forscher, L. K. Kaczmarek, J. Buchanan, and S. J Smith. Cyclic AMP induces changes in distribution of organelles within growth cones of Aplysia bag cell neurons. *J. Neurosci. 7*:3600–3611 (1987).

H. Fujisawa. Persistence of disorganized pathways on tortuous trajectories of regenerating retinal fibers in the adult newt Cynops pyrrhogaster. *Dev. Growth Differ. 23*:215–219 (1981).

M. Hattori, M. Osterfield, and J.G. Flanagan. Regulated cleavage of a contact-mediated axon repellent. *Science* 289:1360–1365 (2000).

D. O. Hebb. The Organization of Behavior. New York: Wiley (1949).

S. P. Hunt, A. Pini, and G. Evan. Induction of c-fos-like protein in spinal cord neurons following sensory stimulation. *Nature* 328:632–634 (1987).

S. A. Jo, X. Zhu, M. A. Marchionni, and S. J. Burden. Neuregulins are concentrated at nerve-muscle synapses and activate Ach-receptor gene expression. *Nature* 373:158–162 (1995).

Y.-J. Lo and M.-M. Poo. Activity-dependent synaptic competition in vitro: Heterosynaptic suppression of developing synapses. *Science* 254:1019–1022 (1992).

L. M. Marshall, J. R. Sanes, and U. J. McMahan. Reinnervation of original synaptic sites on muscle fiber basement membrane after disruption of the muscle cells. *Proc. Natl. Acad. Sci. U.S.A.* 74:3073–3077 (1977).

S. Salmons and F. A. Streter. Significance of impulse activity in the transformation of skeletal muscle type. *Nature* 263:30–34 (1976).

R. W. Sperry. Chemoaffinity in the orderly growth of nerve fiber patterns and connections. *Proc. Natl. Acad. Sci. U.S.A.* 50:703–710 (1963).

J. Walter, S. Henke-Fahle, and F. Bonhoeffer. Avoidance of posterior tectal membranes by temporal retinal axons. *Development* 101:909–913 (1987).

Chapter 19

Recommended reading

L. F. Abbott and S. B. Nelson. Synaptic plasticity: taming the beast. *Nat. Neurosci. (Suppl.)* 3:1178–1183 (2000).

P. A. Getting. Emerging principles governing the operation of neural networks. *Annu. Rev. Neurosci.* 12:185–204 (1989).

S. Grillner and T. Matsuchima. The neural network underlying locomotion in lamprey—synaptic and cellular mechanisms. *Neuron* 7:1–15 (1991).

M. Hastings and E. S. Maywood. Circadian clocks in the mammalian brain. *Bioessays* 22:23–31 (2000).

P. X. Joris, P. H. Smith, and T. C. T. Yin. Coincidence detection in the auditory system: 50 years after Jeffress. *Neuron* 21:1235–1238 (1998).

References

P. D. Brodfuehrer and W. O. Friesen. From stimulation to undulation: a neuronal pathway for swimming in the leech. *Science* 234:1002–1004 (1986).

P. J. Conn and L. K. Kaczmarek. The bag cell neurons: a model system for the investigation of prolonged changes in animal behavior. *Mol. Neurobiol.* 3:237–273 (1990).

P. S. Dickinson and E. Marder. Peptidergic modulation of a multioscillator system in the lobster. I. Activation of the cardiac sac motor pattern by the neuropeptides proctolin and red pigment–concentrating hormone. *J. Neurophysiol.* 61:833–844 (1989).

W. O. Friesen. Neuronal control of leech swimming movements. In *Neuronal and Cellular Oscillators*, J. W. Jacklet (Ed.). New York: Marcel Dekker, pp. 269–316 (1989).

S. Grillner, A. El Manira, J. Tegner, T. Wadden, L. Vinay, and J.-Y. Barthe. Dynamic changes in functional connectivity in a lower vertebrate model. In *Cellular and Molecular Mechanisms Underlying Higher Neural Functions*, A. I. Selverston and P. Ascher (Eds.). New York: John Wiley & Sons, pp. 125–147 (1994).

R. M. Harris-Warrick and R. E. Flamm. Chemical modulation of a small central pattern generator. *Trends Neurosci.* 9:432–437 (1986).

L. K. Kaczmarek. A model of cell firing patterns during epileptic seizures. *Biol. Cybern.* 22:229–234 (1976).

C. M. Macica, L. Y. Wang, R. H. Joho, C. S. Ho, and L. K. Kaczmarek. Knockout of the Kv3.1 gene impairs high frequency firing in auditory neurons. *Soc. Neurosci. Abstr.* 26:1705 (2000).

M. Moulins and F. Nagy. Extrinsic inputs and flexibility in the motor output of the lobster pyloric neural network. In *Model Neural Networks and Behavior*, A. I. Selverston (Ed.). New York: Plenum, pp. 49–68 (1985).

M. P. Nusbaum and E. Marder. A modulatory proctolin-containing neuron (MPN). II. State-dependent modulation of rhythmic motor activity. *J. Neurosci.* 9:1600–1607 (1989).

R. A. Satterlie. Reciprocal inhibition and postinhibitory rebound produce reverberation in a locomotor pattern generator. *Science* 229:402–404 (1985).

R. A. Satterlie, M. LaBarbara, and A. N. Spencer. Swimming in the pteropod mollusc *Clione limacina*. I. Behavior and morphology. *J. Exp. Biol.* 116:189–204 (1985).

A. I. Selverston. *Model Neural Networks and Behavior*. New York: Plenum (1985).

G. S. Stent, W. B. Kristan, W. O. Friesen, C. A. Ort, M. Poon, and R. L. Calabrese. Neuronal generation of the leech swimming movement. *Science* 200:1348–1357 (1978).

Chapter 20

Recommended reading

C. H. Bailey and E. R. Kandel. Structural changes accompanying memory storage. *Annu. Rev. Physiol.* 55:397–426 (1993).

R. L. Davis. Physiology and biochemistry of *Drosophila* learning mutants. *Physiol. Rev.* 76:299–317 (1996).

J. Dubnau and T. Tully. Gene discovery in *Drosophila*: new insights for learning and memory. *Annu. Rev. Neurosci.* 21:407–444 (1998).

R. Levy and P. S. Goldman-Rakic. Segregation of working memory functions within the dorsolateral prefrontal cortex. *Exp. Brain Res.* 133:23–32 (2000).

R. Malinow, Z. F. Mainen, and Y. Hayashi. LTP mechanisms: from silence to four-lane traffic. *Curr. Opin. Neurobiol.* 10:352–357 (2000).

A. J. Shaywitz and M. E. Greenberg. CREB: a stimulus-induced transcription factor activated by a diverse array of extracellular signals. *Annu. Rev. Biochem.* 68:821–861 (1999).

L. R. Squire. *Memory and Brain*. New York: Oxford University Press (1987).

References

B. W. Agranoff, R. E. Davis, and J. J. Brink. Memory fixation in the goldfish. *Proc. Natl. Acad. Sci. U.S.A.* 54:788–793 (1965).

M. F. Bear and R. C. Malenka. Synaptic plasticity: LTP and LTD. *Curr. Opin. Neurobiol.* 4:389–399 (1994).

T. V. P. Bliss and T. Lomo. Long lasting potentiation of synaptic transmission in the dentate area of the anaesthetized rabbit following stimulation of the perforant path. *J. Physiol.* 232:331–356 (1973).

J. DeZazzo and T. Tully. Dissection of memory formation: From behavioral pharmacology to molecular genetics. *Trends Neurosci.* 18:212–218 (1995).

K. P. Giese, J. F. Storm, D. Reuter, N. B. Fedorov, L. R. Shao, T. Leicher, O. Pongs, and A. J. Silva. Reduced K$^+$ channel inactivation, spike broadening, and after-hyperpolarization in Kvβ1.1-deficient mice with impaired learning. *Learning and Memory* 5:257–273 (1998).

E. R. Kandel. *Behavioral Biology of Aplysia*. San Francisco: Freeman (1979).

E. R. Kandel and J. H. Schwartz. Molecular biology of learning: modulation of transmitter release. *Science* 218:433–443 (1982).

K. S. Lashley. In search of the engram. *Soc. Exp. Biol. Symp.* 4:454–482 (1950).

C. Luscher, H. Xia, E. C. Beattie, R. C. Carroll, M. von Zastrow, R. C. Malenka, and R. A. Nicoll. Role of AMPA receptor cycling in synaptic transmission and plasticity. *Neuron* 24:649–658 (1999).

L. Minichiello, M. Korte, D. Wolfer, R. Kuhn, K. Unsicker, V. Cestari, C. Rossi-Arnaud, H.-P. Lipp, T. Bonhoeffer, and R. Klein. Essential role for TrkB receptors in hippocampus-mediated learning. *Neuron* 24:401–414 (1999).

R. A. Nicoll, J. A. Kauer, and R. C. Malenka. The current excitement in long-term potentiation. *Neuron* 1:97–103 (1988).

M. E. Raichle. Behind the scenes of functional brain imaging: a historical and physiological perspective. *Proc. Natl. Acad. Sci. U.S.A.* 95:765–772 (1998).

C. F. Stevens and I. Verma. A model with good CREdentials. *Curr. Biol.* 4:736–738 (1994).

T. Tully. *Drosophila* learning and memory revisited. *Trends Neurosci.* 10:330–335 (1987).

D. Zamanillo, R. Sprengel, O. Hvalby, V. Jensen, N. Burnashev, A. Rozov, K. M. Kaiser, H. J. Koster, T. Borchardt, P. Worley, J. Lubke, M. Fritscher, P. H. Kelly, B. Sommer, P. Andersen, P. H. Seeburg, and B. Sakmann. Importance of AMPA receptors for hippocampal synaptic plasticity but not for spatial learning. *Science* 284:1805–1811 (1999).

Index